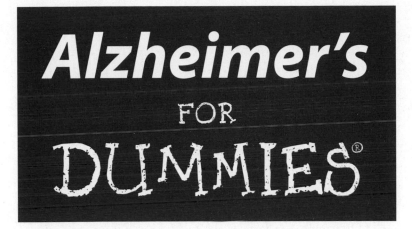

# Alzheimer's FOR DUMMIES®

by Patricia B. Smith, Mary Kenan, PsyD, and
Mark Edwin Kunik, MD, MPH

Foreword by Leeza Gibbons

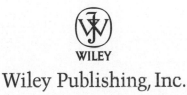

WILEY

Wiley Publishing, Inc.

**Alzheimer's For Dummies®**

Published by
**Wiley Publishing, Inc.**
111 River St.
Hoboken, NJ 07030
www.wiley.com

# *About the Author*

**Patricia Burkhart Smith** is an award-winning health and medical writer. She wrote for *People* magazine for six years. She co-reported a 1998 cover story on breast cancer that won the Society of Professional Journalists' Peter Lisagor Award for Excellence in Journalism. She also co-reported a 1999 cover story on anorexia that won a second place Time Inc. Luce Award. In addition, Ms. Smith serves as a medical reporter for Houston Northwest Medical Center, which for the past two years has been the only hospital in Houston named to the prestigious annual 100 Top Hospitals in America list. In 1984, Ms. Smith lost her beloved mother to Alzheimer's and in 1995, her favorite aunt lost her battle with the disease. The two deaths fueled Ms. Smith's desire to learn as much as she could about Alzheimer's and share that information with people dealing with the same problems and decisions her own family faced. Ms. Smith lives in The Woodlands, Texas with her two children.

**Mary Kenan, PsyD,** is a faculty member with the Department of Neurology at Baylor College of Medicine and is a licensed clinical psychologist. She received her B.A. from the University of Oklahoma and her doctorate in clinical psychology from Indiana State University. She completed her clinical internship and a postdoctoral fellowship in geriatric psychology at the Houston Veterans Affairs Medical Center, where she then served as a staff psychologist. In 1999, Dr. Kenan assumed her current position as the Director of Education and patient/family counselor for Baylor College of Medicine's Alzheimer's Disease Center. Dr. Kenan's clinical interests include the non-pharmacological management of Alzheimer's Disease, issues of adjustment and caregiving in chronic illness, the psychology of health and aging, and personality disorders across the lifespan. Dr. Kenan has served as a member of the Patient and Family Services Committee of the Alzheimer's Association of Houston and Southeast Texas chapter and she currently holds a appointment to the Texas Council on Alzheimer's Disease and related Disorders. She is also in private practice.

**Mark Edwin Kunik, MD, MPH,** is a leading expert on dementia. He is a practicing geropsychiatrist who has conducted extensive clinical and health services research on dementia. Dr. Kunik has done a lot to improve the quality of life for people with dementia, both as a caring physician to his patients and as a researcher who has published more than 40 papers on dementia-related issues alone. The many patients whose lives he's touched since he first joined the Houston Veterans Affairs Medical Center (VAMC) in 1993 would gladly attest to the thoughtful and sympathetic attention Dr. Kunik he has shown to each one. After having served as the Director of the Geropsychiatry Service at the VAMC from 1993–1999, Dr. Kunik received an Advanced Research Career Development Award and moved to the Houston Center for Quality of Care and Utilization Studies (HCQCUS) portion of the Houston VAMC to further his research efforts on behalf of those with dementia. Recently, he was appointed to the position of Associate Director of the HCQCUS, offering leadership and guidance to numerous other researchers, as well. He is also an Associate Professor in the Department of Psychiatry & Behavioral Sciences at Baylor College of Medicine, where he has served as a faculty member since 1992.

# Dedication

To the memory of three of the most important women in my life: my beloved mother, Ruby Nelson Ivey Burkhart, and aunt, Zora Chambers, fondly known as "Aunt Sissy," and my surrogate grandmother, Jeanette Renegar. All three had Alzheimer's Disease, and they inspired me to write this book. And to the memory of my beloved father, Hugh Reginald Burkhart, who suffered with Mom as she battled Alzheimer's Disease.

Finally, to all the researchers, scientists and doctors looking for way to prevent or cure Alzheimer's Disease, may God guide your efforts so that we may soon celebrate your
victory.

— Patricia Burkhart Smith

In memory of my grandparents,
    C. Joe Chatman,
    Lela Fay Naylor Chatman,
    Dan Cummins Kenan, and
    Mitchell Harrison Kenan.

— Mary Kenan

This book is dedicated to Mardi, Max, and Illan.

— Mark Edwin Kunik

# Authors' Acknowledgments

I would like to acknowledge the contributions of my co-authors, Dr. Mary Mitchell Kenan and Dr. Mark Edwin Kunik. Mary poured her heart and soul into reviewing and strengthening the book, and Mark added many salient points as we went along. If Alzheimer's Disease could be cured through compassion and dedication alone, then Mary and Mark would surely already have the cure.

I would also like to thank Natasha Graf and Tim Gallan, two of the best editors I've ever had the privilege to work with. Writing this book was a time-consuming and complex process that tapped into unplumbed wells of emotion and memories of my mother's illness. Both Natasha and Tim helped to smooth the way. And Natasha, thanks for all the funny stories. They really helped to keep my spirits up.

— Patricia Burkhart Smith

I would like to thank the Houston Center for Quality of Care and Utilization Studies, Houston Veterans Affairs Medical Center, whose work and resources contributed greatly to this book.

— Mark Edwin Kunik

I am indebted to my Alzheimer's patients and their families, whose trust in me has enriched my life, and to Rachelle S. Doody, MD, PhD, Director of the Alzheimer's Disease Center at Baylor College of Medicine, for her continued mentorship and support.

— Mary Kenan

## Publisher's Acknowledgments

We're proud of this book; please send us your comments through our Dummies online registration form located at www.dummies.com/register/.

Some of the people who helped bring this book to market include the following:

### Acquisitions, Editorial, and Media Development

**Senior Project Editor:** Tim Gallan

**Acquisitions Editor:** Natasha Graf

**Senior Copy Editor:** Christina Guthrie

**Editorial Program Assistant:**
Holly Gastineau-Grimes

**Technical Editor:** Dr. Joel Levy

**Editorial Manager:** Christine Meloy Beck

**Editorial Assistants:** Melissa S. Bennett,
Elizabeth Rea

**Cover Photos:** © Owen Franken/CORBIS

**Cartoons:** Rich Tennant,
www.the5thwave.com

### Composition Services

**Project Coordinator:** Adrienne Martinez

**Layout and Graphics:** Seth Conley,
Shae Lynn Wilson

**Proofreaders:** David Faust, TECHBOOKS
Production Services

**Indexer:** Aptara

**Special Help:** Jennifer Bingham,
Kristin DeMint, Michelle Dzurny, Tina Sims

### Publishing and Editorial for Consumer Dummies

**Diane Graves Steele,** Vice President and Publisher, Consumer Dummies

**Joyce Pepple,** Acquisitions Director, Consumer Dummies

**Kristin A. Cocks,** Product Development Director, Consumer Dummies

**Michael Spring,** Vice President and Publisher, Travel

**Brice Gosnell,** Associate Publisher, Travel

**Kelly Regan,** Editorial Director, Travel

### Publishing for Technology Dummies

**Andy Cummings,** Vice President and Publisher, Dummies Technology/General User

### Composition Services

**Gerry Fahey,** Vice President of Production Services

**Debbie Stailey,** Director of Composition Services

# Contents at a Glance

# Table of Contents

# Foreword

*U*nless you're a medical student or a doctor, you never expect to become a disease expert, but the minute your family gets a diagnosis, you scramble to get your hands on any and all the information you can find. If you're reading this, you have probably already reached critical mass in your search to become a health-care advocate for yourself or someone you love. You're in luck. Alzheimer's For Dummies will become your constant companion as you battle this illness.

I have always loved the For Dummies books. My own office boasts copies of Philosophy For Dummies, Internet For Dummies, and a couple of other titles that somehow make me feel a little, well, less like a dummy. I never dreamed I would have to add the Alzheimer's book to my collection.

At the young age of 63, my mother — our rock, our steel magnolia — was diagnosed with early stage Alzheimer's Disease. Our family felt alone, frustrated and frightened. To make the ache in our hearts even greater, this news closely followed my mother's painful struggle with her own mother's battle with the same disease. We lost my Granny. I lose a little more of Mom every day. I want so badly to promise my daughter that she will never have to lose me in the same way.

Until I can promise my children that they don't have to worry about me, I fight. I learn. I seek information and I look for ways to help. Recently, I created the Leeza Gibbons Memory Foundation and I am proud to announce the opening of Leeza's Places. Leeza's Place has been designed to give families, who are struggling with this thief, a safe place for education, energy and empowerment. Our goal is to assist with the day-to-day challenges of coping with this disease and to support both those who have been diagnosed and their caregivers.

Education is one of our primary objectives. There is no upside to keeping your head in the sand. This book is a crucial step in your new fight. Arm yourself with the knowledge waiting for you in these pages. It will help you find answers and resources as you adjust to your new reality.

I promised my mother that I would make her story count and use it to help others. She is in the final stages of the disease now, but she would be so proud to be associated with this series. I'd have given anything to have a book like this when we got our diagnosis. I wish you strength, courage and clarity as you read it and hope that you are able to use what you learn to assist you in your fight.

Blessings,

Leeza Gibbons

# Introduction

● ● ● ● ● ● ● ● ● ● ● ● ● ● ● ● ● ● ● ● ● ● ● ● ● ● ● ● ● ● ● ● ● ● ● ● ● ● ● ● ● ● ● ● ● ● ● ● ●

*1*t seems like you can't turn on a TV or pick up a magazine or newspaper these days without seeing something about Alzheimer's Disease. As Baby Boomers age and advances in healthcare continue to push down the death toll from well-known killers like heart disease and cancer, more people are living longer than ever before, meaning that more people are at risk of developing Alzheimer's Disease (AD) than ever before.

Put simply, that increase means that more and more families are dealing with Alzheimer's Disease, trying to provide care for an AD patient while maintaining some semblance of balance in their own lives. If you have a loved one who's been diagnosed with AD, chances are you've got a lot of questions. *Alzheimer's For Dummies* tries to help you find the answers that are right for your particular situation.

Statisticians and epidemiologists can paint a big, frightening picture of what the cold numbers and statistics mean for the economy, the healthcare industry, lost productivity, and a dozen other markers. However, little of that information is likely to hold much meaning for the family that must care for a loved one with Alzheimer's Disease. You want to know how Alzheimer's Disease is going to affect you and your loved one. How will it change your life, and how can you provide the care and comfort your family needs as they deal with the effects of this disease?

*Alzheimer's For Dummies* can help you answer these questions. This book provides a comprehensive look at the current state of research, diagnosis, and treatment of Alzheimer's Disease. It looks at how AD impacts a family and offers solid, up-to-date advice to guide caregivers through the medical, legal, and financial tangles that can develop when caring for an AD patient. You can find out about the different types of care available and their relative cost, and also get some tips on taking care of the caregiver (whether that person is you or a friend or family member) to keep him or her from burning out or becoming ill.

When reading this book, you'll discover that you aren't alone; vast resources are available that are devoted to helping caregivers balance their caregiving responsibilities with caring for the rest of the family and holding down a job. Whether you're a caregiver, a friend, or a family member of an Alzheimer's patient simply looking for additional information, this book is a great place to start.

***Note:*** This book provides the most up-to-date information about Alzheimer's Disease, its diagnosis, and its treatment. The information presented here is intended for educational purposes only and is not meant to replace professional medical evaluation and care.

# About This Book

If you think that Alzheimer's Disease is a hopeless diagnosis, think again. Although no cure is available right now, you can do many things to improve the quality of life both for your loved one with Alzheimer's and yourself, particularly if you're the primary caregiver.

*Alzheimer's For Dummies* takes a realistic look at Alzheimer's Disease, what it is and what it isn't, and offers pertinent, realistic advice for dealing with the myriad of concerns and responsibilities that a primary caregiver must assume when managing an Alzheimer's patient.

# Conventions Used in This Book

This book has a few conventions that we want to point out:

- We refer to the person who has Alzheimer's Disease as "your loved one," and occasionally as "the AD patient."
- We abbreviate Alzheimer's Disease as AD, at times, throughout the book.
- We want the book to be as user friendly as possible. As far as possible, we've used everyday language. If we occasionally have to use a medical term or other important term that may be unfamiliar to you, we *italicize* it upon first mention and then provide a brief definition.
- All Web sites and e-mail addresses appear in `monofont` to help them stand out in the text.
- The sidebars in this book are shaded gray and contain relevant but nonessential info. If you want to read them, that's great, but you won't be missing any important points if you skip them.

# Foolish Assumptions

We assume that you, the reader, have a family member or close friend who's suffering from Alzheimer's Disease and that you bought this book because you're looking for current, helpful information about the disease, its diagnosis, and treatment. We also assume that you want to take care of yourself while taking care of your loved one, so we've included info on getting that topic as well.

Finally, we assume that you understand that although AD is associated with the aging process, it's by no means a normal or inevitable part of aging.

# How This Book Is Organized

*Alzheimer's For Dummies* is divided into five parts. Each part covers a different aspect of dealing with Alzheimer's Disease. It's not necessary to read the book through from cover to cover; however, you may want to read the first part to get a thorough understanding of the basics of Alzheimer's Disease. After that you can use the Table of Contents to look up specific topics of interest and read those sections. Each section flows into the next, but is also written to stand on its own.

Because the book is arranged in a modular fashion that allows you to jump in wherever you want, we provide lots of cross-references within the text to help you find additional topics of interest.

## Part I: Could It Be Alzheimer's Disease?

Part I identifies the symptoms and risk factors for Alzheimer's Disease, and walks you through the diagnostic process. You find out what distinguishes AD from other brain diseases and medical conditions and how to handle the fears that may accompany the diagnosis.

## Part II: Helping a Loved One Manage the Illness

With diagnosis in hand, the next step is understanding the various stages of Alzheimer's Disease and how they impact caregiving. This part helps you evaluate current drug therapies and watch out for scams and quack treatments, and it explains the benefits and pitfalls of participating in a clinical trial. It also covers effective alternative therapies and takes a peek into the future to see what researchers are working on in the hope of finding new treatments, or maybe even a cure.

## Part III: Providing Care for the AD Patient

Part III is a crash course in a book, with valuable information regarding the myriad medical, legal, and financial issues you have to deal with as an Alzheimer caregiver. You discover how to find the best doctors and how to deal with attorneys and CPAs. You also find everything you ever wanted to know about Medicare regulations, evaluating the cost of care, plus you get some smart ideas about what to do if your family doesn't have adequate resources to provide care. The different types of care are evaluated to help you select the care option that best suits your family. And you can find a complete range of information about the requirements of the caregiver's job and how to find reliable people who can sub for you when you need a break.

## Part IV: Respite Care for the Caregiver

Providing care for a person with Alzheimer's Disease can be a daunting task. The demands are many and unrelenting, and the job grows more difficult as your loved one progresses through the stages of AD. Part IV offers some smart ideas to help the caregiver manage stress and cope with the demands of caregiving. You find ideas to take better care of yourself, maintain your own physical and mental health, and enlist help from family, friends, professional caregivers, and support groups. We even show you how to juggle work, family, and caregiving in a productive way. Finally, other family members can find out how to help the primary caregiver, even if he or she lives hundreds of miles away.

## Part V: The Part of Tens

The Part of Tens is a *For Dummies* tradition, featuring quick resources that provide lots of information in an easy-to-digest fashion. *Alzheimer's For Dummies* contains two Part of Tens chapters. We tell you ten ways that caregivers can get a break, and list more than ten invaluable resources for Alzheimer's Disease caregivers.

## Icons Used in This Book

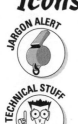

Wherever you see a term, medical or otherwise, that isn't exactly part of everyday vernacular, you'll also see this icon, followed by an explanation in plain language.

Text next to this icon is difficult or complicated medical information. Feel free to skip it.

This icon points out little snippets of information that guide you to interesting Web sites or tell you easier ways to get things done.

 Whatever you do, don't skip paragraphs that have this icon attached. Warnings alert you to scams, dangerous situations, and other pitfalls to avoid. Reading this info can help you protect your loved one and yourself.

We use this icon to flag information that you ought to keep in mind.

# Where to Go from Here

If you don't know a thing about Alzheimer's Disease (or you just can't bring yourself to begin a book in the middle), start from the beginning with Chapter 1. If a loved one has received a diagnosis of AD and you want to know what treatments and care are available, check out Parts II and III. If you need advice on caring for someone with AD, see Part IV.

# Part I

# Could It Be Alzheimer's Disease?

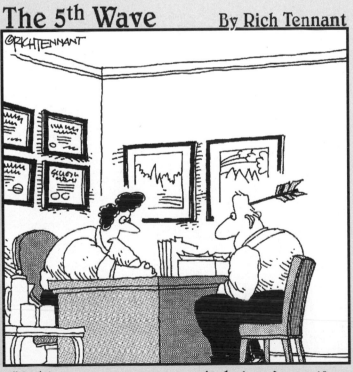

The 5th Wave     By Rich Tennant

"I think we can rule out Alzheimer's as the cause of your memory loss."

## In this part . . .

We identify the symptoms and risk factors for Alzheimer's Disease, and we walk you through the diagnostic process. You discover what distinguishes AD from other brain diseases and medical conditions, and we talk about how to handle the fears that may accompany the diagnosis.

# Chapter 1

# The Facts on Alzheimer's Disease

*T*he last time you visited your elderly mother, she seemed confused and disoriented. She kept asking the same question over and over again and couldn't remember that you'd already given her the answer a dozen times. She laughed uproariously over something you said that wasn't meant to be funny and spent a good deal of your visit staring into space with a blank expression in her eyes. When you got ready to leave, she became quite upset because she couldn't find her purse and accused you of hiding it. None of these behaviors is typical for her, and you can't help wondering — could this be Alzheimer's Disease?

It could be.

An estimated 4 million people are living with Alzheimer's Disease (AD) in America today, with approximately 370,000 new cases diagnosed every year. The incidence of the disease rises dramatically with age, from 3 percent affected in the 65 to 74 year age range all the way up to 47 percent affected in the 85 and older age range. AD patients live anywhere from 5 to 20 years after their diagnosis, and their inability to care for themselves grows more dramatic as the disease progresses, creating profound implications for their families and healthcare providers.

AD causes fewer than 50,000 deaths annually, making it only the eighth leading cause of death. But its impact on families during the caregiving years is overwhelming. Particularly worrisome is that, as America's Baby Boomer population ages, experts are predicting an epidemic of Alzheimer's Disease; that makes continued research even more crucial.

This book is intended to serve as a resource guide to anyone who has a family member living with Alzheimer's Disease. Whether you're a caregiver, a friend, or a family member of an AD patient simply looking for additional information, *Alzheimer's For Dummies* is a great place to start.

# Defining Alzheimer's Disease

AD is a form of dementia. Although all AD patients have dementia, not all dementia patients have Alzheimer's Disease. The Alzheimer's Association defines Alzheimer's Disease as "an irreversible, progressive brain disease that slowly destroys memory and thinking skills, eventually even the ability to carry out the simplest tasks." AD is a fatal disease, ending inevitably in death.

Alzheimer's Disease was named after a German physician, Alois Alzheimer, who first identified the condition in 1906 when he performed an autopsy on the brain of a woman who'd been suffering severe memory loss and confusion for years. He observed plaques and neurofibrillary tangles in the woman's brain tissue and correctly hypothesized that these abnormal deposits were responsible for the patient's loss of memory and other cognitive problems. To this day, AD can only be diagnosed with 100 percent accuracy through an autopsy that reveals the presence of the characteristic plaques and tangles. However, a comprehensive examination and good work-up do provide a reliable diagnosis with greater than 90 percent accuracy.

Abnormal deposits of specific proteins inside the brain disrupt normal brain function and cause the cognitive and functional problems typically associated with AD. Eventually, as the deposits spread throughout the brain, brain tissue starts dying, which leads to further cognitive impairment. The resulting brain shrinkage can be seen in CT scans and MRIs. Current research is focused on trying to determine what causes these deposits and is looking for ways to prevent or reverse them before they cause permanent brain damage.

Healthcare professionals are already sounding the alarm in the halls of Congress, warning that many more resources must be devoted to Alzheimer's Disease research to avoid a catastrophe in the not-too-distant future. The National Institutes of Health and the National Institute on Aging, both agencies of the federal government, are partnering with various universities and research facilities in a concerted effort to foster the search for answers, and perhaps even to find a cure or a preventive agent like a vaccine. Various advocacy groups are calling for national programs to offer training and support for the family caregivers who provide 75 percent of the care for Alzheimer's patients.

Although these efforts are much needed, probably the only things you want right now are answers to some of the following questions: How is Alzheimer's Disease going to affect me, my loved one, and the rest of my family? What can I do to make the experience as positive and painless as possible? Where can I go to get help?

We hope that this book helps you answer these questions.

# Busting the Myths About AD

The preceding section, "Defining Alzheimer's Disease," talks about what Alzheimer's Disease is. Now, allow us to go over what it isn't. Alzheimer's Disease is *not:*

- ✔ Curable
- ✔ Contagious
- ✔ A natural part of the aging process
- ✔ Something you get from using deodorant or cooking in aluminum pans
- ✔ Inevitable if you live long enough

Although certain familial forms of Alzheimer's Disease do run in families, these forms are extremely rare, accounting for less than 5 percent of all cases. So just because your mother or your brother got Alzheimer's Disease doesn't automatically mean that you're going to get it as well.

No test can predict whether you'll get Alzheimer's Disease unless you have the very rare inherited form of AD. A blood test exists that can tell you whether you have a certain form of a cholesterol-carrying protein associated with a higher incidence of Alzheimer's Disease, but that's all that it can tell you. The test can't tell you whether you'll actually develop the condition because at least 50 percent of the people who have the risk factor never actually get AD.

For ethical reasons, healthcare professionals advise against taking this blood test or undergoing other genetic testing because they want to spare their patients unnecessary worry about something that'll probably never happen even if the tests do come out positive. They also recommend against testing because if a person does find that he or she has inherited the gene or the risk factor, this information may negatively impact the person's ability to get health insurance and long-term care coverage.

# Looking at Symptoms and Causes

Doctors and researchers still aren't sure exactly what triggers Alzheimer's Disease, but the symptoms are all too familiar. Part I of this book looks at current theories about causes and reviews the range of symptoms that may be present at each stage of the disease. You can also find information to help you decide whether to take your loved one to a doctor for testing.

As we mention earlier, Alzheimer's Disease has no method of diagnosis that's 100 percent accurate (other than an autopsy at death). But the range of diagnostic tools is so good that most doctors can now diagnose Alzheimer's Disease with about 90 percent certainty. The results of a battery of workups — a physical exam, lab tests, imaging, and evaluations of thinking, memory, and day-to-day functioning — are used to determine the likelihood of Alzheimer's Disease.

# Discovering Treatment Options

Just four drugs are FDA approved for the treatment of Alzheimer's Disease. As we discuss in Part II, the standard of treatment calls for the administration of one of the three drugs still in use, along with a recommended 2000 I.U. of vitamin E daily. Depending upon your loved one's condition, additional medications may be used to treat other behavioral symptoms of AD that can occur at any point in the course of the disease. If your loved one has an underlying condition like diabetes or cardiovascular disease, he may have to take additional medications for those conditions as well. Your doctor will work with you and your loved one to determine which medications and treatment options are best suited to your particular case.

# Tackling Financial and Legal Issues

A diagnosis of AD requires some thoughtful planning from families so that they can manage the complex legal and financial issues that will crop up as their loved one's capabilities diminish. Make your legal and financial decisions as soon as possible, and put plans in place before your loved one becomes incapacitated; otherwise, you may have a court peering over your shoulder every time you try to pay a bill or shift funds to cover expenses. Part III presents practical tips that could save your family thousands of dollars and hours of time.

# Making Medical Decisions and Providing Care

If you don't have a medical background, accepting the responsibility for making medical decisions for your loved one can be a daunting task. You can find out how to determine whether your loved one is receiving the optimum care by comparing the treatments he or she is getting to the Alzheimer's Disease Standard of Care. You'll also gain insight into the process that doctors follow to make a diagnosis of Alzheimer's Disease.

If your family is like most families, you'll opt to provide in-home care for your loved one for as long as possible, particularly in the early, more manageable, stages of the disease. Part III also discusses what care options are available in most communities along with a comparison of the cost, benefits, advantages, and disadvantages of each. You can discover how to find good caregivers and how to share the caregiving burden among various family members. You also find tips for juggling work and family with the responsibilities of caregiving.

# Finding Respite

Even if you're Superwoman (or Superman), you need a break from your caregiving chores sometimes. Caregiving is demanding work. Remember to schedule regular breaks to keep yourself from burning out. In Part IV, you can find lots of creative ideas for relaxing and taking time off that are both time and cost effective. You can find out how to take good care of yourself even as you provide care for your loved one.

# What Should I Do Now?

Losing someone you love is never easy, but losing a loved one to Alzheimer's Disease seems particularly cruel. People recognize each other in so many ways — by voice, by a glance or gesture, by a familiar and comforting touch. But the glue that truly binds loved ones to each other is their shared memories.

Alzheimer's robs all of these. It's a thorough and impartial thief that steals away the landmarks of your most cherished relationships and leaves you lost. It takes mothers, fathers, husbands, wives, sisters, brothers, grandparents, aunts, uncles, and beloved friends and turns them into strangers. And it does so ever so slowly, by agonizing inches and degrees.

In a recent interview, Nancy Reagan simply and eloquently called Alzheimer's Disease "the long goodbye." Anyone whose life has ever been touched by Alzheimer's knows instantly what she means. The person you love is there in front of you but isn't there. You can touch them, but not reach them. Like so many other grieving husbands and wives before her, Nancy Reagan has watched as Alzheimer's silenced her beloved husband, Ronald Reagan, the former President we called "The Great Communicator."

Although researchers have come a long way in their search for the cause of Alzheimer's Disease, doctors still don't have a complete answer. They've identified anomalies in the brains of Alzheimer's victims but don't know what causes them or how to prevent them. Some effective treatments have been developed, but most people with AD never get the opportunity to try one of these medications, or if they do, they only stay on the drug for a short period of time because most physicians misunderstand what the drugs are capable of doing. Unlike some other diseases that may strike and kill relatively quickly, AD allows its victims to live for 4 to 8 years after diagnosis, and cases are reported of individuals living as long as 20 years in a completely dependent state. This obviously creates a tremendous strain on the family that is caring for an Alzheimer's patient.

Families with an AD patient have hundreds of questions, as do AD patients themselves. What causes Alzheimer's Disease? Can it be cured? Is it hereditary or contagious? What are the best treatments?

Although not every question can be easily answered, *Alzheimer's For Dummies* gives you the latest and most up-to-date information available to help you make informed decisions about medical care, prescriptions, care options, and legal and financial issues. And if you can't find the answer in these pages, we'll show you some Internet resources that can point you in the right direction.

# Chapter 2

# Symptoms, Causes, and Risk Factors

*In This Chapter*

▶ Understanding symptoms

▶ Being aware of conditions that mimic Alzheimer's Disease

▶ Uncovering the possible causes of Alzheimer's Disease

▶ Assessing possible risk factors

Although Alzheimer's Disease (AD) may not exactly be the hottest topic of conversation around your office water cooler, talk to any group gathered there or in a restaurant, and you're likely to encounter at least one person with a family member or friend who has been diagnosed with the condition. You may also hear of someone who was afraid he had AD but discovered he was just depressed or stressed out.

Common conditions like depression can cause memory problems that may be mistaken for AD. With all the news about AD on television, radio, and the Internet, along with the many newspaper and magazine articles devoted to the subject, it's easy to panic when you can't find your car keys. This tendency to assume the worst may be especially true as you age or if you have a family member or friend affected by AD. But don't overreact if you or a loved one occasionally experiences forgetfulness. However, you can watch for certain signs that should prompt you to seek a professional evaluation.

This chapter helps you sort out the differences between ordinary forgetfulness and the changes in memory that are associated with AD. Changes in other areas of thinking and day-to-day functioning due to AD are also discussed. In addition to discussing the symptoms that are characteristic of AD, we provide an overview of the known and theoretical changes in the brains of those with AD, and discuss identified and possible risk factors that may make an individual more susceptible to developing AD.

# Getting an Idea of What to Look For

Remember that no one symptom or test shouts, "This is Alzheimer's Disease!" However, a well-established constellation of symptoms, when taken together, allow a physician to diagnose AD with more certainty. Just because a person has occasional bouts of forgetfulness doesn't automatically raise a red flag that she has AD, because many other things can cause temporary forgetfulness — like several sleepless nights in combination with low blood sugar, an unexpected reaction to a new medication, or the use of multiple medications. Forgetfulness is a symptom of AD, but the syndrome of AD extends beyond forgetfulness. To diagnose AD, a person must have impaired memory plus problems in at least one other area of thinking or functioning, whether it's socially, on the job or performing individual tasks. Some signs to watch for are cognitive symptoms, language problems, changes in mood and personality, social problems, and physical symptoms.

## Cognitive symptoms

The cognitive symptoms of AD include any symptoms that affect or impair the patient's ability to think, speak, reason, understand, remember, plan, and exercise reasonable judgment.

AD patients typically display memory problems (described in the next section) along with one or more of the following cognitive symptoms:

- **Forgetfulness and memory problems:** Difficulty recalling previously known information and difficulty learning, retaining, and recalling new information

- **Language disturbance:** Difficulty finding the right word, use of similar sounding words, or inability to put together a coherent sentence. Empty or nonsensical speech, plus difficulty comprehending spoken language

- **Difficulty recognizing everyday objects:** For example, looking at a stove or a toilet and having no idea what it is or how to use it

- **Difficulty in staying oriented to time, place, and location:** Confusing the days of the week, months, seasons, and even years; problems telling time or getting lost in familiar settings

- **Inability to plan, organize, or solve everyday problems:** They may clean up by storing garbage in the refrigerator, or pay bills twice.

### Memory problems

Memory can be affected by AD in more than one way. People with AD may experience problems learning new material or may forget information that they previously knew, or both. Problems learning and retaining new information often precedes the loss of already learned information.

Don't automatically suspect AD every time someone has a memory lapse or exhibits forgetfulness. Everyone has memory problems from time to time; you forget the name of your poker buddy's wife, you forget to pay your cable bill, or you misplace your keys or your wallet. But forgetting doesn't mean that you have AD, even if you have a family history of the condition.

Problems with memory typically start slowly for a person with AD. In fact, researchers now believe that changes in the brain that are associated with AD actually start several decades before the first symptoms are detected. AD is no longer considered a disease of old age, but rather a disease of the life-span. It's *not* a normal part of the aging process.

At first, an AD patient may not remember recent events. As the condition progresses, he may have difficulty recalling a relative's name. You may take your mother to the grocery store in the morning, and later that day, she calls saying she needs to buy food and refuses to believe that you already shopped with her that morning. If she has no memory whatsoever of such a recent event, that is definitely cause for concern.

Perhaps your father has trouble remembering the names of his young grand-children or new neighbors, but his forgetfulness is more than just a brief memory lapse. This is a situation that also calls for further investigation.

Although the memory loss of a person with AD is progressive and irre-versible, with some conditions memory loss is reversible with proper treatment or treatment can stop or help prevent future memory loss. For example, a person who has suffered a series of small strokes may exhibit signs of memory loss, but early intervention and treatment with the appro-priate drugs can prevent additional damage and further loss of cognitive function. If you automatically assume that all memory loss is AD, your loved one may not receive the most appropriate treatment, which in some cases can greatly reduce her symptoms or perhaps even alleviate them altogether. Without a proper diagnostic workup, your loved one can be subjected to unnecessary or incorrect treatment, which can allow the real condition to go untreated. Your healthcare professional is the only one who can determine which treatments are appropriate and beneficial for your loved one's particular condition.

The key point regarding memory loss due to AD is that it's not static. As AD progresses, you realize you're not seeing just occasional forgetfulness but a pattern of steadily worsening memory loss.

With more advanced AD, your loved one may have trouble recalling familiar people and places as well as forming new memories; recent events seem to drift away as soon as they're over.

### Other problems in thinking due to AD

Of course, memory loss is not the only cognitive symptom your loved one may display. As you know, a diagnosis of AD can't be made if *only* memory is affected. Here are some other areas of thinking that may also be affected if your loved one has AD.

- ✔ **Executive functions:** Executive functions include planning, organizing, sequencing, and abstracting abilities. Any loss in executive functions impacts a patient's ability to make decisions, make and follow plans, establish goals, control impulses, think abstractly, and reason and solve problems. Obviously, many safety issues arise because of impairment in these areas. See Chapter 14 for help in protecting your loved one from con artists and Chapter 16 for safety tips for AD patients.

- ✔ **Problems with calculation:** Solving math problems in day-to-day situations is one ability that can be affected by AD. Some patients, even those with mild AD, may have problems making change, calculating tips in a restaurant, or balancing their checkbooks.

## Problems with language (aphasia)

Although memory loss is a key symptom that doctors look for when trying to assess the presence of AD, language impairment, which may also be called aphasia, is another symptom that may be present.

Many people develop language problems early in the course of AD. You may notice someone who used to be an avid talker now has trouble finding the right word. Or you may notice hesitations in their speech that weren't there before or find yourself filling in words for them or anticipating or interpreting their speech. A person with AD may say a similar but incorrect word or give a description of what they're trying to say but never recall the word they wanted to use. Unlike the memory problems that are present in all AD patients, difficulty with speech doesn't affect every AD patient.

As AD progresses, problems with language tend to become more noticeable. Your loved one may have trouble putting together a coherent sentence or start speaking in a nonsensical or fanciful language that is hard to understand. Patients who are particularly sensitive to their language difficulties may withdraw socially, become more passive in social situations, and rely on you because they're frustrated with their inability to express themselves. They may also withdraw because they fear embarrassment or that someone will find out they have a problem comprehending or following conversation.

As language skills deteriorate, so does reading comprehension and the ability to understand what others are saying. Some families find it helpful to label everyday objects to assist their loved one in maintaining some feeling of control over their environment; other families find that signs or labels do no good because their loved one can't understand them.

# Non-Cognitive Symptoms

Non-cognitive symptoms of AD are physical and behavioral symptoms that are not related to the process of thinking. They include a number of mood and personality disturbances that may be seen quite early, as well as physical symptoms that develop much later in the course of the disease.

## Mood problems and personality disturbances

One of the most difficult manifestations of AD that families may have to deal with is drastic changes in their loved one's personality. A person who was mild and sweet-natured may become hostile and aggressive. An open and trusting person may become suspicious to the point of delusion, believing that everyone is out to get her or that her family members are stealing from her. Naturally, these problems are very upsetting to the patient's family members.

An AD patient's personality may remain as it always was or it may radically change, even early on. Someone who was very easygoing may suddenly display bouts of extreme irritability. He or she may appear frustrated, apathetic, disinterested, or depressed and cry easily or for no apparent reason. He may withdraw from social activities or stop working on his hobbies. He may become argumentative, suspicious, or distrusting of his family members and close friends. Less frequently, he may be inexplicably sunny all the time, even when circumstances dictate a more somber mood.

If AD patients become suspicious to the point of delusion, their suspicions may involve one or more of these common themes:

- They believe a stranger is living in the house and going through their things (known as The Phantom Boarder syndrome).
- They believe someone is stealing their personal belongings.
- They believe someone is stealing their money, although they may have actually given it away or misplaced it.
- They believe their spouse is having an affair.

## Apathy

Apathy is the number one non-cognitive behavioral symptom of AD, occurring in 72 percent of patients. The patient loses interest in activities they once enjoyed and doesn't express much emotion. Unfortunately, apathy is frequently mistaken for depression; for effective treatment, distinguishing between the two is critical.

### Anxiety

Some AD patients suffer from periodic bouts of anxiety. Think how you would feel if the world suddenly didn't make sense to you; If you couldn't remember what someone told you just seconds before or even that someone had talked to you; if your familiar surroundings seemed alien and threatening; if the people you have known, loved, and trusted all your life appeared to be strangers; wouldn't you feel anxious?

### Aggressiveness

Some AD patients can become agitated or explode with aggressiveness, so monitoring your loved one's behavior is essential to make sure she doesn't hurt herself or others. If trouble is brewing, the patient's expressions of anger and hostility build as the situation reaches a head. If the patient's behavior can't be modified with appropriate distraction or medication, and the triggers in the patient's environment that set off the aggression can't be modified, relocating the patient or placing him in a hospital temporarily is best until the situation can be brought under control.

As executive functions decline, a patient may no longer understand social norms (see executive functions in "Other problems in thinking due to AD" earlier in this chapter). Inhibitions may disappear, and you may start seeing signs of inappropriate bathroom or sexual behavior, such as your loved one exposing himself, masturbating, or urinating in public. Try to remember the context of this behavior and respond appropriately and without anger. Your loved one truly isn't aware of what he's doing or that his behavior is considered inappropriate.

Maintaining a sense of humor can really help a family make it through the challenges of caring for an AD patient. If you respond to a difficult situation with humor instead of anger, you're gaining two benefits: first, your humor can help defuse your loved one's anger or aggression, and second, your humor helps you avoid becoming overly stressed. So, sign up for a free subscription at:

- ✔ www.jokeaday.com/
- ✔ www.laugh-of-the-day.com/

## Social problems

As AD progresses, your loved one may develop social problems. He may become so disoriented and disconnected from his normal routine that withdrawing just seems easier. He also may withdraw because of an increased awareness of his problems. This self-imposed isolation is a common behavior in AD patients.

AD patients may become embarrassed because they can't keep up with their personal hygiene. Poor personal care may result in social isolation, particularly if the person with AD is living alone. If a family member asks her about her hygiene or whether she has been eating regularly, she may become argumentative, combative, or simply withdraw into silence.

Alzheimer's daycare facilities can help families meet their loved one's social needs by providing structured activities with other AD patients in a controlled, secure environment. Many patients respond favorably to this sort of planned activity. (For more benefits of adult daycare, see Chapter 15.)

# Physical symptoms

Unlike memory problems, which are noticeable almost from the onset of Alzheimer's Disease, with few exceptions early stage patients display almost no significant physical disabilities.

### Extrapyramidal signs

As the disease advances, some patients may display what is known as *extrapyramidal* signs including tremors, rigidity, and slowness of movement. This kind of physical symptom may also indicate the development of another condition or a problem with medications interacting.

More commonly, patients who exhibit extrapyramidal signs early in the disease are at risk for developing non-Alzheimer's dementia, such as that caused by a vascular accident like a stroke. The symptoms may also be caused by Parkinson's Disease or some anti-psychotic drugs like haloperidol (trade name Haldol).

If your loved one has an odd shuffling gait or swings his legs in wide circles from the hip as he walks, have him evaluated immediately. These extrapyramidal symptoms may respond well to treatment if caught early enough.

If you're thinking that extrapyramidal means outside the pyramid, you're almost right. Many of the nerves that control movement and sensation run through a part of the brain stem called the *medulla*, which is shaped somewhat like a pyramid. The nerves running from the medulla to the spinal cord are called the *pyramidal tract*, and they control all voluntary muscle movement like walking or raising your hand. Nerves outside of this main bundle are called extrapyramidal and run from a group of brain structures called the *basal ganglia*. The extrapyramidal nervous system controls involuntary motor movement like posture, balance adjustments, and non-intentional gross motor movements that are part of a more complex act like walking. Damage to the extrapyramidal nerve system can result in a disruption or impairment of motor ability.

Patients with more advanced AD may display extrapyramidal signs; it depends on how the AD progresses in each case. If the neurofibrillary tangles and amyloid plaques that are characteristic of AD (see more about this in Chapter 3) invade the basal ganglia, extrapyramidal symptoms follow because the functioning of this part of the brain is disrupted. Remember that if extrapyramidal symptoms occur, these degenerative changes are more likely to happen in the later stages of the disease.

### Restlessness or agitation

Another significant physical symptom that develops as AD progresses is restlessness or agitation. The patient can't seem to sit still for a moment and is constantly pacing around with no real purpose in mind.

One family tried keeping their father at home after he developed a habit of marching up and down the street with a clipboard, ringing each doorbell as he went. The man had been a successful door-to-door salesman all his life, and the clipboard was where he had recorded his sales. Even though he was no longer employed and had nothing to sell, he remembered that the clipboard was something important to him, so he carried it with him faithfully on his wanderings. As he wandered farther away, he became disoriented and couldn't find his way home. Kind neighbors always brought him back, but the stress of not being able to keep their father safely at home finally caused this family to place him in a residential facility that specialized in caring for AD patients.

Restlessness may also manifest as sleep disruption, occurring in as many as 45 percent of all AD cases. Some patients withdraw and sleep almost all the time, while others barely sleep at all. Many families report that their AD patient roams around all night long, making it impossible for other family members to sleep soundly. In extreme cases, the patient may experience a complete reversal of their nights and days, sleeping all day and staying awake and active all night. In addition to physical aggression and incontinence, families cite sleep disturbances as a major reason why they decide to put their loved one in a residential care facility.

### Other physical symptoms

The following physical symptoms may also be present in AD patients, but they generally don't appear until someone is profoundly affected by the disease.

- **Impaired motor ability:** Even though muscle function remains intact, the nerve signals that initiate voluntary movement may degrade as AD progresses into the sections of the brain that control these movements. When this happens, your loved one may move more slowly or with a marked degree of uncertainty.
- **Difficulty walking**
- **Problems with pacing or poor directions**
- **Trouble maintaining balance, resulting in falls**

Remember that these kinds of physical symptoms generally don't appear until later in the course of AD. If they appear early on, you may be looking at something else altogether, such as Parkinson's Disease, stroke, or Normal Pressure Hydrocephalus (NPH), all of which produce gait disturbances right from the onset of the problem. See Chapter 4 for a complete discussion of conditions that may mimic the symptoms of AD.

# Red Flag or Red Herring?

So how do you decide whether you need to take your loved one to a doctor for assessment? *Any ongoing memory loss requires professional evaluation.* Remember that doctors are looking for memory loss *and* at least one other cognitive deficit or problem in day-to-day functioning in order to make a diagnosis of AD. AD *may* be the cause if memory loss is accompanied by

- Difficulty speaking or comprehending information
- Confusion
- Disorientation (for example, confusing the days of the week or problems estimating or telling time)
- Problems recognizing or identifying objects
- Problems with motor skills
- Personality changes (such as sudden irritability)
- Agitation (such as restlessness, pacing, unprovoked verbal or physical aggression)
- Problems recognizing similarities or differences between ideas and concepts
- Problems planning, reasoning, judging, and other higher-level thinking
- Any significant change in day-to-day functioning that contradicts your loved one's normal conduct

If you suspect AD, start keeping a record of any symptoms and behavioral changes that you notice in your loved one. Gathering this information gives your doctor a leg up as she starts the diagnostic process.

One of the biggest problems healthcare professionals face when diagnosing AD is that other conditions mimic many of its most common symptoms. That's why it's important for you to present the big picture to your doctor; looking at a patient's entire range of emotional and behavioral difficulties along with problems in their cognitive skills helps doctors make a better diagnosis. Any bit of information that you don't include in your comments to your loved one's doctor may be the missing key that prevents an accurate diagnosis or a diagnosis at all. Leaving out information can also prevent a referral to a specialist.

For example, if you forget to mention that your loved one has a thyroid condition but refuses to take the prescribed medication, or if you don't know whether she's taking it, then your doctor may believe that some of the symptoms caused by the thyroid condition are an early manifestation of AD. That's why it's so important to maintain complete healthcare records and to make sure you share *all* the information you have with your doctor, even if it doesn't seem important.

You may be thinking that seems like an awful lot of work, and you'd be right. Some concentrated effort is required to gather all the information your doctor may need to make an accurate diagnosis of your loved one's condition. Write things down as you notice them. The most important thing is to record events as they happen, noting the time of day and whatever incident may have preceded the behavior you're noting.

The idea is to give your doctor as much information as you can about your loved one's symptoms and behavior. Only an experienced healthcare professional can determine whether a particular fact truly raises a red flag of concern or is simply a red herring that can lead in the wrong direction if it's given too much importance. If your doctor isn't familiar with dementia, seek a second opinion.

# Looking at Some Theories on the Causes of AD

When it comes to pinpointing the causes of AD, the jury is still out. Researchers believe several factors may contribute to someone developing the condition. There is definitely a genetic component to the inherited form of AD, but familial AD is rare, accounting for 1 to 5 percent of all cases. In other words, a lot of work still needs to be done before any definitive answers about the causes of AD are known.

Researchers have identified age as the most important risk factor for developing AD. But this isn't to imply that dementia is an inevitable consequence of aging; people who manage their risk factors and are proactive about their health have a statistically significant improvement in their odds of staying both mentally and physically healthy as they grow older.

According to the Alzheimer's Disease Education and Referral Center, for every five years past the age of 65, the number of people with AD doubles.

## Aging theories

Aging increases the risk for developing AD, but scientists are only now beginning to theorize why this may be so. A body of evidence has accumulated over the past 20 years that free radicals (highly reactive molecules produced as a byproduct of metabolism) cause damage to cells throughout the body. Some speculate that this kind of age-related change in brain tissue may be responsible for triggering the onset of AD.

Another theory involves something called messenger RNA. *Messenger RNA* is a class of ribonucleic acid that serves as a template for protein synthesis. As people age, mutations in their messenger RNA lead to mistakes in the amino acid sequences of the proteins they manufacture. Those damaged proteins (amyloid precursor protein and ubiquitin-B) are found in the brains of AD patients along with their corresponding mutated messenger RNA; however, these substances aren't found in the brains of people who don't have AD. Researchers haven't determined if this buildup of protein that can damage other molecules in cell membranes is a cause or a consequence of AD.

Unfortunately, that's as far as research has currently taken us. The proteins have been identified, and it's certain that they appear in the brains of all AD patients. But what causes these proteins to form is not known. What is known is that the chances of getting abnormal protein deposits in the brain increase dramatically with age.

## Genetic theories

Scientists have done a lot of work in recent years with genes, trying to determine if and how genes may increase the risk for, modify the course of, or influence the onset of AD. People who have a family member with AD can take heart in this research. Although several genes have been identified as having something to do with the development of AD, only three (amyloid precursor protein, presenilin 1, and presenilin 2) have been linked to the early onset form of AD, called *autosomal dominant inheritance*. Most people with this inherited form of AD first develop symptoms between the ages of 40 to 60.

### A2M gene

The A2M gene, or the alpha 2-macroglobulin, has been identified as a sort of trash collector in the brain. The A2M's job is to pick up potentially toxic peptides, such as the amyloid precursor protein, and carry them out of the brain to an area of the body where they're degraded and excreted. Researchers now believe that when the A2M gene undergoes mutation, it no longer performs its trash collecting chores as effectively, allowing dangerous deposits of amyloid protein to build up in the brain, perhaps leading to the onset of AD.

Research is underway to find out whether there is a familial component to this mutation or whether the mutation is something that happens randomly throughout the population. Remember that gene mutation is the least common pathological cause of AD.

### E4 variant

The E4 variant of the APOE gene, or apolipoprotein gene, has been associated with an increased risk of developing AD. But the presence of the E4 variant isn't predictive of AD; it's simply another risk factor for developing the condition. Forty to 50 percent of patients with AD have the E4 variant, but half of the people who have E4 never develop AD; so some additional factor must trigger AD.

Long before any clinical symptoms appear, some people with the E4 variant show declines in visual attention that may be suggestive of the eventual onset of AD. This discovery excited researchers because it was the first time they were able to use genes to identify subtle cognitive changes in an at-risk segment of the population that wasn't yet showing any signs of the disease.

## Microbial theory

Some researchers are looking into whether a viral or bacterial infection may trigger the onset of AD. The microbial theory has gained credibility in recent years because of similar studies that have proven a hitherto little-known bacteria *(Helicobacter pylori)* is responsible for many ulcers, and bacterial or viral inflammations are now suspected as causative factors in heart attacks.

Researchers are studying several pathogens (organisms that cause disease). *Chlamydia pneumoniae*, a common bacteria that causes pneumonia or bronchitis and is easily spread by coughing or sneezing, has recently been identified as an underlying causative factor in hardening of the arteries. Researchers have proposed that the same organism may also play a role in the development of such diverse conditions as asthma, arthritis, and even AD. It's interesting to note that as people age, the prevalence of *Chlamydia pneumoniae* infection increases.

## Nutritional theory

A growing body of evidence suggests that people who follow a diet high in essential fatty acids, low in saturated fats and trans fatty acids, and rich in naturally occurring antioxidants like vitamins E and C, may have a lower risk of developing AD. Numerous studies have shown that people who had high dietary consumption of vitamin E had a 67 percent lower risk of developing AD than people who consumed very little vitamin E. Interestingly, the effect was seen only in vitamin E consumed in the diet and couldn't be duplicated with vitamin E supplements.

Another study showed that people who ate primarily fresh fruits and vegetables along with lean fish and poultry had a lower risk of developing AD than people who ate high-fat, high-sugar diets.

Although much more research is needed, the findings certainly are thought-provoking and reason enough for people interested in maintaining long-term health to take a hard look at their diet and make changes to benefit their overall well-being.

## Cardiovascular risk

Some researchers speculate that cardiovascular disease may increase the risk of developing AD. High levels of the amino acid homocysteine increase the risk for cardiovascular disease by increasing inflammation in the heart and arteries. Several studies are underway to determine whether high levels of homocysteine may also increase the risk of developing AD, and whether statin drugs (used to lower cholesterol in cardiovascular patients) may also reduce the incidence of AD in at-risk patients.

## Head trauma theory

A number of studies have found a link between traumatic brain injuries that resulted in a loss of consciousness with an increased incidence of AD. The link is particularly significant in people who have not only suffered a serious head injury at some point during their lives but who also have the E4 variant of the APOE gene.

## Early life education and stimulation theory

Some studies show the more years of education someone has, the less likely he or she is to develop AD. The theory is that the additional years of study force the brain to develop denser networks of synapses, making the brain less susceptible to AD because it has to use a sports term, a "deeper bench" or cognitive reserve of brain cells to draw upon to compensate for any damage caused by early AD.

A *synapse* is a specialized junction or point of connection between two nerve cells or neurons, where one neuron communicates with a target cell by means of chemical messengers known as neurotransmitters.

## Immune system theory

Dr. Zhi-Qi Xiong and Dr. James McNamara of Duke University recently published a study in the journal, *Neuron*, outlining their theory that AD is an autoimmune response to some outside provocation that causes the body to attack itself. They postulate that such a response may follow a seizure, traumatic brain injury, or stroke. Although other doctors disagree with their findings, their theory represents another intriguing idea about the underlying cause of AD.

## Environmental triggers

Some of the most interesting AD research is being conducted by scientists looking for a link between environment and the onset of AD. Preliminary studies suggest that people with a large number of siblings have a higher risk of developing the disease, while people who were raised in the suburbs have a lower risk. Researchers theorize that some unknown environmental or socioeconomic factor that directly impacts brain growth and development in young children may translate to a higher risk of developing AD later in life.

Researchers are examining a plethora of ideas in their attempts to isolate the cause of AD. The most current thinking is that AD has no single cause, but rather a cascade of events that may be triggered by one precipitating event, like an infection or an injury.

# Examining Risk Factors for Developing Alzheimer's Disease

Advancing age increases the likelihood of developing AD, but other risk factors may play a contributing role in the development of the disease as well. Just remember that risk factors don't cause the disease — they just give you a better idea of what your odds are of developing a given condition. A few of the better-recognized risk factors for AD are a family history of the disease, presence of the E4 variant gene, and high blood pressure and high cholesterol.

## Family history

Families that have two generations or more of close relatives (a parent or sibling) who developed early onset AD (ages 65 or under) may have Familial Alzheimer's Disease (FAD). Families that have a history of AD have a greater chance of developing the disease than people who have no family history of the condition. The good news is that FAD accounts for only 1 to 5 percent of all AD cases.

# Counting the cost: Alzheimer's Disease statistics and prevalence

Although AD isn't our most deadly disease (heart disease claims that dubious distinction), it is one of our more expensive ones, mainly because people live with it for so long and require so much supervision and care. AD puts a huge drain on our healthcare resources, and the problem is only getting bigger. In 1900, only 3 million Americans were ages 65 and older; currently, the United States has approximately 34 million senior citizens who make up 13 percent of the population.

By 2040, the year when the last of the Baby Boomers hits age 65, the number of new cases of Alzheimer's Disease is expected to more than double, from an average of 377,000 new cases a year now to more than 959,000 new cases annually by 2040. By the year 2050, experts estimate that about 50 million older Americans will comprise 18 percent of the population, with approximately 14 million cases of Alzheimer's Disease, almost four times the 4 million cases we have now.

Take a look at these interesting statistics regarding Alzheimer's Disease:

✔ Average age at onset: 72.8 years

✔ Average length of time between onset of symptoms and diagnosis: 2.8 years

✔ Average length of survival following diagnosis at age 65: 8.3 years

✔ Average length of survival following diagnosis at age 90: 3.4 years

✔ Number of deaths from Alzheimer's Disease in 2000: 49,558

✔ Alzheimer's rank among causes of death: 8

✔ Alzheimer's relative cost: third most expensive disease

✔ Average cost of Alzheimer's Disease to U.S. economy annually: $100 billion

✔ Annual cost of lost productivity due to work disruptions related to caregiving: $26 billion

✔ Annual cost of caregiver absenteeism to businesses: $7.89 billion

✔ Average annual cost of caregiving per family: $12,500

✔ Average lifetime caregiving cost per AD patient: $174,000

✔ Average length of nursing home stay for AD patients: 2.5 years

✔ Average cost of nursing home care for AD patients: $139,000

## E4 variant

People who have at least one E4 variant gene are twice as likely to develop late onset AD than people who don't have this gene variant. People who have the E4 variant gene and high blood pressure have a five times greater chance of developing the condition; if they also have high cholesterol, their risk is eight times greater. Remember, though, that just having the E4 variant gene doesn't automatically mean that you'll get AD. Having the gene is simply one of the risk factors. The use of genetic testing to determine the presence of the E4 variant in unimpaired individuals isn't recommended.

## High blood pressure and high cholesterol

Researchers are starting to explore the possibility that many of the well-established risk factors for cardiovascular disease, including high cholesterol and high blood pressure, may also be risk factors for AD. A large study conducted by researchers in Finland showed a strong link between elevated cholesterol and high blood pressure and the eventual development of AD. All the more reason to keep these two conditions under control.

# Chapter 3

# Getting a Diagnosis

· · · · · · · · · · · · · · · · · · · · · · · · · · · · · · · · · · · · ·

· · · · · · · · · · · · · · · · · · · · · · · · · · · · · · · · · · · · ·

*P*erhaps you've decided that there's a good chance your loved one is suffering from Alzheimer's Disease (AD). Now you need to get a definitive diagnosis so that you can start planning for the future.

This chapter provides an overview of standardized Alzheimer's Disease diagnostic criteria. In other words, we explain how a doctor diagnoses AD. In many ways, the diagnostic process is something like following a treasure map. The path may not be clear, but if your doctors can make out all the clues, they'll end up at the right destination.

We also give you guidelines to find an appropriate healthcare provider to perform an evaluation of your family member. We discuss the types of tests that may be performed to reach a diagnosis, including an initial screening; a mental status evaluation and a battery of neuropsychological tests that help to determine the patient's current level of cognitive and functional ability; a neurological status evaluation; a general physical exam; various imaging studies; and blood tests.

After you get a diagnosis, you need some good ideas to help you decide if, how, and when to share the news with friends and family members. Many people will step up to the plate and offer to help in any way they can, but be prepared for some surprises. We help you anticipate the range of reactions you may encounter. Finally, we share some clues to identify people who may be willing to help you shoulder the responsibility of caring for your loved one. It's a big job, and you're not going to want to go it alone.

# How Doctors Diagnose Alzheimer's Disease

There is no definitive, 100 percent sure way to diagnose Alzheimer's Disease other than by dissecting the patient's brain after death to look for the presence of characteristic neurofibrillary tangles (see the next paragraph) and amyloid plaques in the brain. However, by applying nationally recognized diagnostic criteria, doctors can and do make the diagnosis of Alzheimer's Disease with 90 percent or greater accuracy. Diagnosis is a two-part process. First, doctors conduct a variety of tests to rule out what the patient doesn't have, for example, to determine that a patient hasn't had a stroke, doesn't have Parkinson's Disease or multiple sclerosis, and has no history of mental illness.

What the heck are *neurofibrillary tangles?* They're abnormal deposits of a protein called tau along nerve pathways within the brain. The body normally uses tau to build and repair structures called *microtubules* that the body uses to transport substances like nutrients and waste products into and out of brain cells. In AD, the microtubules collapse in tangles, which means that the cells of the brain can no longer communicate with each other and the brain can't work the way it's supposed to. As the tangles accumulate throughout the brain, the Alzheimer's patient becomes less and less able to function normally.

Then doctors use standardized diagnostic criteria that outline the behaviors, physical symptoms, and cognitive symptoms that are typical of Alzheimer's Disease sufferers to "rule in" a diagnosis of AD. If your loved one meets the criteria for AD established by The American Psychiatric Association DSM (Diagnostic and Statistical Manual) or The National Institute of Neurological and Communicative Diseases and Stroke/Alzheimer's Disease and Related Disorders Association and no other underlying cause for their symptoms is found during a physical examination, then your doctor should feel assured in making a diagnosis of Alzheimer's Disease.

Cognitive deficits have many causes. Something as readily identifiable as depression, a thyroid problem, dehydration, or even a vitamin deficiency can cause people to act in an impaired manner. It doesn't always have to be AD. Appropriate diagnostic tests can help your doctor determine the cause of your loved one's problem and the best course of treatment.

# Finding Someone to Do an Evaluation

One of the most important decisions you'll make when you start looking for a conclusive diagnosis is who to call. If you live in or near a large metropolitan area, you may be able to find an Alzheimer's Disease or dementia program associated with a medical school, and that's a good place to start.

Before you seek a diagnosis of AD, get long-term care insurance. You can always cancel the policy if you do not have AD; however, if you do have a diagnosis of AD on your medical records, you are no longer eligible to purchase long term care insurance.

Unfortunately, you can't just pick up the phone book and find an Alzheimer's expert. Even in very large cities, the only listings you're likely to see under "Alzheimer's Disease" in the Yellow Pages are ads for home care services, special daycare programs, or the Alzheimer's Association. In smaller communities, you may not even find a listing for Alzheimer's Disease.

Your local branch of the Alzheimer's Association may maintain a list of healthcare providers who treat people with AD.

But don't despair. Although all sorts of medical practitioners deal with Alzheimer's Disease and deciding which doctor to consult can be a daunting task, we guide you through the maze. If you're not familiar with the different types of practitioners who deal with AD — neurologists, gerontologists, psychiatrists, psychologists, even internal medicine specialists and family practitioners — here is where you find the help you need to choose the right healthcare provider for your family and circumstances.

This section lists the various specialists who deal with AD and provides an overview of their particular area of expertise. During the course of diagnosis and treatment, you and your loved one may see many different doctors, so you may meet one or more of the specialists we describe. Why is it important to know the difference between various specialists? Because informed patients ask better questions and get better answers from their doctors.

## Enlisting help from your family doctor

The easiest place to start is with the doctor who knows you and your loved one best: your family practitioner, sometimes called a primary care physician. Even though family practitioners may not be specialists in Alzheimer's Disease, they are specialists in the health of their patients. When a doctor has seen a patient regularly over many years, it's easier for him or her to pick up on subtle changes in behavior and personality that may signal a real problem. Someone who's never seen the patient before doesn't have this advantage.

Family practitioners generally have a network of specialists that they work with on a regular basis. They feel comfortable referring patients who need further assessment to these trusted colleagues. If your primary care physician suspects that your loved one may have Alzheimer's Disease, he may make the diagnosis himself or refer you to a specialist for further evaluation. If you feel that your primary care physician isn't responsive to your concerns, don't hesitate to ask for a referral to another doctor or a specialist.

Unfortunately, research shows that, as a group, primary care physicians aren't very good at diagnosing Alzheimer's Disease, especially early on. One study showed an average of 30 months from time of onset of symptoms of AD until diagnosis by the primary care physician.

## Picking a specialist

Several types of healthcare providers specialize in the diagnosis and treatment of Alzheimer's Disease. We provide an overview to help you understand their different areas of focus. Armed with this info, you'll be able to ask a few savvy questions if your loved one is referred to a specialist for further testing. And remember that the title of neurologist, geriatrician, or psychiatrist doesn't automatically mean that the doctor is an AD expert. Go ahead and ask if you're not sure of a doctor's area of specialization or experience in working with AD patients.

✔ **Neurologists:** A neurologist is a physician specializing in the diagnosis and treatment of disorders of the nervous system, such as strokes, seizures, headaches, multiple sclerosis, other muscle and nerve diseases, nervous system tumors and infections, Parkinson's Disease, and dementias, including Alzheimer's Disease.

If you're picking a specialist out of the phone book, make sure that you call a *neurologist* and not a *neurosurgeon*. A doctor specifically trained in the surgical treatment of nervous system disorders and disorders of the areas surrounding the brain and spinal cord is called a neurosurgeon. If you end up in a neurosurgeon's office, she'll refer you to a neurologist anyway, so save yourself some time and expense by starting out with the appropriate specialist. Fortunately, Alzheimer's patients rarely require any sort of surgery, not unless other health problems that are unrelated to the Alzheimer's diagnosis, such as diabetes or heart disease, are present.

✔ **Geriatricians:** Geriatrics is the branch of medicine that deals with the medical problems of patients ages 50 and older. Geriatricians are physicians practicing this specialty. As you get older, the rate of Alzheimer's Disease rises dramatically — from about 10 percent of adults at age 65 to 50 percent at age 80. Because the incidence of AD increases so significantly with advancing age, geriatricians are frequently called upon to diagnose and treat Alzheimer's patients.

✔ **Psychiatrists:** Psychiatrists are medical doctors who specialize in the diagnosis and treatment of mental illness. Psychiatrists can determine whether a symptom such as agitation is indicative of mental illness or a manifestation of an underlying problem such as pain or infection, or is a sign of a neurodegenerative disorder such as Alzheimer's. Keep in mind that people with Alzheimer's Disease may also suffer from psychiatric problems, such as depression or anxiety, that should be treated.

✔ **Psychologists:** Psychologists aren't medical doctors and, therefore, can't prescribe medications. They specialize in the science of human behavior, including its physical, cognitive, social, and emotional components. Some psychologists specialize in counseling Alzheimer's patients and their families. Psychologists who specialize in AD may partner with a doctor in one of the specialties listed earlier so that a patient's medical as well as emotional needs can be met. They can also help a patient's family members learn how to deal with symptoms of AD.

✔ **Neuropsychologists:** Neuropsychologists practice a specialty of psychology that involves the study of the relationship of functions of the physical body, especially the brain, with emotions, thinking functions, and behavior. Neuropsychologists conduct a battery of diagnostic tests that reveal the reliable cognitive and personality results for various dementia disorders. The tests used are very specific and sensitive in determining the functional status of the part of the brain they're related to. Physicians then factor these findings into their diagnostic decision making.

Try asking friends who may have a family member with Alzheimer's for the names of their healthcare providers. Their advice can be particularly valuable because it's based on personal experience. Other patients and their family members have nothing to gain or lose by providing an honest assessment of a physician. Talking to people who've been down the road before you can save you time and money. Doing so may also help you to avoid wasting your time with a difficult or not very helpful doc.

Although a specialist such as a neurologist or psychiatrist may manage AD, patients still need a generalist or primary care physician to manage their other health needs. For example, some common diseases, such as urinary tract infections, may make the cognitive problems of Alzheimer's Disease more severe. A neurologist may not feel comfortable treating this problem, but the primary care provider and the specialist can really work together in situations like this to provide optimum care for their patient.

## Evaluating your choices

With so many choices, how do you know which doctor to select as the primary healthcare provider for your loved one? Although you must consider several factors, the most important one is to trust your own instincts. Still unsure? Ask yourself the following questions before making your choice. And remember, if you're not happy with the first doctor you choose, there's no law against switching to another doctor who may make you feel less rushed or do a better job of answering questions and calming your fears.

✔ Do you like and trust the doctor?

✔ Does he or she have experience in diagnosing and treating AD patients?

> ✔ Does your loved one feel comfortable with him or her?
>
> ✔ Does the doctor answer your questions and those of your loved one fully and treat you both with courtesy, compassion, and respect?

The answers to these questions are important because they can help you select a healthcare provider who keeps you informed and helps you both to feel comfortable and supported. AD typically progresses at a slow rate, so finding a doctor you can work with over a long period of time is essential.

## Tapping into other resources

If your family practitioner doesn't know a local specialist, try contacting the local branch of the Alzheimer's Association for a physician referral. Can't find the organization in your phone book? Go online to www.alz.org.

Click on Your Chapter at the top of the page and then enter your zip code to find the group nearest you. Volunteers with the local chapter of the Alzheimer's Association should be able to help you find an Alzheimer's specialist in your area.

Many Alzheimer's Disease centers (ADCs), Alzheimer's Disease research centers (ADRCs), and Alzheimer's Disease clinical centers (ADCCs) don't require a physician referral for a patient to be seen. These centers are funded by the National Institute on Aging and located in major medical institutions and teaching centers nationwide. Some maintain satellite facilities to serve rural and minority communities. Call your local Alzheimer's Association for information regarding the availability of such services in your area.

Wondering whether an ADRC or ADCC is located near you? Log on to www.alzheimers.org/pubs/adcdir.html#about and scroll down to the list of states that have these centers. Find your state and then call the ADC nearest you to see whether it offers any services close to your home.

The doctors and research scientists who staff Alzheimer's Disease centers are devoted to better understanding the cause of AD and to finding effective new treatments. And yes, they're also searching for a cure and, better yet, a preventive measure like a vaccine that would spare future generations from the heartbreak of this devastating disease. Because the centers are networked, researchers are able to collaborate on promising treatments; the resulting synergy is producing some exciting advances in the field of AD treatments.

So what does all this mean for you and your loved one? If you're fortunate enough to live close to an ADC, you'll be able to take advantage of the latest diagnostic and disease management resources, as well as tap into a vast storehouse of knowledge and information about AD. You'll find support groups for caregivers; some centers even have support groups for Alzheimer's patients themselves. Private counseling for the patient and his family may be available. In addition, your loved one may have the option to participate in a clinical research trial to evaluate new Alzheimer's drug therapies.

# Before You Seek a Diagnosis: Collecting Medical History

If you've made up your mind to pursue a diagnosis for your loved one, you can do several things to help your doctor determine what's causing the symptoms. If you were a fly on the wall in any doctor's lounge, you'd discover that their number one complaint is that patients don't provide their doctors with enough information to plan a targeted diagnostic assessment.

The first thing any doctor does when seeing a new patient is collect a medical history from that patient. You know those 28-page documents that your doctor's office forces you to fill out when you have a sprained knee and are waiting to see an orthopod for the first time, the documents that make you ask, "What does beriberi have to do with anything?"

Yes, those medical histories. It's most helpful to your physician if you inform him of any other health problems your loved one may be experiencing, particularly chronic problems such as diabetes or emphysema that require ongoing care and daily medications. It's also helpful for your doctor to know whether any other family members have ever suffered from any sort of organic brain disease, because there's a rare type of AD that is genetic and may be inherited. (If you want to find out more about this, flip to Chapter 2.)

## Digging through your roots

Now's the time to compile your family's medical history. You may have to search through old family scrapbooks or obituary clippings to find causes of death for your older family members, or even interview maiden aunts or long-lost cousins you haven't seen in years. But this expedition through your family's medical history is important. A little digging through your roots can produce some valuable clues to help your doctor narrow the scope of his or her diagnostic efforts by providing other possible causes or contributing factors for the symptoms your loved one is displaying.

A complete family medical history can suggest areas of interest to a doctor. For example, if your family has a tendency toward lung problems, perhaps chronic oxygen insufficiency is causing your loved one's neurological symptoms. If the doctor treats the breathing problem, that may help the neurological problems to clear on their own. Or your loved one could be suffering from sleep apnea, a sleep disorder that shuts off the airway, repeatedly depriving the brain of oxygen for periods as long as a minute throughout the night. This asphyxiation "in slow motion" can seriously affect memory and attention.

Please don't hold any information back from your doctor because you think that it's too embarrassing to think about, much less write down. You know what we're talking about — things like psychiatric, gastrointestinal, urinary, or sexual problems. Details help to support or rule out a diagnosis of a particular disorder. For example, impotence in men is frequently caused by high blood pressure, and this same high blood pressure may have significant adverse effects on the brain. So tell your doctor everything you know about your loved one's medical history, even if you don't think it's relevant. You should also include any pertinent information about your family's medical history, particularly if your family has a history of AD or another condition that needs monitoring like diabetes or heart disease.

On the other hand, if your loved one has no underlying health issues and the symptoms seem to exist independently of any other condition, the doctor may suspect that Alzheimer's may be causing the neurological and behavioral problems you're reporting, but only a complete workup will provide a definite answer.

After you've gathered as much family medical history as you can, it's time to construct an individual medical history for your loved one. Make it as complete as possible. You may have to collect medical records from a number of doctors to build an accurate history. Although most doctors readily comply with requests for these records, occasionally, one will make it difficult and try to act like you can't have the information you're seeking.

If a doctor's office gives you an attitude when you request medical records, remind the staff that while the records belong to the doctor, the information contained within those records belongs to the patient and you have a legal right to access it. The doctor's office can charge you a small copying fee, but they can't refuse to provide you with copies of requested records.

No matter how hard you search, some records may be impossible to find. For example, a doctor may have retired, passed away, moved to a different state, or even lost his records. If you can't find complete medical records for your loved one, try to fill in the blanks by talking to family members and friends. Ask whether they can recall any details that may help your current doctor make a good diagnosis.

## Keeping a journal

When you first notice symptoms that make you suspect your loved one may be entering the early stages of Alzheimer's Disease, start keeping a journal. When you think "journal," don't think, "I must have an expensive leather-bound volume with hand-pressed paper and a little brass key and secret password." Not unless you want to. A journal can be something as simple as a 79-cent spiral notebook. The most important thing is to record events in the order they happen. Note specific instances of worrisome or uncharacteristic behavior, and accurately record the date, time of day, and any factors you believe may have triggered the incident and that may help the doctor in his evaluation. For example, record exactly what happened and what your loved one was doing just before and during the event and how long the event lasted.

This sort of information can be invaluable in helping a doctor determine a diagnostic approach. For example, if your journal shows that your loved one is blacking out frequently, your doctor may begin looking at cerebral vascular disease or seizures as the problem. A series of TIAs, or *transient ischemic attacks*, during which the blood supply to the brain is momentarily cut off, can produce neurological symptoms similar to those experienced by the AD patient. If your journal shows that your loved one's symptoms started soon after a new medication was added, the doctor may suspect that the medication could be triggering the altered behavior. This problem is very common in older people, especially if they're going to several doctors and taking many prescriptions, some of which may not be compatible. This problem also highlights the importance of all your doctors being in communication with each other to prevent situations where combinations of various drugs can cause cognitive problems or even actually be life threatening.

If you don't record information in your journal as it happens, and you don't tell your doctor about significant events such as behavioral changes or new physical symptoms, you may put yourself and your family member through an expensive and unnecessary series of tests as the doctor strives to rule out possible causes for the symptoms.

## Looking for other sources of information

While you're gathering records to compile your family member's medical history, don't forget the person's dental history as well. Infections spreading from the gums to the interior of the heart and its valves and even brain infections resulting from oral surgery may cause permanent brain damage that affects day-to-day functioning

Other family members may be able to help if you can't get all the information you need to compile a complete medical history for your patient. If the patient is one of your parents, perhaps your aunts and uncles can tell you where to get additional information. If the patient is your spouse, the employer's insurance company or human resources department may have additional medical history that your family doctor doesn't have. Even an old family Bible that lists causes of death for deceased relatives can provide a valuable clue for your doctor in his search for answers.

## Rounding up medication records

When you're compiling a medical history for your patient, don't forget to include a complete list of any prescription drugs, over-the-counter medications, vitamins, and herbs your patient may be taking. This information is vitally important in order to avoid a potential drug interaction.

For example, if your loved one has a tendency toward blood clots, your doctor may put her on a blood thinner such as heparin or Coumadin. But if you fail to inform your doctor that the patient is already taking aspirin or an herbal remedy that can also act as a blood thinner, such as ginkgo biloba, or even high doses of vitamin E, mixing the medications together could trigger a potentially fatal stroke or lead to a hemorrhage if the patient requires emergency surgery.

Many pharmacies today keep computerized records of their customers' medication histories. If you patronize a pharmacy that maintains such records, simply ask it to print out a copy for you to give to the doctor. But remember, these records supply only prescription drug information; you yourself must supply accurate records regarding any self-prescribed vitamin, mineral, nutritional supplement, or herbal regimen your loved one may be using.

# Understanding AD Diagnostic Tests

We know that not having a piece of paper with a definite diagnosis written on it can be unsettling. This is just one of the many frustrating things about Alzheimer's Disease: You can't be 100 percent sure that's what you're dealing with. But current diagnostic practices do offer a high degree of certainty. And researchers are attempting to develop kits intended for use in doctor's office screenings that would quickly identify Alzheimer's patients through use of gene markers or some other chemical flag.

Although no single definitive test for Alzheimer's Disease is currently available, modern diagnostic procedures can identify the disease with 90 percent or greater accuracy.

In the following sections, we discuss the various diagnostic tools your healthcare provider may use to help diagnose your loved one. We tell you why that particular procedure may be used and what information it provides.

# Diagnostic screening tools

A mental status evaluation (MSE) or mini mental state examination (MMSE) may be one of the first screening tests a doctor performs when trying to arrive at a diagnosis of Alzheimer's Disease. But the mental status examination is only a screening tool and may not be able to detect early symptoms of memory or thinking problems, particularly in high-functioning people.

The MSE exam includes assessment of three types of skills:

- ✔ **Self-care skills:** These skills include the ability to get dressed, prepare and eat simple meals, move about safely without risk of falling, bathe and perform other hygienic routines such as brushing teeth, driving, cleaning house, taking prescribed medications, and using household equipment and supplies appropriately.

- ✔ **Communication skills:** These skills include a person's ability to make himself understood either verbally or in writing, and the ability to read and understand simple written instructions and comprehend and carry out oral instructions consistently.

- ✔ **Simple math skills:** This category includes the ability to make proper change, write checks, pay bills, tell time, balance a checkbook, and manage personal finances.

The MMSE is a 10-minute standardized questionnaire that evaluates short-term memory, concentration, language, and visuospatial skills. Although it's not diagnostic, it quantifies cognitive ability and can track changes in functioning.

After these basic skills start to disappear, you must think about making lifestyle changes to keep your loved one safe, which may include setting up care arrangements. See Chapter 15 for more about choosing care options.

## Assessing your loved one's self-care skills

In order to assess your loved one's ability to care for his or herself, a psychologist or other professional may administer a self-care test that will clearly show whether he or she still is capable of functioning independently.

## But why do I even need a diagnosis?

You're pretty sure that your loved one has Alzheimer's Disease, so why waste time and money getting a diagnosis? What good is that going to do?

Getting an accurate diagnosis is essential because other medical conditions that are more treatable and sometimes even reversible, such as depression, stroke-related dementia, and some drug reactions, can mimic the symptoms of Alzheimer's Disease. If your loved one has such a look-alike but reversible condition and you just assume that it's Alzheimer's, the person won't get the treatment that could restore normal functioning. We discuss more about diseases that can be mistaken for Alzheimer's in Chapter 4.

Your doctor must perform a complete physical exam and comprehensive evaluation of your loved one's cognitive and functional abilities so that he can give you the most accurate diagnosis and create a personalized treatment plan. Doing so helps you avoid unnecessary and expensive tests and procedures that won't help if the diagnosis is incorrect. Ultimately, finding out that your loved one actually has Alzheimer's relieves the stress of not knowing "for sure" and allows family members and their loved one to make reasonable plans for the future. It also gives the patient an opportunity to participate in his or her own future care, which can go a long way toward relieving the anxiety and fear associated with being diagnosed with Alzheimer's Disease. Finally, early diagnosis means early treatment, and early treatment gives your loved one the best chance of maintaining his or her cognitive abilities and usual functioning for a longer period of time.

The person administering the test will note several things:

- Does your loved one's appearance show attention to detail? Is she neatly groomed or disheveled, perhaps even dirty and wearing mismatched clothing, such as two different colors of socks or two different styles of shoes? (Inform the tester if you provide grooming and hygiene services for the patient so that the tester can get an accurate picture of your loved one's level of functioning.)

- Is he remembering to eat regular meals or is he losing weight?

- Can he manage his personal hygiene or does he need help?

- Is she paying her bills and income taxes on time?

- Can she successfully and consistently perform necessary household functions, such as cooking, and basic maintenance, such as garbage removal?

- Does he still know how to operate basic household equipment, such as furnaces, stoves, and faucets? Does he remember to turn appliances off when he's finished using them?

### Assessing communication skills

Communication skills vary widely from one person with Alzheimer's Disease to the next. One person may retain the ability to engage in conversation for quite some time, while another may struggle to find words, express himself, or understand conversations. As AD advances, your loved one is likely to suffer some loss of the ability to communicate. The loss is most often gradual; like all other symptoms we discuss, it varies from patient to patient.

No one can predict how any given patient will be affected as the disease progresses, but speech and communication skills can offer a measure for assessing a patient's current level of cognition. Here are some areas a tester may look at in order to assess your loved one's current level of cognitive functioning:

- ✔ Is his speech normal in tone and pacing?

- ✔ Does she speak in a louder than normal tone of voice?

- ✔ Does he have problems reading?

- ✔ Does she repeat the same statements, questions, or stories over and over?

- ✔ Can he listen to and follow instructions?

- ✔ Does she have difficulty expressing herself or finding the right word?

- ✔ Can he follow and participate in a normal conversation, or does he quickly lose interest?

- ✔ Are his facial expressions relaxed and friendly or guarded and worried?

- ✔ Does she look you straight in the eye or avoid eye contact?

- ✔ How is his mood? Is he depressed? Anxious? Angry? Irritable? Uninhibited? Inappropriately giddy?

### Assessing simple math skills

You may be wondering why math skills are important in assessing the ability to live independently. But think about how many times in the course of your day you use math. Every time you write a check, get change from a $10 bill for lunch, calculate a tip, or even try to figure out how much time you have before your big meeting, all those tasks depend on basic math skills.

When a person enters the early stages of Alzheimer's Disease, difficulty with math skills is one of the first signs that your loved one is having problems. Assessing your loved one's ability to perform simple math problems can give your healthcare provider a surprisingly accurate measurement of the degree of impairment.

Here are some things to watch for that you may want to report to your doctor:

- ✔ Does your loved one have difficulty performing simple math problems?
- ✔ Can she balance a checkbook, make change, or calculate a tip?
- ✔ Can she follow a complex train of thought or perform activities that have many sequential steps, such as cooking?

Your observations help the doctor construct a profile of the patient's current level of cognitive functioning. A skilled examiner can interpret your patient's particular array of symptoms to help the doctor make his diagnosis. Regular assessments of these skills will help you decide when your loved one requires additional care or monitoring. Ongoing reevaluation of cognitive functioning is critical to provide the best possible care for your loved one.

## Competency and capacity tests

We must make it clear from the outset that competency is a legal and not a medical issue. Your doctor's primary concern is the well-being of his patients; he's not interested in their legal status. But because healthcare providers are the ones who perform the tests that lawyers and courts use to make judgments about competence and the need for a legal guardian, you must find someone who's skilled and experienced to assess a person's capacity to provide food, clothing, or shelter for himself or herself; to care for the individual's own physical health; or to manage the individual's own financial affairs.

Capacity testing is another tool to help you assess what level of care your family member requires to stay safe. A competent person uses good judgment and exercises his ability to reason in order to make appropriate decisions. Alzheimer's Disease impairs judgment and reason, which, in the eyes of the law, are necessary for a person to be considered competent. Memory loss also contributes to incompetency. People do learn from their mistakes, and when they can't remember why they're not supposed to do something, they'll do it over and over again and be continually surprised at the negative outcome.

When people can no longer remember basic concepts such as "I should not put my hand on the stove because it's hot," their safety is at risk. In that situation, you must make appropriate arrangements for increased care and monitoring of your loved one as quickly as possible.

Competency also involves the ability to be oriented to time and place. Many Alzheimer's patients don't know where they are or what time of day it is. Some actually get lost in their own homes, unable to find their way from the bedroom to the kitchen or to the bathroom. If they leave their homes, they may quickly become disoriented and get lost.

Finally, competency involves basic eye-hand and motor coordination skills. As these start to erode, it becomes more and more difficult for a person with Alzheimer's Disease to function normally.

### Evaluating memory

An examiner will administer tests to determine whether your loved one is suffering from memory problems, the extent of those problems, and whether they affect immediate memories, recent memories, remote memories, or all three. The examiner will try to see whether the patient has trouble remembering recent events and conversations and whether the person has a tendency to misplace objects. Sometimes, Alzheimer's patients can become quite agitated if they can't immediately put their hands on something, such as their purse or a box of tissues. Even if it's in plain sight, they may not recognize it for what it is.

Don't be surprised or get upset if your loved one accuses you of stealing from him. Although it's distressing, this behavior is normal for Alzheimer's sufferers. Think how frustrated you would feel if you could never find your wallet. You might start to assume some sort of conspiracy was afoot, too. A little humor can help to defuse these situations, but they can be wearing. For tips on how to give yourself a mental health break, see Chapter 17.

### Assessing judgment and reasoning skills

The examiner will present your loved one with a series of problems or everyday situations and ask the person to plan a solution for the problem or give an appropriate response to a given situation. Here are some examples:

- ✔ If your bathroom flooded, what would you do? A person with normal cognitive functioning will tell you that he would lay down towels or some other absorbent material to clean up the water, and then call a plumber. A cognitively impaired person may offer a solution but not the best one; for example, he might say he'd call his doctor. Or he may offer no response at all, look away, and appear to be disinterested, or he may exhibit an inappropriate response, such as loud giggling or anger.

- ✔ If a man rang your doorbell and told you that your roof was damaged but he could repair it if you lent him your debit card to buy materials, what would you do? A cognizant person would recognize an obvious scam and either chase the man off or call the police. A person with impaired cognitive functioning might freely hand over his debit card, if he could remember where it was. If he couldn't remember its location, he may even go so far as to invite the person in to help him look!

As reasoning and judgment skills deteriorate, an Alzheimer's patient may become an easy target for rip-off artists. See Chapter 14 for ways to protect your loved one from fraud.

### Assessing disorientation

People in the early stage of AD have trouble managing time and keeping their appointments. People in the advanced stage often show classic signs of disorientation. They may not know where they are or why they're there, and they may not have any idea of the time of day, day of the week, or date. This disorientation may make them fearful, or they may become inattentive and easily distracted, or show overt signs of confusion by repeatedly asking where they are.

An examiner may ask your family member to say where he is and why he's there. The examiner may ask the patient what month it is or what time it is. Alzheimer's patients may have difficulty in answering even these simple types of questions.

The biggest danger with this loss of ability to remain oriented is that your loved one will get lost. Alzheimer's patients are at greater risk for wandering, so when this becomes a problem, you must consider changing your care arrangements to keep your loved one safe.

### Testing eye-hand coordination skills

Eye-hand coordination is another basic skill that everyone takes for granted. You may be asking yourself, but what that does that have to do with anything? Well, think about trying to feed yourself if you couldn't make your hand pick up and correctly hold your fork whenever you wanted. Or, if you did manage to pick it up, what if you still couldn't figure out how to get food from your plate to your mouth, where your mouth was, or even what a mouth was? That's the state your loved one may find herself in as the Alzheimer's Disease slowly advances.

An examiner may test eye-hand coordination through a series of simple exercises, such as the following:

- ✔ Can your loved one complete a simple task such as stacking a tower of blocks?
- ✔ Can he tie his shoes and consistently put the left shoe on the left foot?
- ✔ Can he button his shirt or use a zipper?
- ✔ Can he handle utensils with enough skill to feed himself?

### Testing motor skills

Your healthcare provider will observe several key points when assessing motor skills.

- ✔ Can your loved one walk steadily on his own without assistance, or is he shaky and disoriented?
- ✔ Can he sit down and get up again without assistance?
- ✔ Is he steady on his feet?

As motor skills start to fail, Alzheimer's patients tend to become more and more sedentary. Family members should try to keep sufferers up and moving for as long as possible because even moderate activity helps to decrease the incidence of other health problems, such as diabetes and heart disease. In addition, after an Alzheimer's patient loses the ability to walk, the loss of other cognitive skills seems to accelerate.

As with the mental status evaluation, your doctor will look at the results of the competency tests and use them to advise you about your loved one's current position. This information will help you to make good care choices for both yourself and for your family.

# Neurological assessment

Some people mistakenly think that a neurological assessment looks only at what's going on inside an Alzheimer's patient's brain. People hear the word *neurology* and tend to think "head." Even though the damage caused by Alzheimer's takes place in the brain, it eventually affects the entire body. A neurological assessment helps the doctor determine how Alzheimer's affects other bodily functions.

Neurology is the scientific study of the entire nervous system, especially in respect to its structures, functions, and abnormalities.

### Checking muscle tone and strength

If Alzheimer's sufferers become sedentary, they may lose a significant amount of their muscle tone and bodily strength. Their reflexes may become sluggish or nonexistent. A loss of muscle tone can then lead to problems with incontinence and even breathing or cardiovascular difficulties. It may also affect a person's ability to get around safely and may lead to falls.

Doctors check strength with a simple grip test and muscle tone using a hands-on "pull back" in the office. For example, the doctor may lightly hold a patient's wrist and ask the patient to pull against his grip as hard as he can. They check reflexes by applying a rubber hammer to the knee joint.

### Evaluating coordination and eye movements

One of the most baffling things about Alzheimer's Disease is that even though motor function remains intact, the damaged brain can't organize the series of commands required to execute a complex activity like walking. As people lose coordination, they may also lose their ability to walk.

The loss of coordination is so profound that it even affects eyesight. As Alzheimer's Disease progresses, it becomes increasingly difficult for sufferers to track moving objects with their eyes.

Doctors test eye coordination by holding up a finger and asking their patient to track the finger with his or her eyes as it moves. They check physical coordination by having the patient walk so that they can observe any abnormalities in the patient's gait or balance. They may also ask the patient to pretend to perform a routine task, asking, "Show me how you would throw a ball, brush your teeth, comb your hair," and so on because difficulty in imitating these everyday chores may indicate a breakdown in executive functions.

### Checking speech

Speech is a fairly complicated activity that requires our brains to coordinate the movement of our lips, tongues, teeth, and vocal cords to produce intelligible sounds. Alzheimer's sufferers may exhibit symptoms of *aphasia,* or the inability to use or comprehend words correctly. After other potential physical causes, such as a stroke, are ruled out, language disturbances are a good indication that someone may be suffering from Alzheimer's Disease.

In addition to neurological testing, which looks at several areas of language, doctors will evaluate patients' ability to understand language and express themselves through a clinical interview. They're looking for problems in understanding commands (for example, "Take this piece of paper, fold it, and place it on the table"), taking directions, and the ability to find the correct word when speaking. In other words, is the patient's speech fluid and cohesive, or does he or she show evidence of problems when speaking?

### Checking sensory abilities

Sensory abilities help people make sense of the physical world around them. Alzheimer's patients suffer a disruption of their sensory abilities that's similar to the language disruption described earlier. They may see a common item and yet be unable to tell what it is. Tests that reveal an inability to recognize familiar items despite the fact that the five senses are still working perfectly may also point to a diagnosis of Alzheimer's Disease.

Doctors must first confirm that the patient's difficulties in identifying common objects aren't caused by an actual physical impairment, such as failing eyesight or hearing. They administer standard visual and hearing checks to rule out this possibility. They also ask the patient and the patient's family if they're aware of any problems with vision or hearing.

Patients are told to arrive for the sensory exam wearing both their eyeglasses and their hearing aides if they require them. If the person has identified hearing problems but no hearing aide, the tester may have him or her wear a sound amplifier or "personal talker" during the test to ensure the best results.

# Physical and psychiatric exams

A physical exam is one of the most important parts of obtaining a diagnosis of Alzheimer's Disease because it can conclusively rule out other diseases and conditions that may be causing the suspicious symptoms. Psychiatric exams are important because early-stage Alzheimer's is frequently accompanied by clinical depression or another mood disorder, while patients with more advanced disease can present symptoms of psychosis. Treating those symptoms as well is important.

## Ruling out other physical causes

The primary purpose of the physical exam is to rule out other possible causes for the symptoms your loved one may be displaying, and also to check for any underlying illness that may require treatment as well. The exam should include the following:

- ✔ A complete physical, including a blood pressure reading

- ✔ A complete blood count

- ✔ Blood chemistry screens to determine blood gases, along with calcium, glucose, vitamin B-12 and electrolyte levels, and also to assess kidney and liver function

- ✔ Chest X-ray

- ✔ Urinalysis

- ✔ Thyroid function text

- ✔ Heavy metal and toxicology screening

- ✔ MRI or CT scans of the brain

High blood pressure is a leading risk factor for stroke. If your loved one has high blood pressure, she may have suffered a stroke that could explain her symptoms. Both kidney and liver disease can alter body chemistry and produce symptoms of dementia, as can variations in blood sugar or glucose, calcium, and vitamin B-12. Even an electrolyte imbalance can mimic Alzheimer's Disease. Certain thyroid conditions and syphilis can produce also similar symptoms; the good news is that those conditions can be treated successfully, and their symptoms reversed.

Brain scans can reveal areas of brain atrophy, stroke, the presence of tumors, or swelling of the brain. However, at present, scans can't detect plaque deposits or neurofibrillary tangles (see the section "How Doctors Diagnose Alzheimer's Disease," earlier in this chapter), the hallmark indicators of Alzheimer's Disease. This technology is currently under development.

### Ruling out other psychiatric causes

Don't get offended when your doctor orders a psychiatric examination for your family member; no one is suggesting that the person is crazy. But many conditions can mimic or contribute to symptoms of dementia and can be treated successfully

Psychiatric exams are important because mild Alzheimer's may be mistaken for clinical depression or another disorder such as anxiety, while some patients can present symptoms of outright psychosis. These conditions can mimic Alzheimer's Disease and/or coexist and make its symptoms worse. Making sure that your loved one gets appropriate treatment for these treatable psychiatric conditions greatly improves the person's quality of life.

Your loved one may also show signs of apathy, which is frequently mistaken for depression. Apathy is a common symptom of Alzheimer's patients and can interfere with your loved one's ability to organize, plan, and carry out normal activities. Doctors hear caregivers say, "He just doesn't do anything anymore. He won't do his hobbies. I keep telling him to get a new hobby, but he won't." Apathetic patients may quit going to their group counseling sessions.

Alzheimer's patients experiencing clinical depression can benefit greatly from an appropriate antidepressant. Your doctor may refer your loved one to a psychiatrist for an exam to rule out other potential causes for his symptoms.

# What to Do When the Diagnosis Is Made

You've been through all the tests and dragged your loved one to multiple doctors. Now it's time to get the results. If your doctor confirms your suspicions and tells you that your loved one most likely is suffering from Alzheimer's Disease, you two have some big decisions ahead. First, you must decide whether to get a second opinion to confirm the diagnosis. After that, you have to determine if and when you're going to share the news with family and friends. A person with Alzheimer's Disease may initially be reluctant to share the diagnosis with anyone, and you should respect that decision. Give it time; this is a normal response to a devastating diagnosis. Now is a good time to seek counseling to help you and your loved one plan for the future. When your loved one is ready, share the news with family and friends, and assess what sort of support you may have in the difficult days ahead.

## Seeking a second opinion

A diagnosis of Alzheimer's Disease can be terribly upsetting for both the patient and his family, so wanting a second opinion is natural. Just be aware that you don't need to go through all the testing and evaluation again; you can simply find a doctor to review and confirm the findings of the first tests.

Both you and your loved one should feel comfortable with the diagnosis and with the healthcare provider who's given it to you. As we state earlier, there's nothing wrong with looking around for a doctor who offers you the kind of comfort and support you need to survive the challenging road ahead. If you don't really like the doctor you started out with, by all means, switch to someone else.

Before you make your decision to either seek a second opinion or skip it, do a risk-versus-benefit analysis. What are the potential benefits if you do decide to get a second opinion, and what are the potential risks? Identifying what you hope to gain from seeing another doctor may help you make the decision as to whether that step is truly necessary.

## Letting the patient know — the pros and cons

How you tell your loved one that she has Alzheimer's Disease depends on a number of factors, particularly her ability to understand the implications of the diagnosis. But remember, "how" and not "if" you should tell your loved one is the question. Most doctors believe patients have a right to know so that they may participate in the decision-making process regarding their care. The simple ability to choose a living arrangement or select among two or three care centers can give Alzheimer's patients a valuable sense of empowerment.

Although sharing the diagnosis may be upsetting, it may also offer relief to the person with Alzheimer's Disease, because it gives the person an explanation for the problems she's been experiencing. It also offers patients the opportunity to find out more about the disease and participate in their medical care so that they can maintain a sense of control over their own lives. It validates their experiences and dispels incorrect beliefs they may have about themselves, such as "I'm crazy." In addition, it opens the door for discussion about treatment options and gives patients the opportunity to talk about the experience of having Alzheimer's Disease.

## Sharing the news with family and friends

Some patients and their families want to share the news with other family members and friends; others feel shame or fear that they may be treated differently. No one can predict how the person with Alzheimer's Disease or his family members will respond to the diagnosis. No matter how you choose to handle the news, you still have some decisions to make about whom you want to tell.

You'll also have to consider carefully when deciding which friends to tell. Some perfectly wonderful people may hear a diagnosis like Alzheimer's Disease and run screaming out the door, never to be heard from again. That's just the way it is. Not everyone can handle bad news with the same degree of calm. Just be prepared for different reactions. Although most of your friends and family members will take the news in stride, a few of them won't.

Some people hide their distress by trying to assign blame for the situation or by lashing out at you for not letting well enough alone. Know that they mean well and are simply acting out their distress in a way that's consistent with their own personalities. But don't let anyone attack you because you stepped up to the plate and got the diagnosis. You did what was right for your loved one, and now that you know the score, you can make informed choices for the future.

## Identifying your allies

Right from the start, certain people will make themselves available to help you in your new role as caregiver for an Alzheimer's sufferer. Other people will make sure that they're overbooked every time you call. Get your support team in place early on because you're definitely in for an extra-innings game.

So how do you identify your potential allies, the people who will be your lifelines as you care for your loved one? Most of them identify themselves by volunteering to help out in any way they can. When someone freely offers their help, grab 'em.

An ally is a person who'll listen to you at any hour of the night or day, who offers not only a shoulder to cry on but also good advice. An ally is a person who will cook supper when you've had a bad day, or even offer to sit with your loved one for a few hours so that you can take a break. An ally is worth his or her weight in gold.

Some potential allies do need a little nudge. It's not so much that they don't want to help as that they're hesitant to interfere. If people like this always seem to be hanging around looking for something to do, welcome them into your circle and assign them a job.

# Chapter 4

# Distinguishing Alzheimer's Disease from Other Medical Conditions

*In This Chapter*

▶ Knowing the difference — clues to a more accurate diagnosis

▶ Recognizing the many faces of dementia

After you've been told that your loved one is indeed suffering from dementia, your doctor still has some detective work to do because so many medical, psychological, and nutritional conditions can trigger dementia. You may be saying, "Well, why is it important to figure all this out? Isn't dementia really just another way of saying Alzheimer's Disease?"

No, it isn't. Although all Alzheimer's patients eventually develop dementia, not all dementia patients have *Alzheimer's Disease* (AD for short). The distinction is important because some dementias are partially or almost completely reversible and respond very well to treatment. That's why a diagnosis of dementia isn't particularly useful; treatments vary widely depending upon the root cause of the dementia, and effective treatment depends entirely upon accurately identifying what type of dementia is present.

This chapter introduces you to the many other conditions that can mimic Alzheimer's Disease. We also discuss what symptoms may help to set them apart and what treatments are most effective for each condition.

## Making Sure that You Have a Reliable Diagnosis

We can't overemphasize the importance of making sure that you have an accurate diagnosis of your loved one's condition. If his or her symptoms are caused by something metabolic, such as a severe vitamin B deficiency, something that could've been cured easily with vitamin therapy won't be cured if that person's been misdiagnosed with AD. The best Alzheimer's treatments in the world would have little or no effect on someone with this deficiency because the illness demands nutritionally based therapy. In addition, depression and delirium must be ruled out as the cause of the symptoms.

You may run into difficulty from your loved one's insurance provider, however, if your doctor pushes for additional tests. All too often, the third-party actuaries who make crucial medical decisions for insurance companies have no medical training whatsoever. If your insurance provider is content to call the problem dementia without being any more specific, but you suspect it may be AD or something more serious, you have to serve as an advocate to get additional testing approved. If the insurance company continues to withhold approval, you may have to reach into your own pocket to pay for the tests. But if you or your doctor believe that you may be dealing with something other than AD, or even something in addition to AD, getting these other tests performed is important in order to nail down the diagnosis. Your doctor can't provide the best possible treatment for your loved one unless he or she's working from an accurate diagnosis.

The reason you may have trouble convincing an insurer to pay for additional tests after an initial diagnosis of dementia is confirmed is that statistically speaking, Alzheimer's does account for the majority of all cases of dementia. Because AD is the most common cause, many insurers are quick to assume that dementia is AD. Read this chapter and you can find out that that equation doesn't always add up.

You may be asking, "Well, heck, I'm not a doctor. How am I supposed to know if my mom or dad has Alzheimer's or another form of dementia?"

*Dementia* is a clinical state characterized by loss of function in multiple areas. Its most common symptom is memory impairment, accompanied by problems in at least one other area — language, movement, the ability to recognize objects, and *executive functioning* (the ability to plan and carry out complex actions). Dementia is not an illness in and of itself, but rather a complex array of symptoms that indicate an underlying disorder. There are approximately 70 to 80 different types of dementia. AD is just one of them. Depending upon which study you believe, overall, 3 to 15 percent of dementias are potentially reversible.

No one expects you to know, but you *do* know your loved one, and you do have the best chance to observe him or her and keep a record of his or her symptoms and behavior, the problems that brought you to the doctor in the first place. If you keep a good record of your loved one's symptoms, you can play a huge role in coming to a correct diagnosis. For instance, symptoms of memory loss alone may tell your doctor one thing, but memory loss accompanied by delirium may lead him to check for substance abuse or underlying psychiatric conditions. The clues you provide in your initial interview with the doctor are incredibly valuable in helping to determine which tests should be ordered and which aren't needed.

Giving your doctor accurate information may save you and your loved one years of suffering. For example, if your loved one is suffering from NPH, or *normal pressure hydrocephalus,* its accompanying dementia, incontinence, and gait disturbances may make your loved one look as though he or she is in the late stages of Alzheimer's Disease. This condition frequently goes undiagnosed, which is tragic, because proper treatment can sometimes completely alleviate the symptoms and restore sufferers to normal or near-normal functioning.

The key here is timing. People in the early stages of Alzheimer's do *not* suffer from gait disturbances; this is a symptom that, if it occurs at all, shows up much later in the disease process after Alzheimer's has attacked the part of the brain that disrupts the gait. NPH sufferers show gait disturbances right from the onset of their disease. Giving your doctor an accurate timetable will help turn his thoughts in the direction of NPH if he knows that the gait disturbances started at the same time as the dementia.

Admittedly, NPH is a dramatic example, and the outlook for recovery is much rosier than the outlook for many other dementias, including Alzheimer's. But you would definitely want to rule out this condition before assuming that your loved one has AD. If your physician has reason to suspect NPH and tests confirm the diagnosis, the placement of a shunt to drain the excess brain fluid can, in a matter of days, restore the NPH patient to near-normal functioning.

That's why doctors are so careful and deliberate and order so many tests when they're trying to establish a diagnosis of Alzheimer's Disease. Think how tragic it would be if an NPH sufferer was misdiagnosed with Alzheimer's Disease, when a simple surgical procedure could relieve the NPH and restore a greatly improved quality of life to the patient.

# It May Be Dementia, but Is It Alzheimer's?

In Chapter 2, we discuss many other conditions that can cause symptoms similar to AD:

> ✔ **Central nervous system conditions:** These conditions, which include *cerebrovascular diseases* (any disease affecting the arteries or blood supply within the brain) such as stroke, Parkinson's Disease, Huntington's Disease, subdural hematomas (blood clots in the brain), normal pressure hydrocephalus (NPH — a brain disorder caused by blockage of the flow of cerebrospinal fluid), and brain tumors can cause dementia along with progressive deficits in memory.

- **Systemic conditions:** *Hypothyroidism* (an underactive thyroid), vitamin B or folic acid deficiency, niacin deficiency, *hypercalcemia* (too much calcium), *neurosyphilis* (a slow and progressive destruction of brain tissue resulting from untreated syphilis), and HIV infection all produce dementia and other symptoms similar to AD.

- **Drug or alcohol abuse:** Long-term drug and/or alcohol abuse can cause brain damage that produces dementia as well as cognitive and motor skills deficits that can be mistaken for AD.

- **Other mental illnesses:** Problems such as severe clinical depression, severe stress, traumatic injury, or schizophrenia can all produce symptoms similar to AD.

According to the Alzheimer's Association, Alzheimer's Disease accounts for 50 percent of all dementias, with *vascular dementia* (caused by problems with the brain's blood supply) responsible for another 20 percent. An additional 20 percent of cases are due to combined causes. So even if your loved one acts like he has AD, don't go jumping to conclusions until you get the test results and a good diagnosis.

# Ruling Out the Usual (and Unusual) Suspects

You may be surprised when you find out how many other conditions can cause dementia, giving the appearance of Alzheimer's Disease to the unschooled eye. Even medical professionals with years of training and experience can sometimes be fooled into thinking that something is AD when it's not.

As we emphasize throughout this chapter and this book, accurately identifying the underlying cause of dementia to determine the proper course of treatment is vitally important. With proper diagnosis and treatment, some people who are severely impaired can be restored to health. Even if the prospect for your loved one doesn't turn out to be so rosy, proper treatment can still alleviate many troubling symptoms and preserve a better quality of life.

In this section, we discuss the many different conditions that present symptoms that mimic Alzheimer's Disease. We also look at how they're different from AD and how their diagnosis and treatment differs from that prescribed for AD patients.

## Neurodegenerative disorders

Neurodegenerative disorders include any physical condition that leads to a decline in cognitive functioning, but do not include psychiatric disorders.

Anything from an infection to an injury to a heart attack to Alzheimer's Disease can trigger a neurodegenerative disorder. The following subsections look at the most common neurodegenerative conditions.

### Huntington's Disease

Fast facts:

- ✔ Strikes 1 in 10,000 people.
- ✔ Average age at onset: 30 to 45. Death occurs 10 to 20 years from onset.

Huntington's Disease is an incurable, progressive, genetic brain disorder that slowly erodes a person's ability to walk, talk, think, and reason. It's named for Dr. George Huntington, who recognized it as a hereditary disorder and first described it in 1872. Everyone who carries the gene will develop the disease, which is invariably fatal. A test is available that can accurately identify who has the gene; however, it can't predict when symptoms will begin. Children who develop a juvenile form of the disease rarely live until adulthood.

Its onset is characterized by forgetfulness, involuntary twitching, slurred speech, mood swings, depression, clumsiness, and a lack of coordination. The forgetfulness sometimes misleads family members into thinking that the problem may be AD, but because of the genetic component of Huntington's Disease, doctors can distinguish between the two fairly easily.

Huntington's patients eventually develop dementia, but it's a type called *subcortical dementia,* which means that the patient has difficulty performing a series of tasks. Huntington's patients might be able to cook a meal, but they couldn't manage running a load of laundry at the same time. People with subcortical dementia are especially vulnerable to distraction. For example, if they're eating and someone turns on a television, they may become so confused that they can't complete their meal.

In contrast, people suffering from more advanced Alzheimer's Disease usually can't complete a task at all, distracted or not, because the dementia they suffer from disrupts their ability to execute a sequence of events. Although new drugs are available that have been clinically proven to help some AD patients maintain cognitive function longer, at present, no effective treatment for Huntington's Disease exists.

In the late stages, patients are unable to walk, speak, or swallow effectively. In fact, choking claims the life of many Huntington's Disease sufferers. Folk singer Woody Guthrie, who wrote "This Land is Your Land," is probably the most famous Huntington's Disease patient. The condition claimed his life in 1967.

If your family has a history of Huntington's Disease, ask your doctor to administer the relevant gene test to your loved one so that you can determine whether Huntington's Disease is responsible for the symptoms or not.

### Pick's Disease

Fast facts:

- ✔ Affects 1 in 100,000 people.
- ✔ Average age at onset: 40 to 60. Death occurs 2 to 12 years from onset.

Pick's Disease is named for Arnold Pick, a German neurologist who first described the disease in 1892. It's distinguished from AD by the fact that, initially, it affects only the *frontal lobe* in the brain, causing a characteristic loss in inhibition, impulse control, and language skills. Pick's Disease patients don't show the memory loss that's typical for Alzheimer's Disease patients until the disease progresses to the *temporal lobe,* at which point it's easily confused with AD, which generally affects the temporal and *parietal lobes* of the brain first. (See the sidebar "The lowdown on lobes" in this chapter for more info on these parts of the brain.)

Pick's Disease patients are more likely than AD patients to be disinhibited and engage in socially inappropriate behavior. They also tend to overeat and overdrink; as the disease progresses, they may grab anything they see, edible or not, and try to stuff it in their mouths. They may be childlike and cry quite easily, and they may seem inflexible and insensitive to other people's feelings.

The key is early intervention, because diagnosis of Pick's Disease is more likely to be accurate when the patient sees a doctor early in the disease process than if he waits until later, when his symptoms are more similar to those of Alzheimer's patients. A recent study showed that 7 percent of patients who'd been diagnosed with AD were shown to actually have Pick's Disease upon autopsy.

Although no effective drug therapies currently exist to treat Pick's Disease, occupational therapy involving music, art, walking, jigsaw puzzles, or basic crafts can help Pick's Disease patients manage their impulsive behavior.

JARGON ALERT

## The lowdown on lobes

What's all this talk about lobes? The front part of the brain or forebrain is divided into four sections, or *lobes.*

- ✔ The *occipital lobe* processes visual information from the eyes.

- ✔ The *parietal lobe* processes information about spatial relationships and structure.

- ✔ The *temporal lobe* processes memories.

- ✔ The *frontal lobe* is the planning center and regulates language, motivation, behavior, and impulse control.

### Frontal lobe dementia or FLD

Fast facts:

- ✔ Together with Pick's Disease, accounts for 5 to 7 percent of all dementias.
- ✔ 50 percent of new cases have a family history of the disease.
- ✔ Average age at onset: 40 to 65. Death occurs 2 to 15 years from onset.

An unidentified mutation on Chromosome 17 can cause some people to develop frontal lobe degeneration that ultimately produces dementia. It's difficult to pick up in its early stages because the onset is slow and produces personality changes such as indifference, disinhibition, and apathy at first. Although those changes may be dramatic, with a formerly outgoing person becoming withdrawn, or a shy person becoming extroverted, most people don't associate such changes with FLD. Like Pick's Disease and Alzheimer's Disease, frontal lobe dementias are progressive and irreversible, but they can usually be distinguished from AD if they're diagnosed early on because of the different behaviors produced by each.

In addition to the personality changes, these patients may show a marked disregard for the feelings of others. They may have expressionless faces, seemingly moved by nothing, or they may go to the opposite extreme, laughing even when such behavior is inappropriate. Their thinking is rigid and inflexible, they may develop ritualistic behaviors, repeating the same action over and over, and may be sexually promiscuous. Their disregard for others and impulsive desire to seize things may lead them to steal, causing them to usually tangle with the law at some point.

Frontal lobe dementia typically has earlier onset than Alzheimer's, prior to age 65, although that's certainly not always the case. The diagnosis is differentiated by noting an initial personality change followed by indiscriminate eating, putting things in the mouth, loss of inhibition, and, finally, restlessness and roaming. The confusion of diagnosis comes in because AD patients also tend to roam, but much later in the course of their disease; early evaluation is recommended because it increases the accuracy of the diagnosis.

As with Pick's Disease, treatment with drugs intended for AD patients isn't recommended. Some antidepressants and occupational therapy provide the best solution for symptom management.

### Frontotemporal dementia or FTD

Fast facts:

- ✔ Affects 15 in 100,000 people.
- ✔ Four times more common in men.
- ✔ Average age at onset: 30 to 65. Death occurs 3 to 17 years from onset.

If dementia affects both the frontal and the temporal lobes, it's called *frontotemporal dementia* or FTD. This progressive, degenerative condition is even more likely to be confused with Alzheimer's Disease than Pick's or frontal lobe dementia because the memory is affected from the outset. However, these patients also display the same distinct early symptoms as frontal lobe dementia and Pick's patients, so if the patient is seen early, doctors should be able to distinguish between this condition and AD.

Unfortunately, early intervention doesn't always happen. In one study, only 14 percent of FTD cases confirmed at autopsy were accurately diagnosed during the patient's lifetime. That figure rose to 43 percent when the diagnosing doctor was a neurologist, and 97 percent when specific clinical criteria for diagnosing FTD were applied. So you can see the importance of using the correct criteria when making a diagnosis.

FTD patients display the common symptoms of Pick's Disease or frontal lobe dementia — language problems, dramatic personality changes, and loss of inhibition — along with the memory loss common to Alzheimer's Disease. But frontotemporal dementia does have one unique symptom called *hypochondriasis,* or a preoccupation with a fear of serious illness. People with FTD are convinced that they have cancer or heart disease or some other dangerous condition, and they fret over it constantly, experiencing a constantly shifting array of physical complaints that reveal no underlying disease upon examination.

Frontotemporal dementia accounts for approximately 2 to 5 percent of the estimated 7 million cases of diagnosed dementia in the United States. As with frontal lobe dementia and Pick's Disease, drugs used for Alzheimer's Disease aren't recommended. However, antidepressants and antipsychotics may help to relieve some symptoms.

### Dementia with Lewy bodies

Fast facts:

- ✔ Up to 80 percent of patients suffer vivid hallucinations.

- ✔ Average age at onset: 60 to 85. Death occurs about 5 to 7 years from onset.

- ✔ Once thought to be rare, dementia with Lewy bodies is estimated to account for 15 to 25 percent of dementia among the elderly.

First discovered and described in the 1970s, Lewy bodies are abnormal areas of brain tissue found in a part of the brain stem called the *cerebral cortex,* sometimes in conjunction with the characteristic plaques of Alzheimer's Disease. The jury's still out as to whether dementia with Lewy bodies is a distinct syndrome or a variant of AD or Parkinson's Disease.

The wavy, snake-like ridges on the external surface of your brain make up the *cerebral cortex,* which determines both your personality and your intelligence and also controls motor functions, planning ability, and your sense of touch.

Dementia with Lewy bodies is a progressive condition characterized by inconsistent attention levels and frequent hallucinations or paranoid delusions. These patients display early gait disturbance along with rigidity of their bodies, slow movement, tremors, and unpredictable cognitive performance interspersed with episodes of confusion. Dementia with Lewy bodies may be confused with AD because patients can also display language and memory problems, trouble following a line of thought, and difficulty locating objects.

Physically, these patients look a lot like Parkinson's Disease patients because of their tremors and involuntary movements. Treatment is tricky because drugs used to control the Parkinson's-like symptoms can worsen hallucinations and delusions, while drugs used to control the psychotic symptoms can make the involuntary movements much worse.

### Normal pressure hydrocephalus

Fast facts:

- ✔ 10 to 30 percent of NPH patients also have Alzheimer's Disease.
- ✔ All NPH patients are subject to higher than normal rates of depression.
- ✔ Average age at onset: 50 to 60. With appropriate treatment, many patients experience a return to good health.

*Normal pressure hydrocephalus* (NPH) is an accumulation of cerebrospinal fluid that causes the ventricles of the brain to enlarge. NPH may be caused by a previous injury such as a hemorrhage, a previous brain surgery, or a previous infection such as meningitis. NPH may also be caused by an underlying condition such as an aneurysm, tumor, or cyst in the brain. The key is that, unlike other types of hydrocephalus, which cause a spike in intracranial pressure, intracranial pressure remains normal with NPH (hence the term *normal pressure hydrocephalus* — see, medical terminology does make sense sometimes). This normal pressure makes diagnosis tricky indeed.

Symptoms of NPH include dementia, incontinence, and problems with walking. This condition is confused with AD, which is unfortunate because proper treatment of NPH can result in a nearly complete reversal of symptoms. According to the Hydrocephalus Association, many cases go unrecognized and are never properly treated. As with most medical conditions, the earlier the diagnosis, the more successful the treatment. Depending upon the degree of brain atrophy present, up to 50 percent of patients may experience significant benefits following the surgical implantation of a shunt to drain excess cerebrospinal fluid before it can build up and cause further brain damage.

If your loved one suffers from incontinence and walking problems along with dementia, consider having him or her tested for NPH.

If you're having trouble convincing yourself that any significant difference exists between the various conditions that cause dementia, visit this Web site (`www.allaboutnph.com/content/Oriana.htm`) to read about a woman's 15-year struggle with undiagnosed NPH. After five years as a total invalid suffering from severe dementia, her cognitive skills started to return within 24 hours of finally receiving appropriate treatment, and today, at age 71, she leads a normal life.

### Vascular dementia

Fast facts:

- ✔ The second most common form of dementia after Alzheimer's disease, accounting for 20 percent of all dementia cases.

- ✔ Untreated high blood pressure causes 50 percent of all vascular dementia.

- ✔ African Americans have higher rates of high blood pressure and dementia due to stroke than Caucasians.

Vascular dementia is caused by problems with the circulation of the blood inside the brain due to either blood clots or a hemorrhage and can also occur as a result of poorly controlled diabetes, high cholesterol, and high blood pressure.

Brain tissue begins to die from a lack of oxygen caused by this disruption of circulation, and cognitive declines result. Vascular dementia usually occurs after a patient has suffered either a stroke or a series of transient ischemic attacks (TIAs). The episodes cause one or more blood vessels in the brain to be temporarily blocked, which may result in a brief loss of consciousness, along with temporary paralysis and visual disturbances.

A *transient ischemic attack* or TIA is a "mini-stroke" caused by a temporary disruption of blood circulation within the brain, which, in turn, is caused either by a blood clot, narrowing of the artery, or inflammation or injury to the blood vessels. Symptoms are similar to stroke symptoms, but not as profound, and may include dizziness; lack of coordination; confusion; changes in speech, comprehension, or vision; and weakness or tingling sensations in one or more parts of the body. Symptoms of TIAs may go away in as little as an hour or may last for almost a day. If you experience TIA symptoms, you should see your doctor as soon as possible; one-third of TIA patients later have a stroke. Symptoms that last longer than an hour indicate that a full-blown stroke has occurred — a medical emergency that requires immediate treatment.

The most common sort of vascular dementia is *multi-infarct dementia* (MID), a condition in which multiple small clots block blood vessels in the brain, destroying brain tissue. This condition is more common in people with high blood pressure and also occurs more frequently as people grow older. Symptoms include stroke, dementia, migraine-like headaches, psychiatric disturbances, problems with recent memory, wandering or getting lost in familiar places, loss of bladder or bowel control, emotional problems such as laughing or crying inappropriately, difficulty following instruction, and problems handling money.

An *infarct* is an area of tissue death in an organ caused when a blood clot blocks circulation of blood to the area.

The damage caused by MID is usually so localized that problems don't appear severe at first. But as more small blood vessels become blocked, the patient experiences ongoing decline. Patients with vascular dementia don't suffer the severe personality changes that the Alzheimer patients experience, and their judgment may be relatively well-preserved.

The good news is that a diagnosis of vascular dementia due to stroke can be confirmed by computed axial tomography, or a CAT scan of the brain, which readily shows the blocked vessels and areas damaged by the infarcts. Appropriate treatment can slow the damage, although areas of the brain that have already been affected cannot be restored.

## Parkinson's Disease

Fast facts:

- ✔ Affects 120 to 180 people per 100,000 among Caucasian populations; for unknown reasons, the prevalence is lower in African Americans.

- ✔ Average age at onset is 60; however, 10 percent of patients experience onset at age 40 or younger.

The initial symptoms of Parkinson's Disease — rigidity, tremors, slow movement, and poor balance — shouldn't easily be confused with Alzheimer's Disease. However, as Parkinson's progresses, some of its victims do show signs of dementia. This dementia is most likely because of degenerative changes in an area of the brain known as the *substantia nigra*. Because Parkinson's patients generally have a long diagnostic and treatment history before they exhibit dementia (if they exhibit it at all), medical professionals don't confuse Parkinson's with Alzheimer's Disease. However, a layperson who doesn't know a patient's history might well confuse the dementia that can occur in late-stage Parkinson's with AD, especially if the patient's tremors were well controlled by medication.

### Subdural hematomas

Fast facts:

> ✔ Affects 1 in 10,000.
>
> ✔ More prevalent in elderly, especially people over the age of 75.

A *subdural hematoma* (SDH) is a large blood clot that occurs underneath the *dura mater,* or the tough, fibrous, protective covering of the brain, but is external to the brain itself. Because your skull doesn't have a square centimeter of extra space inside it, the pressure of an SDH can cause brain swelling, which produces a variety of symptoms including intense headaches, nausea, vomiting for the acute variety, and confusion and combativeness for the chronic variety. The symptoms get worse as the clot grows larger. An acute subdural hematoma is a life-threatening condition. The chronic variety is the type that produces symptoms that can be confused with Alzheimer's Disease.

SDH can be the result of traumatic injury or blunt-force trauma to the head. People who are on aspirin therapy or taking a blood-thinning medication such as Coumadin have a higher risk. Alcoholism also increases the risk.

When doctors know that a patient has had a head injury, diagnosing SDH is as simple as taking a CAT scan that can show the area of the bleed, along with the degree and severity of the accompanying brain swelling. Diagnostic questions can arise when a patient has suffered a prior head injury and presents with confusion or other Alzheimer's-like symptoms but no external evidence of head trauma. Sometimes, particularly if the accident was a minor fall, patients themselves may not even realize that they've suffered a head injury. In this instance, doctors may evaluate the patient for a brain tumor or AD until tests reveal the SDH.

Small hematomas can resolve on their own, but larger ones may require surgical removal.

### Brain tumors

Fast facts:

> ✔ Benign brain tumors affect 97 out of 100,000 people.
>
> ✔ Malignant brain tumors affect 29 out of 100,000 people.
>
> ✔ Highest incidence is between the ages of 40 and 60.

Depending upon their size and location within the brain, brain tumors may cause a variety of symptoms, some of which may mimic Alzheimer's Disease. Although most brain tumors cause intense headaches, nausea, and vomiting, tumors located in the frontal lobe of the brain cause the type of symptoms that mimic AD, including memory loss, personality changes, and impaired judgment.

Whether the tumor is benign or malignant doesn't really matter; its position within the skull is more predictive of the outcome and symptoms produced. Benign tumors in inaccessible locations can be just as deadly as malignant tumors. Treatment may require surgical removal, chemotherapy, radiation, or a combination of the three.

The good news is that brain tumors are readily identified by either a CAT scan or *magnetic resonance imaging* (MRI), which easily rules out a diagnosis of AD.

# Systemic conditions that mimic Alzheimer's

As we mention earlier in this chapter, a number of other conditions can mimic the symptoms of Alzheimer's Disease, including an underactive thyroid, vitamin deficiencies, too much calcium in the blood, and syphilis that's spread to the brain. Dementia can also be induced by abusing drugs or alcohol or show up as a symptom of severe clinical depression, traumatic injury, or schizophrenia.

### Hypothyroidism or underactive thyroid

No matter what the cause, a person whose thyroid gland is underactive can experience symptoms similar to those of Alzheimer's Disease, including memory loss, irritability, and depression. However, hypothyroidism only accounts for a small number of dementia cases. The key to an accurate diagnosis is the presence of other symptoms common to hypothyroidism but not necessarily present in Alzheimer's Disease, including weight gain; coarse, dry hair; hair loss; dry, rough skin; and constipation. Generally speaking, hypothyroidism can be detected with a simple blood test, although certain cases may require more extensive testing to ensure accurate results.

The condition is readily managed with thyroid medication, but it will require lifelong monitoring to make sure that the dose of thyroid is adequate. After the condition is under control, the memory loss and other cognitive symptoms have a good chance of improving.

### Vitamin deficiencies

Some vitamin and nutritional deficiencies can also produce symptoms similar to Alzheimer's Disease. If someone has a severe lack of certain B vitamins, folic acid, or niacin, that person is at risk for having his or her condition misdiagnosed unless the doctor knows to check for these deficiencies.

Although it's rare, severe B-1, B-6, and B-12 deficiencies can lead to dementia. Simple blood tests can establish definitively whether a deficiency is present. That's just one reason why the blood tests your physician orders at the beginning of the diagnostic process are so important; they can rule out more easily treated causes of dementia such as vitamin deficiency.

Niacin deficiency is another nutritionally based condition that can produce dementia, memory loss, and irritability. However, a niacin deficiency severe enough to cause dementia will actually induce a disease called *pellagra,* which causes diarrhea and dermatitis at the same time as the dementia. Diagnosis is made through a physical exam and symptoms. Niacin deficiency is generally rare in people who consume healthy diets, but is more common among alcoholics who may have poor dietary habits.

Folic acid deficiency is one of the most common nutritional deficiencies in the United States. It's particularly prevalent in people who abuse alcohol. It can cause irritability and difficulty in concentrating. However, people who suffer from a folic acid deficiency also have elevated levels of *serum homocysteine* (a chemical byproduct of protein metabolism found in the blood), which is something that Alzheimer's patients don't necessarily have. Blood tests can help establish the correct diagnosis.

Doctors not only have to diagnose the deficiency, but they must also figure out what's causing it. Deficiencies can be caused by inadequate intake, malabsorption, excessive excretion, or an underlying disease. In some cases, the doctor will have to treat the underlying condition as well as supplement the missing nutrient in order to correct the problem permanently.

### Hypercalcemia

Hypercalcemia is an electrolyte imbalance caused by too much calcium in the blood. Elevated levels of serum calcium are generally associated with a tumor or *primary hyperparathyroidism,* a condition that occurs when the parathyroid glands secrete too much hormone. When the level of calcium in the bloodstream gets too high, it may produce an altered mental status and memory problems that are similar to Alzheimer's Disease. A blood test that measures the levels of both calcium and parathyroid hormone can identify the condition. Surgery to remove the parathyroid glands cures hypercalcemia associated with hyperparathyroidism; when the hypercalcemia is associated with a tumor, particularly a malignant tumor, the outlook is less optimistic.

After the parathyroid glands are removed and calcium levels fall back to normal, the accompanying Alzheimer's-like symptoms diminish. In some cases, the patient may have to take calcium-lowering drugs to help manage the condition.

### Neurosyphilis

Syphilis can cause dementia if it spreads to the brain. Although syphilis can readily be cured with antibiotics if it's diagnosed and treated early on, in patients who don't seek treatment, the infection can spread to the brain — although it generally takes at least a decade to do so. This infection can produce mental confusion, difficulty in walking, and dementia that mimics Alzheimer's Disease. If a blood test detects the presence of syphilis antibodies in the blood, the diagnosis can be confirmed with an analysis of spinal fluid.

Syphilis can be cured with a course of antibiotics; however, if the condition has been allowed to go unchecked for a long period of time, the outlook may not be as positive.

# Other possible causes of dementia

You're probably asking yourself, what other causes of dementia could there possibly be? Well, believe it or not, we've got a few more to discuss.

Because of the number of possible causes for dementia, your doctor will want to take a thorough medical history, including what drugs your loved one is taking and the start/stop dates for those drugs. Because so many different conditions can produce symptoms typically associated with Alzheimer's Disease, you doctor must rule out all other potential causes and ensure that your loved one's symptoms fit the criteria for AD before he or she arrives at a diagnosis.

### Depression

Severe clinical depression may be mistaken for Alzheimer's Disease. People who are severely depressed can experience problems in thinking or memory, including difficulty concentrating, recalling information, and keeping track of dates or time, or they may complain that they can't stay focused on a task. They may report difficulty making decisions or starting or completing projects, and they may appear apathetic.

A person *can* have both depression and Alzheimer's Disease at the same time. A good medical and neuropsychological evaluation is needed to determine if your loved one is experiencing one or possibly both of these conditions. If your loved one is suffering from depression and not AD, you can expect your loved one's cognitive problems to respond to proper treatment for depression. If your loved one is treated for depression and shows an improved mood but no improvement in thinking or memory, a diagnosis of dementia (possibly AD) may be appropriate. The bottom line is that your healthcare practitioner must assess whether your loved one is depressed before a diagnosis of AD can be made.

### Delirium

Another condition that can cause dementia-like symptoms is delirium. Delirium is suspected when someone shows a fluctuating change in thinking — particularly problems focusing, maintaining, or shifting attention — that usually starts within hours or days. Speech may be incoherent, and the individual may have problems staying awake or become agitated and restless. Disorientation to person, place, or time; mood shifts; or hallucinations may also come and go.

Delirium is the direct consequence of a medical condition often caused by an illness (for example, a urinary tract infection, congestive heart failure, and so on), a metabolic disorder (dehydration, kidney problems), physical trauma (head injury), or cardiac problems. Many drugs commonly used by older adults to treat pain, infection, inflammatory diseases, gastrointestinal problems, and more can also cause delirium. Delirium is a reversible condition if properly diagnosed and treated.

Dementia or delirium can also result from alcohol or drug abuse, so you need to let your healthcare practitioner know if your loved one has a history of drug or alcohol problems, including abuse of over-the-counter medications.

As with depression, a person can have both delirium and Alzheimer's disease. People who become delirious don't necessarily have AD, but people with AD are more susceptible to delirium than those without it.

### Infections

Dementia can also result from certain viral or bacterial infections, such as encephalitis, meningitis, or HIV, but doctors rarely confuse these acute conditions with AD, even if some of the symptoms are similar.

### Poisoning

Poisoning can be another cause of dementia. A wide variety of poisons can produce dementia, including organophosphates that are used in agriculture and chronic exposure to low levels of carbon monoxide. Heavy metals such as lead and mercury have well-documented neuro-toxic effects and have also been demonstrated to produce dementia.

# Chapter 5

# Identifying Your Fears: For the Patient and the Caregiver

*A*fter the diagnosis of Alzheimer's Disease (AD) is confirmed, you and your loved one may experience a variety of emotions ranging from anger, disbelief, despair, grief, denial, and depression to acceptance. These feelings don't occur in any given order and may vary from person to person. But even after you come to a point of acceptance, you'll still have many fears left to deal with — fear of what the future holds, worries about work and job security, concerns about safety, caretaking insecurities, how the disease will impact family and friends, legal and financial issues . . . the list goes on and on.

In dealing with AD, one of the biggest fears and frustrations for both the patient and his or her family is the unknown. No one can predict how the disease will progress for your loved one or foresee how AD will affect you and those you love. Only one thing is certain: You can do things to improve the quality of life for everyone involved.

Before you can take any positive steps, it's important to identify your fears. Although you and your loved one may find that you share many of the same fears, there are some that are more often experienced by the person with AD and some that are unique to the caregiver. In this chapter, we address some of the more common fears associated with receiving the diagnosis of AD, starting with those most frequently experienced by Alzheimer's patients, followed by an overview of common caregivers' fears.

# Concerns for the Alzheimer's Patient

We've written this section for the person diagnosed with AD and for those who are interested in better understanding the experience of someone living with the disease. Whether you've been recently diagnosed or have known of your condition for a while, you may find that some of the concerns we discuss here are familiar to you. This section is intended to help you understand your own fears and how these fears may be affecting you and your quality of life. We also hope that by discussing these issues, you'll realize that you aren't alone. Some suggestions for coping and management are included along the way.

## Hearing that you have Alzheimer's Disease

A diagnosis of AD carries with it much uncertainty, and everyone reacts to the news differently. For some, an AD diagnosis helps to explain the problems with memory and thinking that you may have noticed and why things you once did easily now require thought or are frustrating to you. It also dispels the belief that you're "going crazy," or that the problems with your memory are the result of "normal aging." You are not crazy, nor is AD a normal part of the aging process.

Some people describe experiencing a sense of relief after diagnosis. They've been aware for some time that something is wrong, but their complaints have gone unheard, been dismissed, or, too often, been attributed to something else (working too much, "old age," stress, and so on). Some people feel empowered when they find out their diagnosis because, along with it, they discover that they have options and that resources are available to them and their families.

Finding out the cause of your problems allows you to educate yourself about your condition and seek appropriate treatment, thereby avoiding unnecessary treatments or workups.

Becoming aware of your condition allows you to take an active part in your treatment and plan for your future. Although some of the things you plan may never occur, doing so ensures that your preferences are heard. It also takes a lot of pressure off your loved ones, who may otherwise struggle making difficult decisions based upon what they *think* you might want. Talk to them in a meaningful way about your preferences regarding long-term care and end-of-life issues, including decision-making preferences (for example, who would you want making decisions regarding your health and/or finances if you were no longer able to do so independently?). Make a thoughtful will and think about the sort of legacy you want to leave for your children and grandchildren.

You should also discuss any fears you may have about living with a chronic, progressive medical condition. As some people with AD have said, these are a few of the "luxuries of time" that people who die suddenly from heart attacks or strokes don't have. Hearing your diagnosis may even allow you to more readily express your love and gratitude to your family members, strengthen ties to others, or "mend fences." The earlier you seek help for your condition, the more time you'll have to continue enjoying those things in life that you love.

Enjoyment of life doesn't end after diagnosis.

Depending on your outlook, personal concept of AD, religious beliefs, and so on, you may have very different ideas about what your diagnosis means for you and your loved ones than someone else who's diagnosed with AD does. Sometimes, a person with AD fears becoming dependent on others or becoming a "burden" to his or her loved ones.

Try to keep in mind that you're not alone and that any fears you have are a natural part of the whole process. Don't let your fear or your diagnosis define you.

## Understanding what's really bothering you

You may find it helpful to ask yourself a few questions to try to better understand how your apprehension or worries are affecting you and, in turn, those who love you. Some people diagnosed with AD struggle with the following:

- ✔ I fear that I will lose my independence and my current way of life. I worry about becoming dependent upon others for my basic needs and/or becoming a "burden" to those I love.

- ✔ I fear that I may have to move out of my home and into a facility for people with AD. I worry about what might happen to me there if I did relocate.

- ✔ I worry that I may have passed my condition on to my children.

- ✔ I worry that others might treat me differently if they knew that I have AD.

- ✔ I worry about the possibility of one day not knowing my relationship to my spouse or my children, grandchildren, or great-grandchildren; that I won't be able to participate in the significant events of their lives.

- ✔ I worry about losing my memory and my sense of who I am in this world.

- ✔ I worry because I have unfinished business. I have things I planned with my family and my work. I have regrets about the way I lived my life and I'm afraid that now I won't have the chance to achieve those things that are so important to me.

✔ I worry how my family and friends who have always relied on me for direction and help will be able to cope.

✔ I worry about practical issues such as finances (for example, how will my spouse or children get by if and when my care costs start to rise?).

In the following subsections, we address each of these concerns individually.

### *I fear loss of independence.*

If you've been diagnosed with AD late in life and start treatment immediately, your condition could remain stable for several years, provided that you're like most people taking one of the currently approved AD prescription medications. You may never experience the more advanced stages of cognitive and functional decline before some other health condition or age-related condition causes your death.

Be proactive about your condition so that you avoid feeling dependent. Make a care plan that includes having someone else oversee the management of your medications to ensure that you get the full benefit of treatment. Far from being an act of dependence, having someone else manage your meds is your first line of defense against AD. You're taking charge of your health and empowering yourself in a very real way to remain as healthy as you can for as long as you can.

Make sure to get regular checkups from your primary care physician to watch for any other problems that may develop. Underlying health problems, even something as simple as a cold or the flu, can make the symptoms of AD appear worse. See your AD specialist at least yearly to make sure that you're receiving the appropriate medications in the correct dosages. Seeing your specialist and perhaps undergoing repeated thinking and memory tests informs you, your family, and your doctor of your response to treatment and areas of stability. This knowledge can reduce your fear of the unknown as well as your fear of dependence, because you have clear evidence that your condition has shown little change or is progressing at a rate that is slower than expected if you weren't on treatments. Give yourself a pat on the back for taking charge of your health and enlisting the services of a medication manager early.

### *I fear moving out of my home and into an AD care facility.*

At some point, you may have to move out of your home; however, you may not. If you accept that you may have to move one day and explore your options now, you have the opportunity to select where you want to live should that day come. (See Chapter 15 for information on current care options.) You can decide what's most important to you in choosing your accommodations, such as the following:

- ✔ Activities offered
- ✔ Rural or urban location
- ✔ Size of apartment (if you move into an assisted living facility first) or room (if you go into an AD facility or nursing home)
- ✔ Cost
- ✔ Level of security provided
- ✔ Level of care provided
- ✔ Whether you can bring your own furniture
- ✔ Secure outdoor amenities, such as a private terrace or walking trail

Making these plans in advance also relieves your family of their guilt and anxiety about having to make these decisions for you. If you discuss these issues early, you can take an active part in the decision-making process.

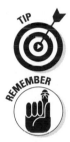

Discuss the circumstances under which you would have to relocate and pick your top three places based on your own and your family's evaluations and resources.

Regarding fear of abuse in a nursing home or abandonment by your family, don't worry. Your family won't let that happen. Even people with no relatives can identify friends they can count on to oversee their care.

### I fear that I may have passed my condition on to my children.

Unless you're part of one of only 200 families in the world known to carry the inherited form of AD (which accounts for less than 1 percent of all cases), you aren't at risk for passing AD on to your children. You may pass on a risk factor for developing AD if you have the version of the cholesterol-carrying protein that's associated with an increased risk of developing AD, but a risk factor is only a risk factor; that doesn't mean your children will develop the disease as a result.

### I worry that others might treat me differently if they know that I have AD.

People who know and love you are already aware of your problem, or at least that you're experiencing difficulties of some sort. Trying to hide your condition won't work and uses too much of your energy. How can you help others if you're always tired or rundown because of the effort you're putting into disguising your difficulties?

Educate yourself about AD, so that you can educate others. When you talk about your health, explain to those you love how the condition affects you, but emphasize that you are not your disease. If your family members and friends are curious and desire more information about AD, invite them to your doctor visits.

We can't stress enough that worries kept silent only multiply. Even if you belong to a family that isn't particularly talkative, after you receive the diagnosis of Alzheimer's Disease, reaching out to each other and sharing your worries and fears openly can help everyone immensely. Your loved ones are your best support system, but they can only help if you allow them to.

### I worry about the possibility of not knowing and being able to enjoy my relationships with those closest to me.

Yes, AD is progressive, and if you live with it long enough, you may not be able to form new memories of events or people. You may have problems consistently knowing your relationship to others, but that doesn't mean you can't enjoy activities or that person in the moment. If the day comes when you struggle to understand your defined relationship to another person, it doesn't mean that you won't be aware of the quality of that relationship.

Make the most of the time you have by planning family get-togethers and outings. Go through old family photo albums and share favorite stories with your children and grandchildren, your nieces and nephews. Write your personal history or memoirs. Draw your family close and frequently express your love in as many ways as you can. Reassure them of your love; it'll help strengthen them for the future.

### I worry about losing my memory and my sense of who I am in this world.

You've probably already lost some memory capacity, but if you're in the early stages of AD, you may be well aware that more severe memory loss is ahead. Worrying about your memory loss may be quite a source of anxiety for you, but anti-anxiety drugs aren't recommended for AD patients because they may make symptoms of AD worse.

If your loss of memory is making you feel sad, an antidepressant may help. You may also benefit from talking to a counselor who can help you work through your fears. Fear is a natural, understandable response to a diagnosis of AD. Don't forget, too, that your family and friends want to do everything they can to make your path easier.

You can also do small things to help yourself. Develop routines and stick to them. For instance, if you have a dedicated place for your house keys, such as a bowl on the table by the door, you'll be less likely to misplace them when you're ready to go out.

The important thing is not to let your fears ruin the time you have left. New medications are helping AD patients retain cognitive, functional, and social abilities for longer periods of time; with good care and a good outlook, you have a strong chance of maintaining a good quality of life. See Chapter 7 for a thorough review of the four currently approved drugs for Alzheimer's patients.

If you've only recently been diagnosed, you may worry about exactly what lies ahead. In Chapter 6, we discuss the stages of Alzheimer's Disease in detail so that you may know what to expect.

### *I worry because I have unfinished business and regrets, and that I may not have the chance to achieve my dreams.*

If you have any unfinished business, now is definitely the time to address it. After you receive the diagnosis of AD, you should discuss your diagnosis with your employer (if you're still working), so that you can make plans for a smooth transition. Depending on the degree of your current impairment, you may be able to keep working for a while longer. Some people with AD find work more frustrating than beneficial; if that's how you feel, you may elect to begin the process of retirement soon after your diagnosis.

If you've never given any thought to retiring or viewed it as a distant event, now is the time to begin anticipating all that you will be able to do after you retire. You can "work" at playing and maintaining your health and well-being.

If you have family issues, such as any estranged sons or daughters or siblings, and you feel like you want to bridge the gap, reach out to them. You can't be sure that they'll respond in the manner you hope for, but you'll at least have the satisfaction of knowing that you made the effort to heal the rift.

Wrapping up unfinished business eliminates at least some sources of worry, and in a time when you'll be facing so many uncertainties, facing and eliminating any fears you can early on is one of the most proactive steps you can take.

### *I worry how my family and friends who have always relied on me for direction and help will be able to cope.*

If you have a family member who's always relied upon you for direction, help, or care, such as a son or daughter who's physically or mentally challenged or who suffers from a chronic illness, now's the time to make care arrangements for him or her. Perhaps one of your other children is willing to take over the responsibility; if not, you must investigate what other options are available, such as home care or residential facilities. Help your dependent understand that your condition doesn't mean you won't be there for him; emphasize that you simply have to make sure that he'll always be well cared for.

If you're having trouble locating long-term care facilities for an adult who's physically or mentally challenged, visit your state's Web site to see what facilities and services are available. If your dependent is a Medicaid recipient, contact your counselor for advice on state facilities.

If you don't make suitable arrangements, your local social services counselor will make the necessary arrangements for housing and care, but generally speaking, it's better if you or a responsible family member takes a hand in making care decisions for your dependent. Knowing where your dependent will be living, who'll be caring for her, and when she'll be making the move to her new home definitely helps to ease your fears about this change.

### *I worry about practical issues, such as finances.*

If you're worried about how your family will make ends meet when you're gone, at the first opportunity, sit down and review your financial situation and make a plan. Depending upon your situation, you may have this discussion with your spouse and your children, your siblings or closest relative, or your significant other or closest friend, or perhaps even an attorney or executor.

If you haven't already done so, meeting with a financial planner is also a good idea (see Chapter 14 for more info on working through financial issues). If you have a long-term care plan already in place, you're ahead of the game. If you don't, you're going to have to face some hard decisions, such as: Do you dig into your retirement account to pay for your care? Must you sell your home? Will you have to rely on the government to provide your care?

No matter what your financial situation, facing it openly with your loved ones can help you all to develop the best possible plan for your particular circumstances. And having a plan in place is an excellent way to defuse financial fears.

## Fearing dependency

If Alzheimer's Disease has any plus side, it's the fact that loss of physical capabilities happens quite late in the process. So you won't likely have to deal with any significant physical problems, such as difficulty in walking or caring for your personal needs early on. AD is typically a slow-moving disease and you may never experience these problems.

Difficulties in performing the basic activities of self care are different from difficulties in performing the activities of daily living, such as balancing your checkbook, making and keeping appointments, shopping, driving, and so on. Although the activities of daily living are affected first, there are strategies you can employ to compensate and preserve your self-reliance. (See Chapter 16 for more information on these strategies.)

Your healthcare provider or counselor can answer any specific questions you may have about your own situation.

# Leaving or losing your job

In today's world, many people take a great deal of pride in their work, and perhaps you're one of those people. A lot of your identity, your conceptions about who you are and where you fit into the world, and what type of contribution you've made may all be tied in with your working life. So when you hear the diagnosis of Alzheimer's Disease, worrying about how that will affect your work, career, and the legacy you may have hoped to leave behind is only natural.

As we mention earlier in this chapter, you may also have financial worries linked to the loss of work. Many families live paycheck to paycheck, and having a breadwinner diagnosed with AD can be a major financial blow. In the following subsections, we discuss job-related fears and suggest some ways to help you face them.

### Feeling unimportant to the world

If your work has always been the way you "connected" to the world, you may fear the loss of your importance in the overall scheme of things. Although you will ultimately be forced to stop working as your condition progresses, try not to focus on that. Think instead of all the valuable contributions you've already made over the course of your career because those ideas, events, big sales, deadlines and quotas met, dragons slain, problems solved, quiet accomplishments, and successful meetings are what your colleagues will remember about you, not your illness. Don't believe it? Think of a colleague who may have recently passed away — from cancer, a stroke, an accident, or whatever. Now, think about how you and the other people at your place of business remembered that person. Sure, for the first few days after the event, you may have talked about what took the person's life, particularly if it was something dramatic or unexpected. But after a very short time, the person is remembered for his or her deeds and accomplishments, not for the particular way that he or she died.

You also have the opportunity to serve as a de facto advocate for people with AD. By example, you can help to break the stereotypes and myths your co-workers may have about AD, and your co-workers will be more informed than most members of the general public about the disease.

So, in the time you have left at work, do the very best you can to continue the good job you've been doing all these years. Your co-workers will admire you for your courage and do their best to help you have a successful transition out of the working world.

After you do stop working, you may find it helpful to think of your AD as a sort of early retirement. Try to make the best use you can of each day, cherishing special moments with your family and friends. Even if you can't hang on to many new memories for yourself, you're helping to create precious life-long memories for the people who love you.

### Finding new meaning in your life

If you do find yourself feeling left out and unimportant after you stop working, consider volunteering someplace. Schools, charities, and other nonprofit organizations are always in need of volunteers. Sure, you may have AD and will need to make that clear when you apply, but while you're in the early stages, you can still do lots of things to help out and serve as a valuable member of the community.

Not sure where to go to volunteer? Call your local Community Service Center or the local United Way. Just be sure not to take on anything that will fatigue you or stress you out. The idea is to enjoy yourself while helping others, not give yourself a new cause for worry! Here are some other ideas to consider:

- ✔ If you've been a teacher and miss being in the classroom with children, perhaps you can volunteer for the children's story hour at the library.

- ✔ If your job was very technical, you may not be able to find a comparable volunteer job available as a substitute, but if you look around your community, you'll see lots of things that need doing. For example, if you've always liked the outdoors and enjoy a brisk walk, take a small trash bag with you on your walks and pick up any trash you see along the trail. Or volunteer to weed the community garden.

- ✔ As AD progresses, walking alone may become a safety issue, especially if you have spatial disorientation. Wear your Safe Return bracelet (see Chapter 16 for complete information) at all times.

- ✔ If you've always liked talking to people, perhaps you can volunteer to help those patients who've been newly diagnosed with Alzheimer's Disease deal with their own fears. No one could possibly make a better spokesperson than you.

## Worrying over losing your income

If you've been the primary breadwinner for your family, no doubt you're worrying about your potential inability to bring in income after your diagnosis. Another one of AD's hidden blessings is that 95 percent of AD patients experience a late onset of the condition, at age 65 or older. If that's your situation, you may have already retired when you get your diagnosis, which will minimize or eliminate any impact on your income.

AD can deplete savings quickly. Home care, paid companions, and assisted living don't come cheap. That's why visiting a financial advisor early on is so important. For more information about financial issues for AD patients, see Chapter 14.

According to the Baylor College of Medicine in Houston, Texas, the average age at diagnosis for an Alzheimer's patient is 70 years, and a study funded by the United States Public Health Service places average age at onset at 72.8 years. If you're among the small group of people who have a rare, genetic form of Alzheimer's Disease, you may start to exhibit symptoms as early as your 40s or 50s, or even more rarely, your 30s. Fortunately, this form of AD accounts for less than 1 to 5 percent of all cases.

If your family does carry this genetic mutation, your chances of getting AD are higher than average. To protect your family against the early loss of its breadwinner, investigate disability insurance programs and invest in the one that seems right for your family and circumstances. You may also want to check out Chapter 14 in this book, which deals with making financial arrangements.

## Handling your fear of loss of control

If you're worried that you might lose your mental and physical abilities before you can make all the necessary arrangements, share that fear with your family. They can help make sure that everything is arranged as you want before you become too incapacitated to make good decisions. If you're worried about having some input into the medical decisions that will be made on your behalf, read Chapter 12 for an overview of issues that your family may have to deal with. Make your wishes known. If you don't want your life prolonged by machines, discuss end-of-life care options, such as a *Do Not Resuscitate* (DNR) order.

If you're concerned about legal issues, read Chapter 13 for guidance through the legal maze. You should discuss legal guardianship and powers of attorney for financial and medical decision making with a trusted family member to determine whom you want to make these decisions should you no longer be able to make them for yourself. And if questions about money are troubling you, read Chapter 14 for some advice about managing your money and preparing for your future and, if necessary, extended care.

You may have a hard time handing over your decision-making power to a spouse or a son or daughter, especially if you've been used to running your own life. Be aware that they have your best interests in mind and that this situation is as difficult for them as it is for you.

Also keep in mind that, as your condition progresses, you may begin to suspect that those who love you the most are untrustworthy. Unfortunately, that's just part of what AD does to your brain; it can make you very suspicious of those closest to you. That's why it's so important to finalize as many arrangements as you can while you still have some capacity to make your wishes known.

## Coping with anger

We mention earlier in this chapter that some people go through a period of anger following diagnosis. You may feel betrayed by your own mind and wonder why you have to deal with this condition. You may be wondering if you could've done something or avoided something to prevent this illness.

This anger is a normal part of the stages of grieving. It may last a few days or a few weeks, but eventually, you'll work your way through it. Remember, though, not to place blame: Alzheimer's Disease is no one's fault; it's just a tragic condition that strikes randomly and without warning.

If your anger lasts longer than a couple of weeks or you feel like it's intensifying or becoming unmanageable, talk to your healthcare provider about getting some counseling.

# Concerns for the Caregiver

If you're responsible for caring for a loved one with Alzheimer's Disease or for planning his or her care, this section is for you. Here we address your fears about losing your loved one and watching his or her memory fail, and we also discuss financial and caregiving considerations.

Some AD patients never acknowledge their diagnosis. As frustrating as this may be, don't try to "force" your loved one to recognize that he has AD. Diminished capacity and ability to understand may truly mean your loved one just can't process the fact that he has AD. His denial that anything's wrong may be a self-protective mechanism that helps him cope.

## Fearing the loss of your loved one

One of the most natural and immediate fears you face when you hear that a loved one has Alzheimer's Disease is your worry over his or her impending death. No one, not even your doctor, can predict how long your loved one will live with this disease or how the condition will progress. The best thing you can do is not to dwell on the idea of loss, but rather make the most of the life you now share with your loved one. Try to find some special moment in each and every day, particularly in the months and years before memory worsens.

The sad truth about AD is that you actually lose your loved one long before he or she dies. Many of the ways you recognize someone you love — the funny stories, crooked smile, or infectious laugh — slip away long before death comes. The most difficult thing to deal with is the day you realize that your loved one no longer knows or recognizes you on a consistent basis.

If you're having trouble dealing with this aspect of AD, by all means seek out a caregiver's support group or some individual counseling to help you cope.

## Watching memory slip away

Problems with learning new information, new routines, and new tasks precede memory problems, which make up the hallmark symptom and often most recognizable sign of Alzheimer's Disease. Dealing with memory loss can be one of the most trying aspects of caring for an Alzheimer's patient, because he or she will ask the same questions over and over and over again and tell the same stories, word for word, without even knowing it.

Try to keep your humor and patience about you and take everything in stride. Keep in mind that AD patients can't help their behavior; they're not misplacing their dentures and asking you the same question repeatedly to annoy you; they're doing it because they can't remember, and their minds are stuck in a sort of endless loop.

Although medication can slow the progress of cognitive loss, don't lose sight of the fact that AD is still an incurable disease. Inevitably, your loved one's memory loss will worsen, and that will make taking care of him or her more challenging.

## Fearing that he or she will forget who you are

AD patients progress in different ways. A rare few may have trouble recognizing their family and friends relatively soon after their diagnosis; others may recognize them for far longer. It depends upon how far along they are in the course of the condition when they're diagnosed.

Although some Alzheimer's patients completely fail to recognize their relatives and friends at some point late in the course of the disease, others continue to recognize them as relatives or at least friendly faces, even if they're not exactly sure of names and relationships.

Don't be discouraged if your loved one seems afraid of you or treats you like a stranger. She's afraid because she doesn't know who you are and is thus unsure of your intentions toward her. Be calm, approach her slowly, and speak softly and reassuringly. Remember that she's acting out of fear and uncertainty and that it's nothing personal directed at you. It's just part of the process of Alzheimer's Disease.

## Building a new relationship

Even if your loved one no longer recognizes you, you can still build a new relationship. If he's living in a long-term care facility, frequent short and pleasant visits may help him to associate your presence with periods of relaxation and fun. If your loved one is still in your home, don't just leave him or her isolated in a room; bring the loved one out to the family room where he or she can be part of the ebb and flow of family life.

Try appealing to the five senses to associate your presence with good feelings. Bring a flower for the loved one to smell, bake some cookies, or bring a small stuffed animal that he or she can hold. Hold your loved one's hands and give lots of hugs and kisses. Let your loved one know that you think he or she is special and loved.

This sort of sensory stimulation can go a long way toward helping you build a new sort of relationship with your loved one. He or she may not remember exactly who you are, but your loved one will happily accept the visit of that nice woman who always has a hug or a smile, or a rose in her pocket.

## Worrying about finances

Unless your loved one had the foresight to make long-term care arrangements ahead of time, one of your next biggest worries may be about where the money is going to come from to pay for all this treatment and care.

Although this question has no easy answers, in Chapter 14 we try to give you an overview of the best available financial advice for providing long-term care and managing your patient's finances (as well as your own).

## Being the primary caregiver

If you're an only child, or the only child still living close to home, and your parent gets diagnosed with Alzheimer's Disease, guess what? You're it. You're going along merrily in your life, dealing with your own issues and goals, and suddenly — WHAM! — this disease gets dropped in your lap and everything goes topsy-turvy. Your plans go on hold, and suddenly you're spending all day every day dealing with your loved one's problems and issues. All you want to know is whether you're going to get your own life back.

Looking for some caregiver's support? Check out this Web site: Caregiver Assistance Network at `www.cssdoorway.org/can/default.htm`.

The good news is that you're not alone in your worries. A number of national organizations are available that are specifically dedicated to supporting, educating, and linking caregivers. Almost every municipality now has some sort of adult daycare available or offers respite care so that a tired caregiver can get out and take a break. Daycare benefits the person with AD as well.

For a complete guide to the types of care available for your loved one, and for help in choosing who'll bear the responsibility for providing care and what challenges are involved, see Chapters 15 and 16.

## Worrying about your loved one

Alzheimer's Disease brings with it a specific list of cognitive symptoms and variable behavioral symptoms, and all the worrying in the world isn't going to change that. Although it's natural to worry about your loved one and want the best for him or her, spending too much time worrying can actually have a negative effect on your ability to provide care — not to mention that the stress of too much worry can have a damaging effect on your own health.

You can't do anything to change a diagnosis of AD, but you can make sure that your loved one feels supported and is living life as fully as possible. You can make sure that he or she has good care and good food and the correct dosage of medication at the right time. You can help your loved one fulfill his or her needs for socialization and stimulation. You can see to it that your loved one stays pleasantly occupied and that his or her living quarters are free from any obvious hazards, such as throw rugs or matches. You can take steps to make sure that your loved one doesn't have access to household poisons or sharp objects, such as knives or scissors.

## Worrying about yourself and your family

Don't feel selfish if you're worried about yourself and your family. Taking care of a chronically ill person, particularly someone with a condition like AD, can be a very frustrating experience for a family. You and your family will have to work extra hard to maintain your relationships and to make sure that you don't let your loved one's condition take over your entire lives.

You may go through times when you feel isolated, particularly if you're the sole caregiver. At other times, financial worries will crowd into your tired head, or in a state of exhaustion, you may worry that your life will never be the same.

Hundreds of thousands of families have lived through this ordeal, and you and your family can do it as well — and perhaps even come out stronger on the other side. Remember to keep the lines of communication open and share whatever is bothering you. If you do start to feel completely overwhelmed, reach out for help from your church, friends, or the community. You don't have to go it alone.

# Part II

# Helping a Loved One Manage the Illness

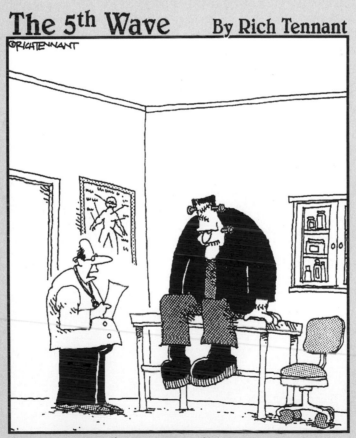

## The 5th Wave — By Rich Tennant

"We've tried adjusting your diet, and prescribing medication for your stress. Now, let's try loosening some of those bolts and see if that does anything."

# In this part . . .

We discuss the various stages of Alzheimer's Disease and how they impact caregiving. This part helps you evaluate current drug therapies and watch out for scams and quack treatments, and it explains the benefits and pitfalls of participating in a clinical trial. It also covers effective alternative therapies and takes a peek into the future to see what researchers are working on in the hope of finding new treatments, or maybe even a cure.

# Chapter 6

# Understanding the Stages of Alzheimer's Disease

*In This Chapter*

▶ Looking at stages as a classification tool

▶ Looking at cognitive and functional impairment as a classification tool

*O*ver the years, doctors and researchers have come up with a variety of ways to classify *Alzheimer's Disease* (AD) as it progresses. Healthcare professionals have found that using stages is a helpful way to describe the expected course a particular illness may take and the array of symptoms that can appear along the way.

Staging a disease not only provides a shorthand that everyone in the medical profession instantly understands, but it may also help to explain the progression of various conditions to patients and their families. It's a way to let them know what they can expect in the way of symptoms at various points during the course of an illness.

Unfortunately, many different groups of experts have developed their own sets of AD stages. Depending upon which set of classifications you're looking at, the condition can be grouped into three, four, five, six, or even seven distinct stages.

To add to the confusion, most healthcare professionals no longer use the numbered stages. Rather, they classify AD patients according to the level of their cognitive and functional impairment — mild, moderate, severe, and profound.

In this chapter, we provide an overview of the staging classifications of Alzheimer's Disease, for informational purposes; you may also find it helpful in evaluating yourself or your loved one. After that, we jump into the four levels of cognitive and functional impairment that are currently being used to describe AD. You can use the information in the chapter to help you better understand the symptoms that your loved one may be displaying.

# How to Use the Classifications

Staging systems provide guidelines that can help patients and caregivers make critical decisions regarding independence, financial and legal issues, and the type of care and supervision that may be required at any given point.

Alzheimer's Disease develops in an unpredictable fashion that can vary widely from one patient to the next. Your loved one may never exhibit certain symptoms, nor cycle through all the expected stages; on the other hand, he or she may experience a textbook progression of symptoms. No one can say for sure how the disease will affect specific individuals. For example, if your mother is 83 years old when she's diagnosed, unless your family is extraordinarily long-lived, she'll probably pass away before she reaches the final stages. Or if your husband was already under treatment for heart disease before his AD diagnosis, that condition may take his life while he's still in the mild or moderate level of cognitive and functional impairment.

As you review the stages, keep in mind that even experts don't agree on these classifications, so you may find some information that seems contradictory or overlapping. AD symptoms don't appear in clockwork order, and you may find your loved one displaying some Stage 2 symptoms when, according to his level of functioning, he's actually still in Stage 1. Every person's AD is different, so don't get hung up on this sort of thing or read too much into it. Alzheimer's Disease is far too complex a topic and there's still too much that simply isn't well understood about the condition to be able to make any blanket statements about how the disease will develop in any given patient. Please keep that caveat in mind.

# Three Stages

One of the earliest attempts to classify Alzheimer's Disease simply divided it into three stages — mild, moderate, and severe, or early, mid, and late, or first, second, and third, or even just simply Stage 1, Stage 2, and Stage 3. No matter what it's called, the symptoms described for each stage are similar.

## Mild

The mild stage of Alzheimer's Disease may last from two to four years or longer. The symptoms may be apparent only to the patients or their families. The person with AD may try to cover up their forgetfulness and deny that anything is wrong. Patients may exhibit any of the following symptoms:

- Repetitive speech patterns. They may say the same things over and over again, or ask the same questions repeatedly.

- Memory deficits. They may misplace things or forget names of friends, relatives, and familiar objects.

- Disorientation — confusion about dates and time.

- Personality changes. They may exhibit changes in social behavior, such as passivity or agitation.

- Loss of interest in normal daily activities and hobbies.

## Moderate

The moderate stage of Alzheimer's Disease is the longest stage, lasting from two to ten years. At this stage, the patient exhibits more severe impairment that he can't cover up or hide. Patients may exhibit any of the following:

- Increasing confusion about recent events

- A tendency to get lost or disoriented, even in familiar places such as their own homes

- Increasingly severe problems with memory

- Problems with normal daily activities, such as dressing, using the phone, microwave, TV remote, bathing, basic personal care and toileting

- May be moody or argumentative

- Speech may ramble

- Increase in anxiety, apathy, and/or depression

- New or additional problems with behavior, such as restlessness or wandering, poor impulse control, verbal or physical aggression, screaming, and sleep disturbances

## Severe

The severe stage of AD may last from one to three years or longer. Patients are essentially totally incapacitated. Their symptoms include the following:

- Severe disorientation or confusion

- Wandering

- Incontinence (the inability to control bladder and bowel functions)

✔ Motor problems, such as difficulty getting into or out of a chair

✔ Swallowing difficulties

✔ Agitation

✔ Hallucinations, delusions, paranoia

✔ Failure to recognize themselves or family members consistently

✔ Inability to use or understand language

✔ Unable to care for themselves at basic levels

✔ Increased susceptibility to infection because of problems communicating pain or discomfort

Even though AD was first identified by Dr. Alois Alzheimer in Germany in 1906, it wasn't widely recognized or diagnosed in clinical practice until the late 1970s and early 1980s. So little was known about the condition that researchers working independently came up with many different ways to classify progression of AD, hence the confusion about the number of stages.

# Four Stages

As doctors and researchers continued to gather more information and observations about the progression of Alzheimer's Disease, some of them became convinced that the three-stage model didn't offer enough differentiation. So they developed a four-stage model that offered more detail about symptoms that could accompany each stage and essentially added a "profound" classification to the description of AD progression.

## Stage 1

The symptoms of Stage 1 may be tricky to pin down. Patients and their family members often try to explain them away and may fail to seek professional evaluation until Stage 2 symptoms appear. Patients in Stage 1 may exhibit the following symptoms:

✔ Memory loss, unable to remember familiar names or everyday information, such as home phone number or street address

✔ Inability to find the right word when speaking, may hesitate or act with uncertainty when speaking

✔ Impaired judgment — dressing in short sleeves during freezing weather, for example

- Desire to stay close to home due to increasing confusion, can still function in familiar surroundings

- Wearing the same clothing over and over despite having many other outfits to choose

- Personality changes, becoming more irritable or more passive, exhibiting uncharacteristic rudeness or lack of social grace

- Acting defensively or minimize their problems

- Loss of interest in current affairs and usual activities

- Restlessness or agitation, lower tolerance for frustration

# Stage 2

When patients enter Stage 2, symptoms become more obvious and more difficult to overlook. Safety concerns related to impaired functioning may force families to decide whether to let their loved one continue to live on his or her own. The following symptoms are characteristic of patients in Stage 2 of the disease:

- Increased memory problems. Patients may not remember to pay their bills, take their medication, or complete routine household tasks. Laundry may mildew in the washer; food may burn on the stove. At this stage, it may be dangerous to allow the patient to continue to live without a caregiver's supervision.

- Inability to retain new information. For example, you may tell them about an upcoming family celebration and five minutes later they will have no recall of the event.

- Loss of ability to perform simple calculations. Balancing the checkbook becomes an impossible task.

- May become more withdrawn as confusion increases.

- Diminished interest in other people, even close family members.

- Loss of ability to plan and execute complex behaviors. Driving is an example of a skill that's no longer possible.

- Deterioration of personal hygiene. They may forget to bathe or brush their teeth or shave.

- Sleep disturbances. Restlessness and agitation may occur, making it hard to fall and stay asleep.

- Wandering. Patients may get lost in familiar surroundings or in new places.

# Stage 3

By Stage 3, patients require more care and supervision to keep them safe and maintain optimum physical condition. Stage 3 patients may exhibit the following symptoms:

- Seriously impaired judgment — giving away money or valuables, for instance
- Decline in or loss of orientation to time and place
- Loss or deterioration of speech and language skills

    This deterioration can be one of the most frustrating for caregiver, family, and friends. Patients repeat things over and over, asking the same questions and telling the same stories without realizing it. Also, patients may no longer understand or respond to simple instructions.

- Increased confusion
- Increased lethargy or restlessness
- Paranoia, aggression, hostility, or delusions
- Loss of self-care abilities, needs a lot of help to bathe, dress and eat
- Requires round-the-clock supervision and care

# Stage 4

By the time an AD patient reaches Stage 4, he or she requires total supervision and care around the clock. This is the most difficult stage for caregivers to manage. The following symptoms are common for patient in Stage 4:

- Further loss of language skills; patients are unable to conduct conversations or understand spoken or written language
- Obsessive repetition of single words or actions like rocking or tapping
- Inability to recognize anyone, including themselves
- Confusion, delusions, hallucinations, aggression, or violent outbursts
- Apathy or withdrawal
- Difficulty chewing and swallowing
- Bladder and bowel incontinence
- Seizures
- Complete loss of ability to walk, may become bedridden if other illnesses are a factor

# *Five, Six, and Seven Stages*

The idea of classifying Alzheimer's Disease into five, six, or seven stages all evolved around the same time, and in many instances, the various classifications are simply different interpretations of the same information. For example, *The Global Deterioration Scale for Assessment of Primary Degenerative Dementia* was developed by a group of psychiatrists and published in *The American Journal of Psychiatry* in 1982. It lists seven different stages, but Stage 1 is "Normal with no cognitive deficits." People who omit Stage 1 end up with a six-stage Alzheimer's Disease model.

Healthcare providers who follow (or followed) the five-stage model of Alzheimer's Disease classify AD in two different ways. One model uses Stage 1: Mild Cognitive Impairment, Stage 2: Mild Dementia, Stage 3: Moderate Dementia, Stage 4: Severe Dementia, and Stage 5: Profound Dementia. The other uses Stage 1: Early Confusional Stage, Stage 2: Late Confusional Stage, Stage 3: Early Dementia, Stage 4: Middle Dementia, and Stage 5: Late Dementia. However, both models describe a similar array of symptoms, and follow the symptom progression laid out in the seven-stage model.

To avoid repetition, we discuss only the seven-stage model. However, keep in mind that this info covers the five- and six-stage models as well.

- ✔ **Stage 1:** No cognitive decline; normal functioning.

- ✔ **Stage 2 or "Forgetfulness Stage":** Very mild cognitive decline. Patients begin to forget names of family members, friends, and common objects. They still function well in social and work situations. They may express worry about symptoms.

- ✔ **Stage 3 or "Early Confusional Stage":** Memory problems become noticeable and start to affect work performance. People may get lost traveling to an unfamiliar location, and try to hide or deny memory problems. Problems with language and finding the right word increase. They misplace items, can't concentrate, and can't retain new information. They may develop mild to moderate anxiety as symptoms worsen.

- ✔ **Stage 4 or "Late Confusional Stage":** Cognitive decline continues with decreased recall of recent events; patients may lose memories of some of their own personal histories. They have trouble handling their own affairs, especially finances and can no longer manage complex tasks. They're still oriented to time and place, recognize themselves and familiar people and places. They may become very defensive about increasing cognitive deficits and deny vehemently that anything's wrong. They may withdraw from challenging situations rather than try to cope.

✔ **Stage 5 or "Early Dementia Stage":** Cognitive decline becomes more severe. Patients require assistance to function, and can't recall or may make up basic facts about their own lives, such as where they live and work, or the names of friends and more distant family members. They still know their own name and names of close family members such as their spouse and children. Math abilities decline sharply. Patients may still feed and dress themselves and use the bathroom without assistance, but due to impaired judgment, they may require close supervision.

✔ **Stage 6 or "Middle Dementia Stage":** Patients exhibit severe cognitive decline. They no longer remember names of close family, but can still distinguish familiar people from strangers. They need help with all activities of daily living. They have a total lack of awareness of current events but may still exhibit some memory of their distant past. Patients may become incontinent; both bowels and bladder may be affected. They show severely impaired judgment and may exhibit dramatic personality changes with episodes of delusion, anxiety, aggression, and even violent outbursts that are completely contrary to their original personalities.

✔ **Stage 7 or "Late Dementia and Failure to Thrive Stage":** Patients show very severe cognitive decline. They can't speak or understand speech and can no longer follow instructions. They're incontinent and require round-the-clock care and supervision. They also lose basic motor skills, including walking and the ability to sit up.

# The Current Thinking: Assessing Alzheimer's Stages Via Cognitive and Functional Impairment

Although some healthcare practitioners do still refer to the various stages of Alzheimer's, most researchers, doctors, and clinicians classify Alzheimer's Disease according to the level of cognitive and functional impairment that the patient displays. As we mention at the beginning of the chapter, the levels used to classify this functioning are *mild, moderate, severe, and profound.*

*Cognitive skills* relate to your ability to think, make and carry out reasonable plans, make judgments, be aware, and learn and retain new information. *Functional skills* relate to your ability to take care of yourself and carry out the activities of everyday life. Doctors and researchers use cognitive and functional skills as a way to classify AD patients because this provides a more reliable indication of where a patient is in the course of the illness. and they use this information to make assessments of a person's current needs.

Patients may show a notable decline in cognitive skills and still display a relatively normal range of functional skills, or vice-versa. No one can say for sure how your loved one's illness will progress or predict the rate of decline because experts still don't know what causes Alzheimer's Disease, and what factors contribute to either an accelerated or relatively slow rate of decline.

The following sections describe the way most medical professionals stage Alzheimer's Disease today, by the degree of cognitive and functional impairment that the patient exhibits.

# Mild

Early symptoms of AD may go unnoticed as patients can be quite adept at covering up any problems they're experiencing. Patients may exhibit the following symptoms:

- ✔ Forgetfulness
- ✔ Difficulty with complex math problems, such as balancing the checkbook, doing taxes
- ✔ Inability to plan and execute a complex series of actions, such as that required to prepare a three-course meal
- ✔ Inability to stick to a complex schedule, such as that required by certain prescriptions
- ✔ Confusion or disorientation about time, date, or place; wandering toward a specific goal, such as a friend's house, that results in getting lost

## Mild Cognitive Impairment or MCI

To this mix, researchers are now considering adding a new classification called MCI, or *Mild Cognitive Impairment,* that's distinct from the mild category mentioned previously. MCI is characterized by memory impairment without impairment of other cognitive or functional abilities to an extent beyond that expected for the patient's age or educational background.

Even though statistics suggest that 80 percent of patients with MCI develop Alzheimer's Disease within ten years at the rate of 10 to 15 percent of the patients per year, researchers still can't agree if it's a distinct condition or an early manifestation of Alzheimer's Disease, especially since there's no consensus that all people with MCI develop Alzheimer's Disease.

Disagreements aside, MCI is currently being investigated to determine whether it could be useful as a predictive tool to help determine who might develop Alzheimer's Disease later in life. Studies are underway, but few solid conclusions have emerged and work on the subject is ongoing. Drug researchers are hopeful that they can develop a medication to help delay the progression of MCI into more profound cognitive and functional decline or dementia.

## *Moderate*

By the time a patient reaches the moderate stage of AD, symptoms have become so noticeable that trying to hide the fact that a problem exists is impossible. The majority of diagnoses are made when a patient has reached this stage. Patients with moderate decline may exhibit the following:

- More pronounced memory problems; may interfere with daily activities
- Difficulty with basic food preparation, such as brewing a cup of tea
- Inability to perform routine household chores and yard work
- Decline in personal hygiene, requiring reminders or assistance to use the bathroom, shave, fasten clothing, and choose appropriate clothing
- Increased wandering behavior that's not goal-directed, getting lost
- Agitation, pacing, increased irritability more likely
- Confusion that often becomes worse in evening

The following symptoms can occur in both the moderate and severe stage, and may become more noticeable as the patient enters the severe stage.

- Increased irritability and agitation, verbal and physical aggression
- Symptoms of psychosis, including delusions, paranoia, and hallucinations

For unknown reasons, many AD patients in the moderate stage of cognitive and functional impairment become increasingly confused as evening approaches. This phenomena is known as *sundowning*.

## *Severe*

By the time a patient enters the severe stage of AD, her care needs may be so overwhelming that her family chooses to put her one in a nursing home or other long-term care facility rather than continue to care for her at home. Patients may exhibit the following symptoms:

- Need for extensive assistance with personal care, including eating, hygiene, grooming and toileting
- Increased irritability and agitation, verbal and physical aggression
- Symptoms of psychosis, including delusions, paranoia, and hallucinations
- Unsteadiness and reduced ability to walk
- Incontinence
- Disorientation

## Profound

The profound stage of AD is the last or *terminal* stage in which patients may suffer from a variety of physical complaints. Not all patients reach this stage, particularly those who have another underlying disease or who were diagnosed at a much older age. Patients may exhibit the following:

- ✔ Complete lack of awareness of surroundings
- ✔ Total dependence on caregivers for feeding, hygiene, and everything else

When AD patients reach the terminal stage, they may become bedridden and will certainly require around-the-clock care. At this stage, many Alzheimer's patients succumb to opportunistic infections, such as pneumonia.

# Chapter 7

# Evaluating Drug Therapies

*In This Chapter*

▶ Reviewing currently available drugs

▶ Considering other drugs your loved one may require

housands of researchers across the globe are devoting their entire professional lives to discovering new, effective drug therapies to slow,
halt, or reverse the devastating effects of *Alzheimer's Disease* (AD). Up to
this point, their efforts have yielded just four drugs — Aricept, Reminyl,
Exelon, and Cognex — currently approved by the United States *Food and
Drug Administration* (FDA) for use in the treatment of AD. All four drugs
boost the levels of the neurotransmitter, acetylcholine, in the brain. In
practical application, they've been shown to slow the rate of cognitive and
functional decline in Alzheimer's patients with mild cognitive impairment.

In this chapter, we talk about how these four drugs were developed and how
they're used, and we review their effectiveness. We also look at expanded
drug trials now underway that are investigating new uses for the currently
approved drugs, such as seeing whether a drug approved for use in people
with mild cognitive impairment could also prove beneficial for people with
moderate cognitive impairment.

Finally, we look at other sorts of drugs that may be prescribed for your loved
one — drugs that don't actually treat the AD itself but rather relieve some of
the more troublesome symptoms of the condition, such as depression,
insomnia, anxiety, and agitation.

# A Little Background on Brain Chemistry

The four FDA-approved Alzheimer's drugs, Cognex, Aricept, Reminyl, and
Exelon work by boosting the levels of *acetylcholine* in the brain. In plain
English, these drugs slow the body's normal chemical process that breaks
down acetylcholine, thereby boosting available levels of this important neurotransmitter in the brain.

A *neurotransmitter* is a chemical that carries messages from one nerve cell or neuron to another in the brain, enabling your brain cells to communicate with each other. These messages are sent across a tiny space between the brain cells called a synapse. Depending upon what neurotransmitters are released, messages either stimulate target cells to initiate an action (excitatory) or inhibit target cells to stop or slow down an action (inhibitory). There are about 100 neurotransmitters in the brain; each performs many different jobs. For example, acetylcholine stimulates muscle fibers to initiate movement. Gamma-aminobutyric acid or GABA reduces anxiety. Some neurotransmitters work together to accomplish specific tasks. Electrical pulses known as action potentials stimulate the release of neurotransmitters.

Researchers didn't just haphazardly decide to start investigating every known brain chemical in the vain hope that they'd stumble across something that may help AD patients. Like any good scientists, they had lots of clues telling them where to start, and all the early clues pointed to acetylcholine.

## Following a thread

In a normal brain, as soon as a neurotransmitter finishes its job of conducting a chemical message from one neuron to another, it's "released" so that it can circle back and do its job again and again. While it's in this released state, traveling back across the synapses from the target cell, the neurotransmitter is like a taxicab circling the streets of a city with its "available" light on; any neuron that needs it can reach out and grab it. SSRIs work by selectively reducing the re-entry of serotonin back into the nerve cells, thereby allowing a buildup of serotonin in the synapses of the brain. When researchers discovered that this build-up greatly reduced the negative emotions associated with depression, they realized that they'd found a new family of very effective antidepression medications.

As soon as scientists knew that they could successfully manipulate the levels of one neurotransmitter in the brain, the next logical step was to look at other conditions that might respond favorably to this sort of manipulation. It was a short jump across a narrow creek that sent researchers on the road to discovering reversible *cholinesterase inhibitors* and the benefits they could provide to AD patients.

## Focusing on acetylcholine

Acetylcholine was the first identified neurotransmitter, discovered way back in the 1920s. At that point, scientists weren't even quite sure exactly what a neurotransmitter was, or how it worked in the body. The first studies of acetylcholinesterase inhibitors actually began in the 1960s. You may be wondering what made AD drug researchers focus their attention on acetylcholine in the first place. Their interest was spurred by findings in several clinical studies that showed that Alzheimer's Disease patients had much lower than normal levels of acetylcholine in their brains and cerebrospinal fluid. This discovery led researchers to try to come up with a drug that would reliably boost levels of the neurotransmitter in the brains of AD patients — the idea being that the increased levels of acetylcholine would somehow alleviate some of the cognitive symptoms of the condition. When clinical trials proved that this hypothesis was correct, the rush was on to formulate, patent, and market the first effective drugs that could help slow the progress of Alzheimer's Disease.

Patients with a history of heart disease, ulcers, liver disease, asthma, or chronic obstructive pulmonary disease should use cholinesterase inhibitors with caution. Also, patients receiving nonsteroidal anti-inflammatory drugs (NSAIDS), such as aspirin or ibuprofen, should be watched closely for signs of gastrointestinal bleeding.

Acetylcholine is used as a messenger to send an impulse from one neuron to another. After it's released, an enzyme called *acetylcholinesterase* breaks it down and prepares it to be used as a messenger again. When someone has Alzheimer's Disease, the neurons that use acetylcholine as a messenger are either damaged or destroyed, which results in lower levels of acetylcholine in the brain. A cholinesterase inhibitor prevents acetylcholinesterase from breaking down the acetylcholine, which produces higher levels of the neurotransmitter in the brain, resulting in an improvement in cognitive functioning. In this way, the drug may help to temporarily compensate for the lower number of properly functioning brain cells.

Acetylcholine plays a vital role in the stimulation of muscle tissue. Although the exact significance of acetylcholine in Alzheimer's Disease is unclear, researchers believe that it's involved in thinking, judgment, attention, reasoning, and learning, and also in the recording and storage of memories. By making more acetylcholine available in the brain, cholinesterase inhibitors help AD patients retain a clinically proven higher level of functioning for a longer period of time than might be expected if the patient weren't taking the medication. Why is that important? Because treatment with these drugs may result in a delay in placing the patient in a nursing home, which alone can save families thousands of dollars.

The downside of cholinesterase inhibitors is that in addition to increasing the levels of acetylcholine in the brain, they also increase the production of stomach acid, which can lead to a whole host of side effects related to the gastrointestinal tract, including nausea, vomiting, loss of appetite, and increased frequency of bowel movements. As with any drug, older people don't eliminate cholinesterase inhibitors from their systems as quickly and reliably as younger people do, so they must be monitored for signs of liver toxicity while they're taking this class of drug.

Keep in mind that although these drugs may improve cognitive functioning for a while, they don't alter the course of the underlying disease nor do they alter its inevitable outcome. As Alzheimer's Disease progresses, cholinesterase inhibitors become less effective because fewer and fewer neurons that respond to acetylcholine remain intact. That doesn't negate the importance of these drugs, however. In a progressive disease like Alzheimer's, any drug that improves symptoms, stabilizes behavior, or slows the rate of decline is valuable and should be employed without hesitation.

# Reviewing Current FDA-Approved Drugs

The four FDA-approved Alzheimer's Disease drugs work by boosting the levels of acetylcholine in the brain. Three drugs, Cognex, Aricept, and Reminyl, are reversible cholinesterase inhibitors, and the fourth, Exelon, is a pseudo-irreversible cholinesterase inhibitor. Doctors don't necessarily believe that any one of these medications is more efficacious for cognition or behavior than any other. It is a more a matter of finding the one that works for an individual patient and that takes patience and a willingness on the part of the patient and the caregiver to experiment with different doses and medications until the best fit is found.

Although cholinesterase inhibitors do help slow cognitive and functional decline for many AD patients, these drugs DO NOT CURE the disease. Some 10 to 20 percent of patients do show noticeable improvement while taking one of the approved Alzheimer's drugs, but they're not for everybody; up to 50 percent of patients show no improvement whatsoever in their cognitive functioning, but the drugs do help slow the rate of decline. Other people experience side effects that cause them to discontinue use. Your doctor may try different drugs and different dosages until he finds one that provides noticeable benefits.

## Cognex

Cognex, or tacrine hydrochloride, was approved by the FDA in 1993 and was the first prescription drug made available for the treatment of Alzheimer's Disease in the United States. It was developed by Warner-Lambert and went through repeated clinical trials and a difficult series of rejections by the *FDA's Peripheral and Central Nervous System Drugs Advisory Committee* before it was finally approved.

Although its appearance was greeted with great enthusiasm, Cognex is no longer prescribed because of the frequency of reported side effects, including toxicity resulting in irreversible liver damage. In addition, because of its relatively low bioavailability of 17 to 37 percent, and relatively fast elimination, Cognex had to be administered four times daily to maintain therapeutic levels, which proved to be impractical and undesirable for facilities caring for large numbers of patients with dementia.

*Bioavailability* is the degree and rate at which a drug or other substance like a vitamin is absorbed into a living system or is made available for use by the body.

# Aricept

Aricept, or donepezil hydrochloride, was approved by the FDA in 1996 and was the second reversible cholinesterase inhibitor to make it to market in the United States. Of the newer generation medications, it has been around the longest. Manufactured under a joint agreement between the pharmaceutical giant, Pfizer, and the Japanese pharmaceutical company, Eisai, Aricept is the number one drug prescribed for the treatment of symptoms in AD patients with a mild to moderate level of cognitive impairment.

Aricept is popular for two reasons:

- ✔ It's the only AD drug that has 100 percent bioavailability.
- ✔ It remains in a person's system much longer than Cognex.

Patients can receive the maximum benefits of the drug with just one dose per day, a big advantage for caretakers who often have to fight with their patients to get anything swallowed.

## Dosage

Aricept is available in 5 mg (white pill) and 10 mg (yellow pill) doses, with the drug's name embossed on one side and the dosage strength embossed on the opposite side. Patients take it in the evening before retiring, and they may take it with or without food. Doctors start patients off on the 5 milligram dose for four to six weeks. If a patient can tolerate the drug and shows improvement, he or she may then be switched to the 10 milligram regimen to see if it gives the patient any additional benefits. If patients develop noticeable side effects, they may go back down to the lower dose regimen. It takes 15 days for patients to achieve a steady therapeutic level of Aricept in their bodies, and they must take the drug daily in order for benefits to continue.

A study presented at the annual American Academy of Neurology meeting in April 2003 suggested that Aricept may also prove beneficial for the 1.3 million people with vascular dementia. (See Chapter 4 for more information about vascular dementia.) This development is an important one because no drugs are currently approved for treatment of vascular dementia. Researchers believe that vascular dementia patients given Aricept may demonstrate the same significant improvements in cognition, behavior, and the activities of daily living as Alzheimer's patients.

### Side effects

Alas, Aricept isn't perfect. Possible side effects include nausea, diarrhea, insomnia, vomiting, muscle cramps, fatigue, and loss of appetite. These side effects occurred in approximately 7 to 19 percent of patients receiving the 10 milligram dose, and in 3 to 8 percent of patients receiving the 5 milligram dose. Although you should notify your doctor of any side effects that your loved one may experience, in clinical trials, these effects were temporary, lasting an average of one to three weeks, and resolved quickly on their own as the patient's body adjusted to the medication.

## Exelon

Exelon, or rivastigmine tartrate, was approved by the FDA in 2000. It was developed and is marketed by the huge pharmaceutical house Novartis AG of Switzerland. Exelon has bioavailability of approximately 40 percent at the 3 milligram dose.

Exelon isn't quite as popular with healthcare providers and caregivers because it causes significantly more gastrointestinal side effects than Aricept and also because it requires two daily doses to maintain therapeutic benefits instead of just one. To compensate for this shortcoming, Novartis developed an oral solution of Exelon for patients who have difficulty swallowing pills.

### Dosage

To help reduce the potential for side effects such as nausea, vomiting, and diarrhea, patients should take Exelon with food and start off on a very low dose, 1.5 milligrams twice a day. The 1.5 milligram capsule is yellow and is marked with the brand name and the dosage strength on the side of the capsule. Exelon Oral Solution is supplied in the exact same dosages as the capsules and comes with a dosage syringe so that caregivers can easily measure out the correct dose.

## The long road to approval

According to the FDA, it takes an average of ten years of research, development, and testing to successfully bring a new prescription drug to market. For every 100 new drugs submitted to the agency for review, about 70 will pass through Phase 1 clinical trials successfully and go on to Phase 2 trials. Thirty-three of the original 100 will make it from Phase 2 to Phase 3, and 25 to 30 will successfully complete Phase 3 trials. Of those drugs who make it all the way through the clinical trial process, only 20 of the original 100 applicants will ultimately be approved by the FDA for sale in the United States.

If a patient tolerates the 1.5 milligram dose and doesn't exhibit any side effects, the doctor will double the dosage to 3 milligrams twice a day. The goal is to reach a daily dosage of at least 6 milligrams to a maximum of 12 milligrams, as patients show distinct improvements in their cognitive functioning at these higher dosage levels.

Keep in mind that side effects occur more frequently with higher doses, so keep an eye out for any signs of gastrointestinal distress in your loved one.

The 3 milligram capsule is orange, the 4.5 milligram capsule is red, and the 6 milligram capsule is orange and red. All the capsules, regardless of the dose, are marked with the brand name and dosage strength on the side of the capsule.

### Side effects

Because of the frequency and severity of gastrointestinal side effects that may accompany treatment with Exelon, if your loved one has to be taken off the drug for more than a few days, dosing must start again at the lowest level. Patients who've been taken off Exelon for a long period of time for reasons unrelated to the drug itself have suffered such severe bouts of vomiting when Exelon was inadvertently started back at full dosage strength that some of them even suffered esophageal rupture.

As with Aricept, patients must be watched for signs of ulcers, liver toxicity, and gastrointestinal bleeding. Patients taking Exelon also seem to experience more frequent problems with loss of appetite and weight loss.

# Reminyl

Reminyl, or galantamine hydrobromide, was developed by Janssen Pharmaceutica and approved by the FDA in 2001. It followed a rather checkered path to FDA approval. At one point, the name Reminyl was associated with another compound, sabeluzole, a calcium channel blocker and nonspecific nerve cell stimulant that was purported to protect the brain against further damage from amyloid plaques (covered in Chapter 3) and stimulate the growth of new neurons within the brain. Janssen quit working on sabeluzole after early tests showed no measurable benefit to patients. Because Janssen had already registered the trademark Reminyl and hated to let a good name go to waste, the company simply transferred the trademark to galantamine.

The discovery of galantamine has a really interesting history. Back in the 1950s, a Bulgarian pharmaceutical researcher noticed that people in a local village rubbed a flower called a snowdrop on their foreheads to relieve headaches (snowdrops are part of the daffodil family). He isolated an alkaloid extract of the snowdrop that he believed was the active relief-giving ingredient and dubbed it *galantamine*. For decades, the substance was used throughout eastern Europe in a variety of applications, but its actual use dates back thousands of years in a variety of folk remedies.

## Let the drug taker beware

Don't assume that just because the FDA has approved a drug for sale automatically means that it's safe. In the past ten years, the FDA has recalled 11 drugs that were responsible for more than 1,000 deaths and more than 250,000 adverse side effects. Here are just a few examples:

✔ The popular diabetes drug Rezulin was recalled in March of 2001 after it was reported to have caused almost 400 deaths from liver toxicity.

✔ The cholesterol-lowering drug Baycol was recalled in August of 2001 after it was implicated in more than 40 deaths due to muscle breakdown and organ destruction.

✔ The heartburn drug Propulsid was recalled in July of 2000 after more than 300 people died from heart attacks or cardiac arrhythmias after taking the drug.

Be sure to tell your doctor immediately if you start experiencing any unusual symptoms or side effects after starting a new prescription drug.

By the time researchers started looking at galantamine as a possible treatment for Alzheimer's, the available supply of Bulgarian snowdrops had dwindled to almost nothing, certainly not enough to supply demand. Researchers went looking throughout the daffodil family to find another genus that contained significant amounts of galantamine and found what they were looking for in a common daffodil, *narcissus pseudonarcissus L.* Janssen patented the substance and, after FDA approval, started marketing it as Reminyl.

For reasons that are not yet entirely understood, Reminyl appears to hold Alzheimer's patients at a higher level of cognitive functioning slightly longer than either Aricept or Exelon, an average of 12 months for Reminyl as opposed to an average to 6 to 9 months for Aricept and Exelon. Perhaps it's because the drug has a dual action. However, the medications have not been compared to each other in the same study, which is necessary before drawing firm conclusions about the relative benefits or risks of each drug.

Like the other cholinesterase inhibitors, Reminyl acts to prevent the breakdown of acetylcholine, thereby raising the available levels of the neurotransmitter in the brain. But unlike the other approved drugs, Reminyl also acts upon something called the *nicotinic receptors* in the brain, making them more responsive to acetylcholine. This action is thought to increase the release of acetylcholine.

Nicotinic receptors come in two varieties. N1 receptors are concentrated in the brain and spinal cord, and N2 receptors are concentrated in muscle tissue. The N1 receptors in the brain appear to be involved with cognition, pain perception, and neurodegeneration. Reminyl acts upon the N1 receptors.

Importantly, preliminary research has shown that Reminyl seems to delay the appearance of some of the more troublesome behaviors associated with advancing Alzheimer's Disease, including agitation, aggression, apathy, hallucinations, delusions, and a lack of inhibition. This is important because the ability to hold patients at a higher level of functioning with more desirable behavior reduces the burden on the caregivers by reducing the amount of time that they have to directly assist and supervise their loved ones.

### Dosage

Reminyl comes in 4 milligram white tablets, 8 milligram pink tablets, and 12 milligram orange-brown tablets, as well as in an oral solution for patients who can't swallow pills. The tablets are marked with the manufacturer's name on one side and tablet strength on the other. Patients take the medication twice a day, with their morning and evening meals, along with plenty of fluid. Doctors start their patients on the 4 milligram tablet and then switch them to the 8 milligram tablet after four weeks if the 4 milligram dose has been well tolerated. After four weeks at the 8 milligram dose, doctors evaluate whether their patients should increase to the 12 milligram dose.

Like Exelon, if administration of Reminyl is interrupted for a period of time, the patient should be started back at the lowest dose and progressed back to a higher dose after a period of four weeks on the lower dose.

### Side effects

Patients with severe liver disease shouldn't take Reminyl. Doctors and caregivers should monitor their patients for gastrointestinal bleeding. Patients switching from a lower dose to a higher dose may experience nausea for five to seven days following the switch. Giving the medication with food and adequate fluid reduces the likelihood of nausea.

# Considering Other Types of Drugs

During the course of Alzheimer's Disease, your loved one may need other types of drugs to help control certain symptoms that may accompany the illness, such as agitation or insomnia. He or she may also need drugs to treat the symptoms of other diseases, and even drugs for simple things like pain relief.

The difficulty with administering a variety of drugs to people who are in their 50s or 60s or older is that as they age, their ability to metabolize and excrete drugs and their by-products decreases. That means that a pain drug given three times a day without incident to a healthy 30-year-old can build to dangerously toxic levels in the body of a 65-year-old whose body excretes excess quantities of the drug much more slowly. Because of this problem, doctors are reluctant to use medications to control the behavioral problems of advanced AD patients because overmedication can lead to liver toxicity and kidney failure, as well as many other undesirable and perhaps even fatal complications.

But does that mean that Alzheimer's patients shouldn't receive any other drugs at all? By no means. In fact, some research suggests that one of the main reasons that some AD patients may become aggressive or combative is because of chronic untreated pain.

The important thing to keep in mind is to make sure that all the healthcare providers treating your loved one know exactly which medications, including vitamins and herbs, the patient is taking.

For example, if you take your mother who has AD to see a psychiatrist because she's depressed, your physician's choice of medication to relieve the depression is quite dependent upon which of the Alzheimer's drugs your mother may be taking. The antidepressant Paxil increases serum levels of Reminyl by about 40 percent, while the antidepressant Elavil decreases the body's ability to metabolize and excrete Reminyl by about 25 percent, which can also lead to a buildup of the drug in the system. Without changing the dosage of Reminyl that you're giving your loved one, her actual effective dose could be dramatically increased by the addition of an antidepressant. But other drugs, such as the anti-ulcer medication Zantac, don't affect the metabolism of Reminyl at all.

You can see why your doctor and pharmacist must know all the medications your loved one is taking. They also need to know if your loved one drinks because alcohol consumption can also cause problems when mixed with medications. Although Reminyl is generally considered to be a safe drug when administered appropriately, an accidental overdose caused by the administration of another drug that increases the actual effective dose of the Reminyl can lead to serious complications and side effects, including convulsions and even death.

The following sections look at some of the other types of drugs that your loved one may take.

## Sleep aides

One of the biggest problems families face in dealing with an AD patient is the fact that people with AD often get their days and nights mixed up and wander around the house startling and disturbing other family members who are trying to sleep. This behavior frequently leads to family members asking their doctors to prescribe a sleep medication and is cited as one of the most frequent reasons why families finally decide to place their loved one in a nursing home.

The use of prescribed or over the counter sleep medications in AD patients leads to increased falls, confusion, and daytime sleepiness, so most doctors aren't really wild about the idea of freely handing out sleep aides to this particular patient population. Instead, they prefer to work with behavioral modifications, such as establishing a comforting bedtime routine, engaging in calming activities as bedtime approaches, and sticking to the same schedule for daily naps and bedtime.

## Sedatives

Way back in the Dark Ages (about ten years or so ago), the treatment of choice for AD patients was to sedate them heavily and stick them in a chair in front of a TV so that they wouldn't bother anyone or cause any trouble. We now know that oversedation of older people can have many detrimental side effects, including daytime drowsiness, dizziness, and falls to name a few.

Most older people don't react well to ongoing treatment with sedatives. In AD patients, these drugs should be reserved for use only in emergency situations.

Never try to manage your loved one's medication regimen all by yourself. Only a highly trained and experienced physician or pharmacist is qualified to know what drug interactions may occur if any two particular drugs are administered together. Healthcare professionals are also aware of the special needs of older patients and use that awareness to prescribe medication regimens that provide maximum benefit with minimum risk. You know the old TV warning: "Don't try this at home!"

## Anti-psychotics and antidepressants

When administered properly, antipsychotic medication and antidepressants can be effective for the relief of some of the more distressing symptoms of AD. Antipsychotic medications are useful to manage aggression and other severe behavioral problems while anti-depressants are beneficial for both anxiety and depression. Your doctor will take care to tailor the dose to the age, weight, and physical condition of your loved one, but you should still watch for side effects such as dry mouth, constipation, dizziness, depressed blood pressure, nasal congestion, retention of urine, and impotence. Furthermore, your doctor will help look for underlying causes (such as frustration, relationship problems between the patient and the caregiver, boredom) and non-pharmacologic interventions. More serious side effects include irregular heartbeat, blurred vision, eye pain, and even hallucinations. Antipsychotic medications can also increase symptoms of mental confusion and disorientation. You should report any side effects you notice to your loved one's doctor immediately.

Be aware that antipsychotic medications and anti-depressants take at least three to four weeks to reach a therapeutic level in the body, so your loved one may become discouraged if he or she doesn't see or feel the results of the medication right away. Encourage your loved one to keep taking the medication until he or she can feel its benefits.

## Other medications

Your loved one may be required to take daily medications for conditions unrelated to Alzheimer's Disease, such as diabetes, hypertension, or heart disease. Just be sure to let the doctor or specialist know that your loved one's also being treated for Alzheimer's Disease and what other medications he or she is taking. That way the doctor can take care to prescribe medications that won't interfere with each other.

Some Alzheimer's medications and treatments are not only ineffective, but may be downright dangerous. In Chapter 8, we look at ways you can avoid Snake Oil and other ineffective treatments.

# Chapter 8

# Avoiding Snake Oil and Other Ineffective Treatments

*In This Chapter*

▶ Protecting your family from scams and quackery

▶ Avoiding self-diagnosis

▶ Separating good treatments from the bad

*W*hen the subject is incurable illness, con artists and snake oil salesmen seem to come slithering out of the woodwork. They prey upon people's hopes and fears and promise the moon, not to mention an instant cure. But when you get right down to it, they deliver nothing but heartbreak and disappointment, all while doing their best to empty your wallet. Worse yet, some of these spurious "cures" can even lead to permanent injury or death.

Desperate people make prime targets for quacks promoting bogus cures, and few people are more desperate than those who've just been told that they or a member of their family have an incurable illness. When traditional medicine offers little hope, people naturally go looking for anything else that may help their loved one.

The advent of the Internet has been both a blessing and a curse for the families of Alzheimer's Disease (AD) victims. It's been a blessing because it allows families to access information about the condition and its diagnosis and treatment, but it's a curse because the Internet may not provide the latest and most accurate information and gives con artists an easy way to come right into your home and lure you with hope-filled e-mails promising miraculous results if you send them hundreds, or maybe even thousands, of dollars.

In this chapter, we introduce you to some of the most widespread scams related to AD. But because snake oil salesmen are slippery and tend to move around and come up with new bogus cures as soon as authorities catch on to them, we also clue you in on some savvy tricks to figure out if a new treatment holds real promise or is yet another scam.

# Treatments and Tests That Aren't Worth Your Time or Money

You obviously want the very best and latest treatments available for AD to help your loved one. But how do you know what's going to help and what might hurt? In this section, we tell you about some known scams, devices, therapies, and treatments for which promoters make outrageous claims, including the assertion that their gizmos or special secret formulas cure Alzheimer's Disease. Don't fall for these scams! We also look at the self-diagnosis tests, which aren't scams but still aren't a very good use of your healthcare dollar.

## The Zapper

Just when you think that you've heard everything, along come some people claiming that they can cure everything from cancer to AD with a simple electrical unit called *The Zapper*. The device was originally designed by the controversial Dr. Hulda Clark and her son Geoff to kill a sort of parasite called liver flukes. The units she offered for sale were relatively inexpensive ($68 to $139).

Recently, some other people have jumped on the Zapper bandwagon with much more expensive units, ranging in price from $150 to $300. In addition, they claim that the purchase of electronic "keys" tuned to different electrical frequencies have the power to wipe out various diseases entirely, including AIDS, cancer, and Alzheimer's Disease. The keys cost $10 to $15 each. They work by delivering a 13- to 15-volt jolt of electricity that supposedly kills all viruses, bacteria, and parasites in the body.

You may notice a theme among the conditions that The Zapper is supposed to cure: They're all chronic — and some, like Alzheimer's, arthritis, and AIDS, are incurable — and no single treatment works well for every patient. Although many types of cancer can be cured, in the minds of a lot of people, a diagnosis of cancer represents an automatic death sentence, and that makes them as ripe for cancer cure scams as Alzheimer's patients and their families are for AD cure scams.

The U.S. Federal Trade Commission (FTC) didn't take long to step in and take action to prevent companies from making these outrageous claims in regard to The Zapper. In June 2001, the FTC filed a complaint against a company called Western Herb & Dietary Products, alleging that they'd sold various "cure packages" from their Web site which claimed that a person using their herbal combinations and The Zapper could be immediately cured of Alzheimer's Disease, any sort of cancer, diabetes, and even AIDS.

According to the "theory" promoted by Western Herb in their advertising, all these conditions are caused by an underlying parasitic infestation that responds instantly to their proprietary combination of herbs and precisely modulated square electrical waves delivered via The Zapper.

The final judgment prohibited the company from making any claims for their products that can't be supported by reliable scientific evidence. What happened in practice is that The Zapper is no longer sold in the United States, but it's still widely available over the Internet. A Canadian Web site calls The Zapper the "First Aid Kit of the Future," while slyly stating that according to an agreement with The Department of Health Canada, they're only representing The Zapper as a consumer product intended for use in relaxation and the promotion of well-being. U.S. companies that still offer the device strictly avoid making any claims for it on their Web sites; however, European sites show no such restraint, widely advertising The Zapper as a miraculous device.

What's really miraculous about devices like The Zapper is that the folks who promote them can separate so many otherwise sensible people from their money. If you want to avoid getting zapped, don't waste your money on The Zapper.

## Nutritional supplements

Nutritional supplements may provide measurable benefits for a variety of conditions. In Chapter 7 we discuss how vitamin E is now being used to help AD patients. However, numerous ads now blast across the Internet with claims that some nutritional supplements "cure" AD and restore patients to normal functioning. Such claims are simply not true.

---

### Why do we call 'em "quacks"?

So where did the term "quack" come from? Well, it has nothing to do with ducks. Renaissance doctors battling an epidemic of syphilis found that the only thing that seemed to have any effect on the condition was mercury, commonly known as "quicksilver." Some enterprising street vendors mixed quicksilver with salve to make a "miracle" ointment that they claimed could cure every known disease. Although people were quick to buy initially, after it was discovered that the concoction really had very little effectiveness and indeed had some potent toxic effects, the men who sold it became known as "quacksalvers," which was later shortened to simply "quacks."

Once brain cells die, no known therapy can bring them back to life. No combination of nutrients, vitamins, minerals, or secret ingredients can accomplish this miracle. The day that someone does stumble across such a miracle cure, you can be sure you'll hear about it on every TV news show and read about it in every newspaper.

We're not trying to say that you shouldn't continue to support good general health by taking a multivitamin or some other specialized supplements with proven benefits, for example, glucosamine for joint pain. But if you see an ad for a nutritional supplement that claims to cure AD, particularly if the product in question seems expensive, keep your wallet closed.

## Chelation therapy

In most clinical settings, *chelation therapy* is performed by slowly diffusing *chelating agents* (ethylene diamine tetraacetic acid or EDTA is most widely used) into the patient's bloodstream, where they bind the metal toxins into metal chelates that can be excreted. The average course of therapy is 20 to 30 treatments given one to three times per week.

The word "chelate" is derived from the Greek word *chele,* which means *claw.* Chelating agents "grab" toxic metal ions in the bloodstream and bind them to themselves, creating new structures known as *metal chelates,* which are water soluble and easily excreted in the urine.

Some Web sites are now promoting *rectal chelation* in which the chelating agents are introduced directly into the rectum, and others advocate *oral chelation.* Neither of these modalities has been tested for effectiveness in the way that intravenous chelation has, so beware. One Web site charges well over $300 for ten doses of its chelating agent.

Chelation therapy is a topic that creates a lot of controversy because for more than 60 years the treatment has had an actual medical application: to increase the urinary excretion of lead when a child has been exposed to toxic levels of the metal. But even this application isn't free from controversy, because many pediatricians think that simply removing the lead from the child's environment or taking the child away from the source of the lead contamination is just as beneficial. Getting a child away from the lead is also easier, safer, a lot less expensive, and less traumatic to the child and eliminates the risk of potentially fatal side effects, such as renal failure, that can occur with some chelating agents.

Even though chelation has been proven to increase the rate of lead excretion by as much as 25 to 30 percent, the treatment reduces blood lead concentrations only, and when chelation therapy is stopped, lead levels have a tendency to rebound to toxic levels as the absorbed metal is leached out of the bones back into the blood and soft tissues.

### How chelation relates to Alzheimer's Disease

Given what's known about chelation — that it can reduce levels of heavy metals in the blood — it was only a matter of time before someone proposed that the therapy might be beneficial for AD patients. The belief was especially prevalent during the late 70s and early 80s, when some experts believed that excess concentrations of aluminum might be responsible for triggering the condition, and reared its head once again when some alternative practitioners hypothesized that high concentrations of mercury might cause the diseases.

More recently, researchers at Massachusetts General Hospital reported that a buildup of copper and zinc in the brain triggers deposits of the beta-amyloid plaques that are characteristic of the damage caused by AD. In a well-controlled study with mice, the researchers used a chelating agent known as clioquinol, which reduced the abnormal accumulation of beta-amyloid plaques by half. But clioquinol is so toxic that most experts are deeply concerned about the safety of the drug for use in humans. When clioquinol was used to treat amoebic dysentery in Japan, it caused thousands of cases of blindness.

Unfortunately, the poor clinical results didn't stop many alternative practitioners from claiming that chelation therapy could halt and even reverse the effects of AD. Following close on their heels came the quacks and con artists. Because chelation therapy is an FDA-approved application, consumers easily can take claims made for the therapy at face value. In an area where the science is murky and confusing, the public finds it especially difficult to make informed choices.

### Contraindications and side effects

Patients with underlying heart, liver, or kidney disease and pregnant or nursing women should *never* undergo chelation therapy. People with compromised immunity, such as HIV/AIDS or conditions affecting their blood cells, should avoid it as well.

Despite claims that chelation therapy is absolutely 100 percent safe, in reality, it can cause many side effects — some of them severe and potentially life-threatening. The risk of side effects increases if the therapy isn't administered by a trained medical professional. Among the most dangerous side effects are

- Severe kidney damage
- Dangerously low blood pressure
- Severe allergic reaction that may cause death
- Interference with the body's ability to make new blood cells, resulting in low white blood cell and low platelet counts
- Abnormal heart rhythms, including *tachycardia,* or rapid heart rate
- Dangerously low calcium levels in the blood
- Increased risk of bleeding or blood clots

Less serious side effects include headache, fatigue, fever, nausea, vomiting, gastrointestinal upset, excessive thirst, and sweating.

### Does it work?

Here's the real scoop on chelation therapy for Alzheimer's Disease: Despite what you may read on the Internet or hear from some practitioners who claim to be able to cure AD with chelation therapy, no controlled clinical human studies have been conducted to prove the effectiveness of any particular chelation therapy in Alzheimer's Disease (at least not at the time of this publication). The practitioners answer that by saying that it's impossible to administer a double-blind chelation study, and that we should believe their claims simply because so many people improve after receiving chelation therapy. The difficulty comes in when researchers try to identify these "cured" and "vastly improved" patients, and they can't find any of them.

In a *double-blind study*, neither the subjects receiving the drug nor the doctors and researchers administering the study know which group of patients is receiving the real medication and which is receiving the placebo. This is done to make sure that the study results aren't influenced by anything that could prejudice the accuracy of the results.

If someone tries to convince you that chelation therapy will cure your loved one's Alzheimer's Disease, don't listen to him or her.

## Self-administered tests for AD

Although self-administered tests that are supposed to diagnose Alzheimer's Disease don't strictly fall under the heading of bogus cures, we include them in this chapter because of the absence to date of any single accurate test to diagnose AD.

In general, screening tests are valuable diagnostic tools that save many lives every year. They're designed to identify patients who need follow-up testing to reach a definitive diagnosis. For example, if a woman has a Pap smear that shows abnormal cells, further testing may reveal the presence of an early cancer that will respond favorably to treatment. A man whose colon cancer screening reveals the presence of blood in his stool undergoes additional testing that reveals the presence of a small, localized tumor that's removed surgically. These tests are ordered by the patient's doctors, who then interpret the results and order any additional tests and treatment that may be required.

Self-administered AD screening tests have the potential to cause a great deal of psychological distress and harm.

AD screening tests available for use by individual consumers are offered on a self-referred basis. *Self-referred* means that the patient himself has decided to take the test, and it was not ordered by his doctor. It also means that the patient must pay for the test all by himself because few insurance companies reimburse for self-referred tests. Finally, self-referred test results are reported directly back to the consumer who bought and paid for the test. Because most consumers have little or no medical training or background, they may be unable to correctly interpret the test results and have no way of knowing if the results are accurate or if they need additional testing or treatment.

Here are overviews of two self-administered Alzheimer's Disease tests that are currently being marketed directly to consumers.

### Early Alert Alzheimer's Home Screening Test

The *Early Alert* test, marketed by FMG Innovations, Inc., sells for approximately $20. It's available in drug stores nationwide and via the Internet. The test kit contains an instruction booklet and 12 "scratch and sniff" test strips impregnated with various strong odors, such as cinnamon and garlic. Strips are held under the nose of the person being tested, and he or she is supposed to identify the odor. People with four or more incorrect answers are advised to consult a physician for further testing.

Although researchers have been looking into whether or not loss of smell may be indicative of the onset of Alzheimer's Disease, currently accepted diagnostic criteria doesn't include evaluation of the loss of smell. In addition, many other conditions can lead to a loss of smell, including lifelong smoking, medical conditions such as a tumor in the olfactory gland, or even certain drugs.

## Genetic testing: Another controversy

Although genetic testing isn't a self-administered test like Early Alert or MCAS, it's still a subject embroiled in controversy. Many healthcare professionals think it's wrong to give genetic tests to healthy people who don't display any symptoms of the particular disorder in question. At one point, experts thought that gene testing might prove valuable in determining who may develop Alzheimer's Disease.

That idea has pretty much fallen out of favor because correctly interpreting a positive gene test result is next to impossible. Many people who have the gene variation never develop AD, while others who don't have any gene variations whatsoever end up getting it. Many healthcare practitioners have decided that telling someone that he or she has a higher risk for developing Alzheimer's Disease on the basis of gene testing, when it's not known if that risk will ever have any significance in the real world, is unethical.

Despite the fact that it's widely available, the Early Alert test hasn't been approved for marketing by the Center for Devices and Radiologic Health (CDRH), the branch of the FDA that regulates the sale of such products.

### Minnesota Cognitive Acuity Screen

The *Minnesota Cognitive Acuity Screen* (MCAS) was developed as a risk-management tool to help insurance companies avoid selling policies to patients who were likely to develop dementia. That should tell you something right there. It was developed by CareLink, a firm that specializes in geriatric assessment. It's sold by phone and over the Internet and costs $95.

The test consists of a 15-minute telephone interview administered by a registered nurse. The test is designed to measure an individual's level of cognitive functioning by asking for her name, address, birthday, and so on, asking her to follow a series of commands and perform simple tasks such as tapping on the phone when asked, and finally asking her to respond to a question that requires executive planning, such as, "What would you do if there were a fire in your home?" People who don't achieve a certain score are considered to have "failed" the test and are identified as people who require supervision and monitoring because of their impaired cognitive status. Translated into English, they don't get the long-term care insurance policy.

After CareLink figured out just how lucrative a product their MCAS was, they started marketing it fairly aggressively over the phone to a targeted audience of older people. Their pitch is designed to make you think they're doing you some sort of favor, when in reality, they're gathering information that keeps you from being able to purchase long-term care insurance if you don't pass the test. Despite the fact that no solid clinical guidelines exist for the use of the test, CareLink encourages its customers to submit to the test on an annual basis.

# Sniffing Out Scams: Five Warning Signs to Look For

Because new scams pop up all the time, you need to arm yourself with some good, basic information to help you determine if a particular treatment has merit or is simply a new member of the "Bogus Alzheimer's Treatments Hall of Shame." Here are some things to look out for:

✔ **Outlandish claims:** A manufacturer claims that its product or device cures "everything" or cures a wide variety of unrelated conditions, such as, "Completely reverses the debilitating effects of Alzheimer's arthritis, diabetes, ingrown toenails, and the heartbreak of psoriasis." There's no such thing as a magic bullet. No one product can treat every condition effectively.

✓ **Exaggerated language:** The advertising uses phrases such as "miracle cure" or "revolutionary breakthrough" or "the secret that doctors don't want you to know." The reason doctors don't want you to know about bogus treatments is that they're afraid that you'll waste your hard-earned dollars and valuable time pursuing treatments that have no measurable effect except the ongoing slimming of your wallet.

✓ **Undocumented testimonials:** People who've supposedly tried the cure claim amazing or miraculous results, such as, "My brother had advanced Alzheimer's Disease, was bedridden, bald, and hadn't recognized me as his sister for two years, but just two weeks after starting Dr. Codswallop's Amazing Herbal Alzheimer's and Baldness Cure, he's out of bed, dancing, singing, calling me Sis, performing his normal chores, and all his hair has grown back!!!" Of course, you have no way of contacting Miss T. Rosen of Los Angeles, California, so you can't check out these wondrous claims for yourself.

✓ **Emphasis to buy right away:** The call for an order creates an exaggerated sense of urgency and implies that if you don't order right away, you might miss out. "Limited supply," "Reserve your supply now," or "This offer might not last" are favorite ploys. By the way, "This offer might not last" is probably as close to the truth as you'll ever get with people advertising fraudulent treatments, because as soon as the FDA moves in to stop their scam, the offer does end — at least until they can set up a new post office box.

✓ **Money-back guarantees:** A company may swear to hold your uncashed check for 30 days until you can see how miraculous its product is for yourself. If you fall for this one, maybe you need a dose of that Dr. Codswallop's stuff. Your check will be cashed less than one nanosecond after they rip open the envelope.

Don't get sucked in by products that are advertised as "all-natural" or that claim to be some ancient cure that's only recently come to light after archaeologists finally interpreted Hammurabi's Code correctly. Rest assured that when a truly effective treatment or real cure for Alzheimer's Disease is found, the news will blare from every television, newspaper, and radio station in the world. Unless you're living in a sensory deprivation tank, you'll hear about it. If the information about a particular product or treatment is buried deep in an obscure Web site that keeps moving around, chances are the information isn't all that valid, and the product more than likely doesn't work as advertised.

Some treatments for Alzheimer's Disease, although not fraudulent, are nonetheless fraught with medical, legal, and ethical issues. These treatments are only available in clinical trials. In Chapter 9, you can find out about the ins and outs of clinical trials and get some guidelines to help you determine if a clinical trial is right for your loved one.

# Chapter 9

# Taking Part in Clinical Trials

*T*he search for more effective treatments for Alzheimer's Disease — and maybe even a cure — is an ongoing quest for thousands of researchers all over the world. New drugs and therapies have to pass through several levels of screening and testing before they're approved by the FDA for clinical trials in human patients. Then they have to successfully pass through three phases of clinical trials before receiving final approval for marketing from the FDA.

Taking part in a clinical trial is a big decision. Although many layers of protection are built into trials to protect patients, participants are still human guinea pigs of sorts — the first ones to take a drug or receive a treatment that may either provide unknown benefits or trigger unforeseen consequences, including potentially dangerous side effects.

Participants in clinical trials who actually receive the investigational drug or therapy being studied may benefit enormously. That's the lure that encourages thousands of people to sign up for clinical trials every year. Sometimes, a clinical trial is the only place a person with a difficult or incurable condition can find any real hope.

In this chapter, you find out what's involved in a clinical trial and what you can expect if your loved one participates in a trial. We help you figure out where to find clinical trials, what to look for to help you determine which trials may be beneficial for your loved one's situation, and how to make an informed, educated decision about participating.

Who knows? You just might be part of a history-making event if the researchers conducting your loved one's clinical trial happen to hit upon a real cure for Alzheimer's Disease.

# What Is a Clinical Trial?

The National Institutes of Health describes a clinical trial as the following: "A research study designed to answer specific questions about vaccines, new therapies, or new ways of using known treatments. Clinical trials (also called *medical research* and *research studies*) are used to determine whether investigational drugs or treatments are both safe and effective. Carefully conducted clinical trials are the fastest and safest way to find treatments that work in people."

Basically, the purpose of a clinical trial is to obtain more information about an investigational drug or therapy in a carefully controlled setting, so that the information gained provides credible, verifiable scientific evidence of the claims made for the new therapy. Researchers are looking for information about how well a particular treatment works, or if it works at all, and what risks may accompany the use of the therapy. Other researchers who repeat the clinical trial should be able to duplicate the findings of the original researchers.

The government oversees clinical trials as a way of regulating the development of effective new drugs, devices, and therapies. Without carefully considered *protocols* (rules and regulations) governing the design and conduct of clinical trials, patients enrolled in those trials would be exposed to a higher level of risk, and more products with the potential to cause harm to patients might make it to market.

There are a number of different types of clinical trials designed to test the effectiveness of various treatments and devices. The most rigorous clinical trials are randomized, double-blind, and placebo controlled. The National Institutes of Health lists the following types of trials:

- **Treatment trials:** These trials test new treatments, new combinations of drugs, or new approaches to surgery or radiation therapy. A number of AD trials are currently underway to test new investigational drugs, the effectiveness of combining two or more existing drugs, and the effectiveness of certain vitamins as AD treatments.

- **Prevention trials:** Researchers who conduct these trials are looking for better ways to prevent disease in people who've never had the disease or to prevent a disease from returning. These approaches may include drugs and medications, vitamins, vaccines, minerals, or lifestyle changes. AD investigators are currently looking into antioxidant therapy and vaccines to see if they're effective in stopping the onset of AD.

- **Screening trials:** These trials provide the best way to detect certain diseases or health conditions. Screening trials are generally not used for AD, unless they're part of an epidemiological study to determine the prevalence of AD in certain groups of people.

✔ **Quality of life trials or supportive care trials:** Trials of this sort explore ways to improve comfort and the quality of life for individuals with a chronic illness. Trials are underway to determine the best way to provide community support for AD caregivers.

So what exactly is a *placebo?* It's a harmless substance with no treatment value whatsoever that's used in controlled experiments to test the effectiveness of an investigational drug. A placebo may be in the form of a pill, liquid, or powder. To guarantee impartiality, both the placebo and the investigational drug are made to look alike, so neither the researchers nor the patients know which is the real investigational drug and which is the placebo. Patients who are given the placebo are known as the *control group.* The people overseeing the clinical trial know which group is which, but when the doctors, researchers, and patients participating in the trial don't know, it's called a *double-blind trial.* This ensures impartiality in the results.

# Weighing the Benefits and the Risks When Participating in a Clinical Trial

Before your loved one decides to join a clinical trial, you should sit down with him and weigh the possible benefits against the potential risks to determine if you both think that the level of risk is acceptable. For example, if your loved one is in the very early stages of AD, drugs that do a fairly good job of holding people at a higher level of functioning for a time are currently available. Would you be willing to risk that known benefit in the hope that an unproven drug might provide better results, even knowing the investigational drug could have some as yet unknown but potentially far more serious side effects?

## Looking at the good

Patients who volunteer to participate in clinical trials are essentially pioneers in medicine, and with that title comes some perks. For instance:

✔ They may receive effective new treatments long before those treatments are made available to the general public.

✔ They're helping others by participating in valuable research that can help doctors discover new ways to treat particular conditions.

✔ Trial participants receive expert medical care at major medical facilities free of charge while participating in the trial. But be aware that the care is only related to the clinical trial; patients and their insurers still have to pay for any medical care received that's not part of the trial protocol.

## Facing the bad

Participation in clinical trials certainly isn't easy or free from risk. Here are some downsides to keep in mind:

- Unpleasant or even potentially life-threatening side effects may result from the treatment. The potential for side effects is, after all, one of the reasons researchers conduct clinical trials in the first place. They need to find out whether the benefits offered by a particular treatment outweigh the risks.

- A patient may go through all the trouble of participating in a clinical trial only to discover that the treatment is ineffective, or that she was placed in the control group and didn't actually receive the investigational drug or therapy.

- Participation in clinical trials requires a big commitment over an extended period of time. Patients may have to commit to multiple trips to the study site, overnight hospital stays, and exacting medication schedules. They may also be seen by a variety of healthcare providers over the course of the study, particularly if the study is being conducted at a large teaching hospital or research facility.

## Regulating clinical trials

Even if you're the most famous doctor or researcher in the world, you can't just wake up one day and decide to launch a clinical trial. Clinical trials are regulated by the FDA. Every clinical trial conducted in the United States must first be approved by what's known as an *IRB,* or *Institutional Review Board.* The IRB assesses the risk-benefit ratio of the trial and reviews the trial protocols to make sure that adequate safeguards are in place to ensure patient safety and that the stated purpose of the trial is worth investigating.

IRBs are local, independent committees comprised of physicians, researchers, community and patient advocates, and others who make sure that all clinical trials proposed for their community follow accepted ethical and research standards and protect the rights and safety of the study participants.

The teams that design and carry out clinical trials may include doctors, researchers, scientists, pharmacists, technicians, medical technologists, nurses, statisticians, medical writers, clerical and support staff, and many others. Long before a clinical trial is approved, researchers may spend years testing potential new therapies in the lab and in animal studies. Therapies that show the most favorable results in these early laboratory trials are then considered for clinical trials in human subjects.

Clinical trials are sponsored by a variety of governmental agencies, pharmaceutical companies, medical institutions, volunteer groups, charitable foundations, and even individual physicians. Trials may be conducted in many different locations, such as hospitals, community clinics, universities, and doctors' offices.

## Making an informed decision

On its Web site, www.clinicaltrials.gov, the United States federal government suggests that patients considering enrolling in a clinical trial ask the following questions:

- What is the purpose of the study?

- Who is going to be in the study?

- Why do researchers believe the new treatment being tested may be effective? Has it been tested before?

- What kinds of tests and treatments are involved?

- How do the possible risks, side effects, and benefits in the study compare with my current treatment?

- How might this trial affect my daily life?

- How long will the trial last?

- Will hospitalization be required?

- Who will pay for the treatment?

- Will I be reimbursed for other expenses?

- What type of long-term follow-up care is part of this study?

- How will I know that the treatment is working?

- Will results of the trials be provided to me?

- Who will be in charge of my care?

They advise that the answers to some of these questions may be found in the informed consent document that all study participants are required to read and sign prior to enrolling in any clinical trial. If you still have unanswered questions, ask the people conducting the study to provide any additional information you desire.

Also know that if patients have health problems not related to the subject under investigation in the trial, they must still visit their own doctors for treatment for those conditions.

## Keeping a few other points in mind

Just because a drug causes a side effect in one patient doesn't mean that every patient who takes that drug is going to suffer the exact same side effect. Everyone reacts a bit differently to individual drugs; one person may feel nauseous while another complains of headaches. Interestingly, even patients receiving placebos often report these sorts of mild side effects when, in fact, they've been taking nothing more than a little sugar pill.

When you and your loved one are in the process of deciding whether to join a trial, be sure to ask for a copy of the trial consent form. Read through it thoroughly and ask questions if you don't understand some of the details or sections. Having all the necessary info will help you and your loved one determine if participation is worthwhile.

While you're both weighing the risks and benefits, remember that there are no guarantees that your loved one will be given the investigational drug. In clinical trials, researchers must establish that any observed benefit truly derives from the investigational drug and not simply from the patient's desire to get better. Your loved one may well be randomly assigned to the control group that receives placebos instead of actual medicine. Even if he's part of this group, your loved one may show improvement due to something called the placebo effect.

Many patients who are given placebos do show improvement, even though they aren't receiving any medicine developed to treat their particular illness. This well-documented phenomenon is called the *placebo effect*. Scientists believe that this sort of improvement springs from the patient's belief that she's taking a new miracle drug and will get better as a result. It just goes to show the power of mind over matter.

# Finding Clinical Trials

The federal government spent an estimated $600 million on Alzheimer's Disease research in 2002, which means that at any given time, dozens of FDA-sanctioned clinical trials are going on across the country. The trick is finding out if a trial is taking place anywhere near you, and then determining whether that particular trial is right for you or your loved one.

Depending upon how a trial is structured, it may be carried out in one location or at dozens of geographically diverse locations at the same time. When trials are conducted from one location, all the information is gathered and processed at that location, and is then distilled into a study report that's submitted to the FDA for review. If the findings are encouraging, the research team then applies to conduct the next phase in the clinical trial process.

If you have Internet access, finding a clinical trial is easier than you may think. The federal government sponsors a clinical trials Web site (www.clinicaltrials.gov) where you can search for a trial for a particular disease or a trial being conducted in a particular location. The Web site www.centerwatch.com maintains a list of more than 41,000 clinical trials currently underway all over the world. You can also look for information about current clinical trials on the Alzheimer's Association Web site at www.alz.org/ResourceCenter/ByTopic/Research.htm or search ADEAR's AD Clinical Trials Database at www.alzheimers.org/trials/basicsearch.html.

When a trial is conducted simultaneously at several locations, patients take part at the trial location most convenient to home. The information gathered from these individual studies is sent to a central location where it's processed and correlated with data from other study centers. The research team heading up the trial then assesses all the data to see if the treatment under investigation is safe and effective. If the team members determine that the treatment isn't as safe or effective as they'd hoped, they may halt testing.

# The phases of clinical trials

Three phases of clinical trials precede the approval and marketing of a new drug — Phase I, Phase II, and Phase III. An additional phase, Phase IV, is conducted only after a drug has been released for sale. Each phase of a trial has a different purpose and helps the researchers conducting the trial to answer different questions that have been posed in their protocol.

✔ **Phase I:** Researchers test a new drug or treatment in a small group of about 20 to 80 people to evaluate its safety, determine a safe dosage range, and identify possible side effects. Phase I studies determine the metabolism and pharmacological actions of drugs in humans, the side effects associated with increasing doses, and may include healthy participants and/or patients to provide early evidence of effectiveness.

✔ **Phase II:** The investigational drug or treatment is given to a larger group of people (about 100 to 300) to verify its effectiveness and to further evaluate its safety. Phase II trials are tightly controlled clinical studies conducted to evaluate the effectiveness of the drug for a particular indication or indications in patients with the disease or condition under study, and to determine the most common short-term side effects and risks.

✔ **Phase III:** The investigational drug or treatment is given to large groups of people (anywhere from 1,000 to 3,000) to confirm its effectiveness, monitor side effects, compare it to treatments currently in use for the condition being studied, and collect information that will allow the drug or treatment to be used safely. Phase III trials consist of expanded controlled and uncontrolled trials after preliminary evidence suggesting effectiveness of the drug has been obtained in Phase I and Phase II trials. They're intended to gather additional information to evaluate the overall benefit-risk relationship of the drug and provide an adequate basis for physician labeling. When Phase III trials are successfully completed, the research team members submit their results to the FDA. That agency then considers all the information submitted and the results of all the trials to determine whether a new treatment should be approved for sale to consumers.

✔ **Phase IV:** Phase IV trials are post-marketing studies conducted to gather additional information about an approved drug's risks, benefits, and optimal use.

# Enrolling in a Clinical Trial

Just because you decide that you want to enroll your loved one in a particular clinical trial doesn't automatically mean that he will be selected for participation. A lot depends upon what the team conducting the trial is looking for.

## Understanding exclusion and inclusion criteria

Clinical trials often have certain *exclusion criteria,* meaning that certain conditions, if present, prevent an individual from participating in the study. For example, a research team's protocols may specify that no one with underlying kidney disease may participate in their trial because they already know that the investigational drug they're testing would place an undue strain on a diseased kidney but pose no threat to a person with normal kidneys.

On the other hand, even if your loved one doesn't have any of the exclusion criteria, she still must meet the *inclusion criteria* — the medical and social standards that the research team is using to determine whether an individual may participate in a particular trial. Inclusion criteria may include such factors as age, gender, other medical conditions, treatment history, and the type and stage of condition your loved one has.

Researchers determine the type of patient they're looking for to participate in clinical trials based on what sorts of questions they're trying to answer. Some trials require patients in specific stages of specific diseases; some require patients who are entirely healthy. It all depends on what the researchers are trying to prove or disprove with the trial results.

## Understanding informed consent

After you and your loved one have reviewed and signed an informed consent document, your loved one goes through an initial screening for the clinical trial to see if he's an appropriate subject. The informed document describes the rights of the patients participating in the study, and it explains the purpose of the study, how long it will last, and any procedures the patients will be required to undergo in order to participate in the study. It should clearly explain the potential risks and benefits the patients may experience. It should also provide the names and contact information for the key investigators of the study, and you should be given the opportunity to ask them any questions you may have.

The purpose of an informed consent document is to provide patients with the information they need to decide whether they really want to participate in a particular study or not.

If a patient is unable to provide informed consent because of a decreased level of cognitive functioning, an authorized representative (usually a family member) may give permission for the patient to participate in a clinical trial. For more information about legal issues for AD patients, check out Chapter 13.

Informed consent also requires the research team to give you any new information that comes to light during the course of the trial that may affect your willingness to continue participating in the study. For example, if a much higher than usual number of study participants suddenly develop gastrointestinal bleeding, the research team conducting the study is required to share that information with you.

An informed consent document is not a contract or a legal document, even after you have signed it. Your rights are preserved, and you may withdraw yourself or your loved one from the clinical trial at any time if you so desire.

# What Happens During a Trial

After you or your loved one have met the initial inclusion and exclusion criteria for a trial and signed the informed consent document, the research team schedules a complete physical to check you or your loved one's current health status and ensure that you or your loved one is truly able to participate in the trial without incurring any undue risks. During this initial meeting, you and your loved one will be given specific written instructions for participating in the trial and will be informed of the schedule of appointments you'll be expected to keep during the course of the trial. Be aware that your loved one may have more doctors' appointments and tests than normal while participating in the trial.

Because the research team doesn't know exactly how individual patients may respond to the investigational drug being studied, participants are closely monitored during the entire course of the trial to watch for signs of side effects that may require additional treatment or a change in the medication dosage or schedule.

Some clinical trials require an enormous commitment of time. If you do decide to enroll your loved one in a trial, be aware of the time required for transportation, doctor visits, tests, therapies, administration of medication, patient interviews and examinations, and paperwork. The research team may want to keep in touch with you for several years, even after the actual trial ends, to monitor the health of your loved one. If you work, you may find the commitment overwhelming, so be sure to factor in all the time requirements before you make the decision to participate.

## Keeping good records

The more accurate and reliable the information that researchers are able to gather during a trial, the more accurate and reliable their study results. This need for accurate and thorough information may require that you keep good written records of the medications you give your loved one, along with your observations of side effects and possible improvements. Although it's not your job to gather clinical data, you can help the research team by keeping good records.

For example, if you're supposed to give your loved one a pill three times a day, but you skip a week of medication because you're on vacation, doctors examining your loved one might not find their expected result. Letting the research team know if you've skipped doses of medication or failed to comply with the study protocols in some other way is important, so that they don't draw erroneous conclusions based upon incomplete or inaccurate information or assumptions.

Remember, for drugs intended to stabilize the symptoms of AD, researchers are looking for no increase in symptoms and no further loss of functioning, rather than actual improvement. Being able to stabilize the symptoms of AD would be considered beneficial.

As part of a clinical trial, you may be asked to keep a log to record when you give medication, or as the study progresses, you may also be asked to fill out several questionnaires at each visit to provide additional necessary information to investigators.

## Bearing the cost

Policies for covering the costs of clinical trials vary from study to study. This is one of the most important questions that the research team must answer before you decide to join a study because patients may incur costs not covered by the trial that their insurance companies won't reimburse because they consider clinical trials experimental in nature. Before you decide to participate, you should figure out what additional costs might be involved and who will cover those costs.

One of the big problems facing individuals wanting to participate in trials, as well as researchers who design and conduct trials, is the wild inconsistency in payment policy among insurance companies. Although most companies assert that they will not pay such claims, in actual practice, they do reimburse for routine patient care costs incurred during the course of a clinical trial. According to a recent American Society of Clinical Oncology study, such claims for routine patient care are denied in fewer than 10 percent of cases.

 Despite the fact that the elderly experience a disproportionate share of illness, very few older people participate in clinical trials. In the hope of encouraging more clinical trial participation by older people, Medicare adopted new guidelines in September 2000, under which they agree to pay for routine costs incurred by patients enrolled in clinical trials that aren't covered by the trial itself. Trials must meet Medicare guidelines to be eligible, so be sure to ask your research team whether the trial you're considering is approved by Medicare or not.

Formulas for reimbursement tend to be secret and applied in a somewhat random and arbitrary manner, making it difficult for people trying to reach a decision about participating in a trial to figure out what their additional costs may be.

Generally speaking, all tests, medication, examinations, and medical care directly related to the study will be provided free of charge to the patients. Some studies offer travel reimbursement, and a few offer additional compensation paid to patients after they complete the study as an inducement to participate.

Offering patients large sums of money to participate in a clinical trial is considered unethical.

Most people enter a clinical trial because of the superb level of care they'll receive for their particular condition, and not because of a financial inducement. They look forward to interacting with doctors and nurses who are working toward finding better treatments, and they also enjoy the healthcare education provided to study participants by the research team. However, they *don't* want to find themselves stuck with thousands of dollars worth of medical bills for routine care expenses that never get reimbursed. So be sure to check all the facts before you decide to enroll your loved one in a trial.

## Knowing when to call the doctor

Even though researchers take every possible step to safeguard the health of patients who participate in clinical trials, don't forget that one of the reasons clinical trials are conducted in the first place is to determine what side effects, if any, a particular study, medication, or therapy may cause. Although study participants are given a list of the most common side effects, individual patients may have unexpected reactions — some of them severe.

Anytime you experience a sudden, dramatic onset of symptoms, such as chest pain, difficulty breathing, severe headache, or extreme dizziness, you should seek emergency medical care immediately! Do *not* waste time calling the doctors involved in your clinical trial; dial 9-1-1! If you're taken to an emergency room, make sure any healthcare provider is aware that you're currently participating in a clinical trial.

Let your doctor know of any unusual symptoms you may be experiencing; the symptoms may be an indication of something relatively simple, or they may indicate something serious enough to require you to withdraw from the clinical trial. Only your doctor can help you make this determination, so be sure to call her immediately when you experience a side effect, particularly if it's something that doesn't appear in the list of expected and usual side effects given to you when you enrolled in the study.

## Potential conflicts

There's a perception in the pharmaceutical industry that it's becoming more difficult to enroll participants in clinical trials. This has led to some new tactics that create a potential for a conflict of interest.

Many pharmaceutical companies are now hiring outside companies to find and solicit study participants and bring a study in on time and on budget. Some of these companies may have weak or questionable credentials. Drug companies are also offering doctors payments for each patient they manage to enroll in a clinical trial. This is a troubling development that sets up the potential for a conflict of interest because physicians are supposed to counsel their patients according to what's in the patient's best interests without being influenced by the opportunity for personal profit.

Finally, in an effort to speed up the protocol approval process, some drug companies are now hiring for-profit ethical review committees in place of the volunteer IRBs, which have no vested interest in the outcome of the study — a practice that's raising eyebrows among medical ethicists.

# Current Alzheimer's Trials

The Alzheimer's Association maintains a list of current clinical trials investigating drugs, devices, and therapies for the treatment of Alzheimer's Disease. You can review trials that are currently underway and trials that are recruiting participants by visiting the association's Web site at www.alz.org and clicking on "Clinical Trials" under "Shortcuts."

What follows is an overview of some current AD clinical trials. By no means is this a complete listing of current trials investigating various treatments for Alzheimer's Disease. New trials are always underway. Ask your doctor or look on the Internet to get information about clinical trials near you.

## Anti-inflammatory therapy

In a study published in the September 23, 2002, issue of the journal *Neurology*, a group of researchers reported that long-term use of nonsteroidal anti-inflammatory drugs (NSAIDs) may reduce the risk of developing Alzheimer's Disease. But several questions still need to be answered before doctors can routinely recommend the use of NSAIDs for this purpose.

A Phase II clinical trial is underway at UCLA, sponsored by the NIH, to help determine whether anti-inflammatory drugs can help delay the onset of age-related mental decline. Another trial sponsored by the National Institute on Aging and Johns Hopkins University is investigating the same thing with different NSAIDs. For more information, visit www.clinicaltrials.gov/ct/gui/show/NCT00007189;jsessionid=A73EED39C4FFDD7FF2613D30D0F8765F?order=1.

## CATIE trial for psychiatric Alzheimer symptoms

The *National Institute of Mental Health* (NIMH) is sponsoring a four-phase, multilocation trial to compare the benefits of three antipsychotic drugs — olanzapine, quetiapine, and risperidone — designed to help AD patients who are suffering from delusions, hallucinations, and agitation. Some study participants may also receive an antidepressant, citalopram. In addition, the patient's caregiver will be offered an educational program about Alzheimer's Disease. Visit www.clinicaltrials.gov/ct/gui/show/NCT00015548; jsessionid=A73EED39C4FFDD7FF2613D30D0F8765F?order=2 for information about study locations and enrollment.

## COGNIShunt

COGNIShunt is an investigational device that drains *cerebrospinal fluid* (CSF) from the skull into the abdominal cavity. COGNIShunt is similar to the shunt used to manage *hydrocephalus*, a condition in which an accumulation of excess CSF in the skull puts pressure on the brain.

The theory behind the use of the COGNIShunt in the management of Alzheimer's Disease is that as we age, the body's ability to refresh CSF naturally declines, potentially resulting in a buildup of toxic byproducts, including beta-amyloid protein fragments and abnormal tau proteins, that may contribute to the brain damage associated with Alzheimer's Disease. COGNIShunt is designed to drain CSF along with these toxic elements, thereby forcing the body to manufacture new, fresh CSF that, in theory, wouldn't have these toxic elements present. Early results have been inconclusive, primarily because the sample size was so small, and more research is underway.

A multilocation study sponsored by Eunoe, Inc., the manufacturers of the COGNIshunt device, is currently underway. For more information visit `www.clinicaltrials.gov/ct/gui/show/NCT00056628;jsessionid=51C2CDB5 5FD9878680F5819969D3AC65?order=1`.

# CX516 (Ampalex)

CX516, also known as Ampalex, is currently under development at Cortex Pharmaceuticals, Inc. It belongs to a new class of drugs called *ampakines* that enhance neurochemical signals involved in memory. CX516 enhances the functioning of *AMPA receptors,* which are thought to be essential in the formation of memories. AMPA receptors are docking sites on the surface of brain cells for a neurotransmitter known as *glutamate* that plays a critical, though not yet clearly defined, role in memory and learning. When the cells that release glutamate are damaged, a breakdown in cell-to-cell communication occurs.

Phase I clinical trials have been completed for CX516. The drug appeared to be well tolerated, and it enhanced memory and learning in small groups of healthy adults. Phase II trials are currently underway where the drug is being tested for safety and effectiveness in AD patients and in people with mild cognitive impairment. For more information about the Alzheimer's Disease Phase II study, visit `www.clinicaltrials.gov/ct/gui/show/NCT00001662; jsessionid=DA26738DC00B48B6BEE1ECF78FB51730?order=3`.

For more information about the Mild Cognitive Impairment Phase II study, visit `www.clinicaltrials.gov/ct/gui/show/NCT00040443;jsessionid= DA26738DC00B48B6BEE1ECF78FB51730?order=1`.

# Statins

Statins are a class of drugs that lower the levels of *low-density lipoprotein* (LDL) in the bloodstream. Elevated levels of LDL cholesterol are strongly associated with coronary artery disease and stroke. Statins work by blocking a liver enzyme that's essential for the production of cholesterol.

Researchers working in the field of heart disease noticed that people who'd been taking statins had a decreased occurrence of Alzheimer's Disease, which was surprising because many previous studies had shown that individuals with high risk factors for heart disease also had an increased risk for AD.

Research is currently underway to clarify the relationship between taking statins and a reduced risk of AD. In the meantime, it certainly wouldn't hurt anyone to keep his cholesterol within recommended levels.

Two statin trials are currently underway. The NIMH is sponsoring a Phase IV study to determine the effects of short-term statins and NSAIDS on the levels of beta-amyloids in the cerebrospinal fluid. Participants will be randomly assigned to take either the statin, lovostatin, or the NSAID ibuprofen for 3 months. For more information, visit www.clinicaltrials.gov/ct/gui/show/ NCT00046358;jsessionid=7963151D932AD5580D10436C3DD949B8?order=1.

The CLASP (*cholesterol lowering agent to slow progression*) of Alzheimer's Disease study is a multilocation Phase III study sponsored by the National Institute on Aging. For more information, visit www.clinicaltrials.gov/ ct/gui/show/NCT00053599;jsessionid=7963151D932AD5580D10436C3DD 949B8?order=2.

# Estrogen trials

Three estrogen trials are currently underway to assess the potential benefits of estrogen therapy to AD patients and those at increased risk of developing the condition. Each study is structured a bit differently, according to what questions researchers are trying to answer.

### PREPARE Alzheimer's Disease Prevention Trial

The National Institute on Aging is currently sponsoring a multilocation Phase III clinical trial to assess the effects of estrogen and estrogen taken in combination with progesterone to determine whether the administration of these hormones can delay the onset of memory loss in elderly women with a family history of AD.

For more information, visit www.clinicaltrials.gov/ct/gui/show/ NCT00000176;jsessionid=91D1D0FC1FF3E6E3A877E666EC5F0574?order=2.

### AD and aging: Therapeutic potential of estrogen

The Department of Veterans Affairs Medical Research Service is currently conducting a Phase II study to evaluate the potential benefits of estrogen on the cognitive function of women with Alzheimer's Disease.

For more information, visit www.clinicaltrials.gov/ct/gui/show/ NCT00018343;jsessionid=91D1D0FC1FF3E6E3A877E666EC5F0574?order=1.

### Estrogen effects on memory functioning in post-menopausal women and patients with AD

The National Center for Research Resources is currently conducting a Phase II clinical study to determine if estrogen given concurrently with the cholinesterase inhibitor Donepezil will enhance the system in the brain that involves memory and learning.

For more information, visit www.clinicaltrials.gov/ct/gui/show/
NCT00006399;jsessionid=91D1D0FC1FF3E6E3A877E666EC5F0574?order=3.

## Vitamin E and selenium

Normal cell metabolism results in compounds called *free radicals,* which can damage cells and DNA. Normally speaking, the body's own defense mechanism uses antioxidants, including vitamins E and C, to prevent this sort of oxidative stress or damage. But as we age, the body's ability to fight off free radicals slowly degrades. Researchers started to wonder if damage to brain cells caused by oxidative stress might play a role in the development of AD.

Results of an early trial reported in the April 24, 1997, issue of the *New England Journal of Medicine* suggested that vitamin E might slow the progression of Alzheimer's Disease. The National Institute on Aging is co-sponsoring a multilocation Phase III trial with the National Cancer Institute to see if vitamin E given concurrently with the mineral selenium can help to prevent memory loss and the onset of dementia associated with AD. For more information, visit www.clinicaltrials.gov/ct/gui/show/NCT00040378;
jsessionid=7963151D932AD5580D10436C3DD949B8?order=1.

# Chapter 10

# Promising New Drugs and Diagnostic Tools

*T*he clinical trial process that we discuss in Chapter 9 has spawned a plethora of experimental drugs for the treatment of *Alzheimer's Disease* (AD) — some designed to treat specific symptoms and others aimed at slowing the progression of a patient's decline or even preventing the development of symptoms altogether. As researchers learn more and more about what causes AD, they keep coming up with new ideas about how to attack and treat the illness.

The research couldn't be more crucial. As the Baby Boomers age, statisticians, researchers, and clinicians fear that an all-out epidemic of Alzheimer's Disease may erupt, with devastating economic consequences for both the healthcare delivery system and the families of AD patients. According to the National Institute on Aging, the cost to society of caring for AD patients, both direct and indirect, is as much as $100 billion annually, and that's just for the estimated 4 million patients we have now. In addition, families have an emotional burden to bear — one that all too often results in severe health problems for the caregiver. All this rather depressing information provides a very good incentive for AD researchers to keep pushing for answers.

In this chapter, we take a look at the threads of interest that researchers are currently pursuing. Research is eclectic and far-ranging because we still don't know what causes Alzheimer's Disease in the first place. We also evaluate some of the most promising new experimental agents currently under investigation for the treatment of Alzheimer's Disease, and we look at the significance of emerging new imaging techniques that may prove valuable as diagnostic and staging tools.

# The Current State of Affairs

The state of Alzheimer's Disease research is constantly in flux. Treatments that look promising based on early animal studies may prove disappointing during clinical trials with humans. Problems can also come to light with widespread use. New information emerges all the time that can send researchers off in whole new directions, some of which are productive and some of which aren't. And doctors conducting research on entirely unrelated ailments may discover that the therapy they're investigating has possible benefits for AD patients, perhaps helping to relieve some of its symptoms or reducing people's chances of getting the disease.

What we do know is that Alzheimer's Disease develops as a result of a complex cascade of events — some biochemical, some neurodegenerative, some perhaps even environmental. We don't yet have all the pieces to the puzzle. Whatever doctors believe to be the cause of Alzheimer's Disease, combined research efforts are focused on finding new treatments or a combination of treatments — a drug, vaccine, procedure, or device that can provide real help. For families caring for AD patients, that day can't come soon enough.

# Promising (and Not-So-Promising) New Drugs

A number of promising new agents that have potential as treatments for Alzheimer's Disease are currently in clinical trials. The developers of these drugs are coming at Alzheimer's Disease from a number of different directions. Some are vaccines; others are inhibitors that work on different brain chemicals from the cholinesterase inhibitors, the drugs currently approved for the treatment of AD. Others help the body fight off or delay the build-up of plaques, and others may even help the body break down and eliminate plaques already deposited. Some of these agents are years away from FDA approval and commercial availability; others are very close. In this section, we look at the ones that have gotten the most notice.

## Memantine

One drug that's close to FDA approval is *memantine*. Already approved for marketing by the European Union and widely available throughout Europe, memantine, if approved, would be the first medication specifically approved for use in AD patients with moderately severe to severe disease.

## Keeping up with the latest AD information

Because of the high level of interest in healthy aging today, promising new therapies for Alzheimer's Disease are widely reported in the media. It's hard to pick up a newspaper or magazine or turn on the TV or radio without hearing something interesting about AD research.

Organizations such as the Alzheimer's Association serve as clearinghouses for breaking news and research updates on AD research. Visit its Web site (www.alz. org/AboutUs/AboutSite/New.htm#news) for the latest consumer news.

In a study published in the April 3, 2003, edition of the *New England Journal of Medicine,* memantine was shown to produce significantly superior results to a placebo in three areas: clinical global impression, cognitive performance, and activities of daily living. On average, patients receiving memantine required 45 fewer hours of caregiver time per month than patients receiving a placebo — a result that would potentially ease the care burden on both family and paid institutional caregivers.

The Clinical Global Impression scale or CGI is a tool developed to measure the efficacy of investigational drugs being tested in clinical trials. The three-item scale rates the severity of illness from 1 (normal) to 7 (extremely ill); global or overall improvement (compared to a baseline condition) from 1 (very much improved) to 7 (very much worse); and efficacy from 1 (none) to 4 (outweighs therapeutic effect.) Although CGI is very useful, if the patient's clinical history isn't available for comparison, CGI can't be used.

Because memantine and cholinesterase inhibitors have different methods of action and work on different receptors within the brain, researchers are currently investigating whether giving AD patients both medications at the same time may be beneficial. In a small German study reported in the March 25, 2003, issue of *International Clinical Psychopharmacology,* the drug combo was well tolerated by most patients. Results suggested that giving AD patients both of these medications could enhance therapeutic benefits. More studies are planned.

Memantine is the first of a new class of AD drugs called *NMDA-receptor antagonists.* (NMDA stands for N-methyl-D-aspartate). Glutamate is the most important excitatory neurotransmitter in the brain, regulating up to 70 percent of all excitatory reactions. (See Chapter 7 for more information on excitatory and inhibitory neurotransmitters.) When the process for regulating glutamate in the brain breaks down, excess calcium builds up in the neurons, resulting in a condition called *excitotoxicity* that actually kills brain cells. Researchers now suspect that mild but chronic malfunctioning of the glutamate receptors may play a key role in many neurodegenerative diseases, such as Parkinson's Disease, Alzheimer's Disease, vascular dementia, and others.

Forest Laboratories has acquired an exclusive license from the German manufacturer Merz (the drug's creator) to market memantine in the United States. Forest submitted memantine for FDA approval in December 2002, and the process normally takes about one year to complete. Although it's impossible to predict with 100-percent accuracy, barring any unforeseen snags, the drug should be available by prescription in the United States by the early part of 2004.

## Beta-secretase inhibitors (memapsin 2)

Accumulation of amyloid plaques (See Chapter 3 for definition) in the brain is linked to neurodegeneration, or the gradual loss of properly functioning brain cells. Some researchers think this is one of the primary causes of AD. *Beta-secretase* is one of two "protein-cutting" enzymes, or proteases, in the body. It works with the other protein-cutting enzyme, gamma-secretase, to cut long proteins known as *amyloid precursor proteins*. The by-product of this process is called *beta-amyloid*. When beta-amyloid accumulates in the brain, it causes the plaques and neurofibrillary tangles that are present in AD.

Because overproduction of beta-secretase is thought to play a crucial role in the formation of amyloid plaques, researchers are looking for ways to "inhibit" the release of b-secretase inside the brain. The theory is that this inhibition might prevent amyloid plaques from being formed and deposited.

Two known variants of the b-secretase enzyme exist in the human body: memapsin 1 and memapsin 2. A series of studies in mice has suggested to researchers that it's possible to block memapsin 2 to reduce production of the precursors for amyloid plaques without causing any significant side effects.

In April 2000, researchers at the Oklahoma Medical Research Foundation announced they had come up with a beta-secretase inhibitor that acts as a sort of combination decoy and chemical chewing gum. First, the inhibitor "attracts" the beta-secretase away from the amyloid precursor proteins. When the memapsin 2 tries to cut the decoy, thinking that it's cutting the protein, it adheres to the sticky inhibitor and is disabled, rendering it unable to create the chemical conditions required for the production of amyloid plaques.

The Oklahoma researchers were quick to point out that they hadn't come up with a drug, only a process. They're currently working with several pharmaceutical companies to develop experimental AD drugs based on their discovery, so don't look for FDA approval of any beta-secretase inhibitors any time soon. Researchers believe, however, that this is one of the most promising avenues of current AD research.

## Your brain as an electrical circuit

Did you know that the human brain is basically one big electrical circuit? In much the same way that a rheostat controls the voltage flow in a piece of electrical equipment, *neurotransmitters* help regulate electrical impulses in the brain by exciting or inhibiting the rhythmical amplitude of the neurons' signal output. This exquisitely modulated flow of excitatory and inhibitory neurotransmitters allows the brain and the central nervous system to initiate and carry out an almost infinite variety of activities. Alzheimer's Disease disrupts this finely tuned intercellular communication, producing an array of cognitive and behavioral symptoms.

## *Alzhemed (anti-amyloid)*

On February 19, 2002, a Canadian company called Neurochem received a U.S. patent protecting its amyloid inhibition technology. The technology not only prevents amyloid plaques from being deposited, it also protects the body from the toxicity associated with them. Amyloid fibril deposits are associated with a number of inflammatory conditions, including AD, hemorrhagic stroke, Crohn's Disease, and rheumatoid arthritis.

Neurochem used its proprietary technology to develop a drug called *Alzhemed* that has successfully completed Phase I clinical trials. Alzhemed is part of a new class of "disease modifying" drugs that, if approved and found to work as supposed, will truly provide an exciting breakthrough in AD treatment.

Alzhemed prevents the formation and deposit of amyloid fibrils in the brain and also inhibits the inflammatory response associated with amyloid buildup in AD. In studies in mice, Alzhemed not only reduced levels of amyloid protein in the brain by as much as 30 percent, but it also reduced concentrations of amyloid in plasma by as much as 61 percent.

The company's *investigational new drug* (IND) application was approved by the FDA last September, and they've submitted study protocols for a multi-center, randomized, double-blind Phase II clinical trial, which are currently under review. As soon as Neurochem receives approval for the study, the trial will begin. You can check www.clinicaltrials.gov to see if the trials are underway. As of the writing of this book, no information about Alzhemed was yet listed on that site.

A *double-blind* study is a clinical trial in which neither the doctors administering the study nor the patients participating in the study know who's receiving the investigational drug and who's receiving a placebo. The purpose of a double-blind study is to eliminate any chance that prejudice might influence the study results.

## Neotrofin: One that didn't work out

Not all drugs that initially appear to hold some promise for the treatment of AD pan out. Neotrofin, or leteprinim, is a nerve growth factor developed by NeoTherapeutics, a drug company in California. It was being tested to see if it could repair damaged nerve cells and regenerate destroyed nerve cells in patients with spinal cord injuries, chemotherapy-induced nerve damage, Parkinson's Disease, and Alzheimer's Disease. Initial clinical trials were hopeful, but further testing revealed that patients taking Neotrofin for AD fared little better than patients taking a placebo — a result that precluded any further testing for this purpose. The drug is still under development for use in the other named conditions.

Alzhemed still has a long way to go before it reaches the consumer prescription drug market, and no one knows what turns may be in the road along the way. However, if the results of the Phase II and Phase III clinical trials are as promising as Phase I results, doctors may have a powerful new drug to use to fight AD sometime within the next four to five years.

# An Ounce of Prevention: The Hunt for an Alzheimer's Vaccine

There was great excitement in 1999 when early trials of an AD vaccine called AN-1792 showed that it prevented the formation of plaques in the brains of mice genetically engineered to produce human amyloid. Phase I human trials were also successful. However, in January 2002, the developers of the drug voluntarily suspended human trials after 4 patients in the group of 300 developed inflammation of the brain and spinal cord. Results and analysis of the data are still under review. The latest news is that the vaccine does seem to be effective in preventing the formation of plaques, but researchers must first determine what's causing the brain and spinal cord inflammation before work can resume on developing the vaccine for use in humans.

Despite the disappointment caused by the suspension of the AN-1792 AD vaccines trials, researchers are pursuing other avenues in the search for a safe and effective vaccine to prevent the onset of Alzheimer's Disease. Researchers at New York University have been immunizing mice with a nontoxic A-beta homologue. Early results show a reduction in the overall number of amyloid plaques and even some improvement in cognitive performance.

Other scientists disagree with this approach, saying that introduced A-beta homologues could possibly contribute to existing plaques or even serve as "seed" to encourage the deposit of plaques. Researchers restructured their

formula to address these concerns and recently concluded that animal studies produced reductions in plaques ranging from 81 percent to 89 percent.
Perhaps even more significant is that the new formulation seems to interfere
with the inflammatory processes that some think contribute to AD pathology
(although many researchers think that AD causes inflammation and not the
other way around).

Many years may pass before a safe and effective vaccine is available for AD.
And truthfully, doctors and researchers may never find something that works
well. After all, look at where we are after almost two decades of searching for
an AIDS vaccine. It's a very complex problem, and solving it won't be easy.
Fortunately, researchers are making much better progress in other areas with
other sorts of drugs.

# Drugs and Therapies Already Approved for Other Uses

We mention in Chapter 9 that even after Phase III clinical trials are successfully completed and a drug is approved for marketing by the FDA in the United
States, Phase IV clinical trials still must be conducted to make sure that the
approved drug is as effective as first believed, and that it accomplishes its
stated goal with a minimum of side effects. When researchers review the
results of these later trials, they sometimes observe unexpected effects.

For example, an overview of statin trials showed that, for some unknown
reason, people who take statins to lower their HDL cholesterol also significantly decrease their odds of getting Alzheimer's Disease. But each new finding of this nature must be verified independently, using the same rigorous
scientific standards employed in the initial approval process, before it can
become part of standard practice parameters.

Just because a medication has been approved for one use doesn't mean that
a doctor can't prescribe it for another condition. This type of prescribing is
known as *off-label prescribing*. For example, statins aren't currently approved
for use with Alzheimer's Disease, but if the weight of current clinical evidence
started to overwhelmingly support their benefits for AD patients, many physicians might choose to start prescribing statins for their AD patients off-label
rather than waiting the few extra years required for the FDA to formally
approve this new use.

Although no official position exists on whether off-label prescribing of prescription drugs is a good or a bad thing, most experts agree that a physician's experience and familiarity with ongoing research determines his or her
ability to safely participate in this practice.

Drugs that have long been approved to treat some other condition often undergo clinical trials to test their effectiveness in treating AD. Several cholesterol-lowering drugs, including Lipitor, are currently being tested to see if they are beneficial for AD patients. When evidence points to a different use for a drug, researchers must still study it under carefully regulated conditions to confirm its effectiveness and figure out what dosing rates and schedules are most beneficial for the new application. The advantage to running this type of trial is that scientists already have a good idea about the drug's safety. They simply need to make sure that the drug is, in fact, producing a notable benefit for AD patients and experiment with dosages in order to reap maximum therapeutic benefits with minimum risk.

In this section, we look at some of these familiar drugs and discuss how they're being used in the fight against AD. Be aware that many drugs that were thought to have some potential therapeutic benefit for AD patients didn't perform as expected in tests and, therefore, won't be used to treat AD patients in the future. However, that in no way diminishes the drug's value in treating the condition that it was originally developed to address.

## High-dose vitamin E

So many studies investigating the seeming ability of vitamin E to slow cognitive decline are underway that it would take practically an entire chapter to list them. Early studies concluded that only vitamin E taken in with the diet was of any benefit, but later studies have shown a benefit from high doses of vitamin E administered as an oral supplement. Regardless of the differences in results and findings, researchers do know the following: In a number of studies, high doses of vitamin E did slow progression of AD patients from the moderate to severe stage of the disease by an average of 8 months — a finding that has huge implications for caregivers. It's now standard of care to prescribe vitamin E to treat AD.

Although researchers don't entirely understand how vitamin E works to slow AD progression, they do know that vitamin E is an antioxidant that scavenges and neutralizes free radicals that damage cells and DNA and cause the oxidative stress in the brain, which may be a precursor of progressive neurodegenerative conditions such as AD.

 Like any other substance you put into your body, you can get too much of a good thing if you start pumping yourself full of vitamin E. Moderate overdose may produce nausea, diarrhea, dizziness, blurred vision, and headache; higher sustained levels may produce a risk of uncontrolled bleeding, especially in people with a vitamin K deficiency. So be sure to follow the most important rule of healthcare: Before you add anything to your diet or medication regimen, be sure to consult your doctor.

If you're interested in following the progress of current vitamin E trials for AD, visit the Alzheimer's Disease Education and Referral Center's Web site (www.alzheimers.org).

## Estrogen

Women have been taking *hormone replacement therapy* (HRT) for more than 30 years as a way to ease hot flashes and other uncomfortable physical symptoms of menopause. In the past, the medical establishment believed that HRT didn't have any notable side effects and that it was actually beneficial, serving to stave off heart attacks in older women whose risk shot up after they stopped producing protective levels of estrogen. The decision about whether or not to take hormones isn't quite so easy these days, however. Apparently, the cardio-protective effect is nonexistent, and long-term HRT has plenty of side effects that are just now coming to light.

Researchers, however, hypothesized that regular estrogen supplementation did appear to do one thing, at least in early clinical trials — it seemed to provide some measure of protection against Alzheimer's Disease. However, results of early studies have been mixed. In some studies where women were given estrogen alone, their mental performance improved; in other studies, it had no measurable effect.

Researchers conducting a large study, The Women's Health Initiative Memo Study (WHIMS), stopped giving women an estrogen-progestin combination when clinical data suggested that the hormone combo actually doubled the risk for AD, as well as increased the risk for stroke, heart attack, blood clots, and breast cancer.

Although the belief has been widespread that estrogen does help, results from tests recently conducted by the Alzheimer's Disease Cooperative Study at the University of California at San Diego (UCSD) concluded that, unfortunately, it does not. Although estrogen is not an effective treatment for AD, what has not been determined is whether it provides some protective benefit.

## Erythropoietin (EPO)

*Erythropoietin* (EPO) is a kidney hormone that regulates the production of red blood cells. It's used to treat anemia and was once prized by athletes who took it just prior to a competition to enhance performance (athletes are now disqualified from competition if they take EPO). When researchers realized that EPO has a neuro-protective effect and is produced within the brain following injury or stress, they hypothesized that the substance may have some ability to keep neurons from committing cell suicide. (Cell suicide occurs when the normal brain environment is damaged or has become toxic.)

Research on using EPO for the treatment of AD eventually was dropped because it was the equivalent of swatting a mosquito with a cannon. EPO is a powerful drug that can produce significant side effects and is only available as an injection. It simply didn't offer enough benefits to the AD patient to overcome its disadvantages or to justify further research.

## Statins

*Statins* are a class of drug used to lower levels of *low density lipoprotein* (LDL) cholesterol in the blood. LDL is commonly known as "bad" cholesterol because it's the one that clogs up your arteries. Researchers reviewing data from clinical trials of various statins noticed a smaller-than-expected incidence of Alzheimer's Disease among patients taking the statins to inhibit cardiovascular disease. Two groups of researchers concluded that the likelihood of developing AD was anywhere from 60 percent to 73 percent lower among patients taking certain statins. Other types of cholesterol-lowering drugs did not have the same effect.

Researchers are uncertain whether the benefit is a result of the overall improvement in health due to lowered HDL cholesterol, or if the statins act in some unknown way to alter amyloid metabolism. Clinical trials are currently underway to gather more data about statins and how they work in AD; much more study is needed before anyone can draw any solid conclusions.

One concern about using statins in patients who don't have high cholesterol is that they might cause levels of *high density lipoprotein* (HDL), or "good" cholesterol, to fall dangerously low. Researchers are looking at different dosing schedules to try to determine a therapeutic dose that avoids this side effect.

## Huperzine A

Huperzine A is an extract of Chinese club moss that the Chinese have used for thousands of years to treat fever and inflammation. They call it Chien Tseng Ta. It turns out that Huperzine A is also a potent natural cholinesterase inhibitor. Several well-controlled Chinese studies showed that Huperzine A improved memory in older adults with age-related memory decline, Alzheimer's Disease, and vascular dementia. Other studies suggest that Huperzine A may protect brain cells from toxic levels of the neurotransmitter glutamate that may play a role in the death of brain cells. Although no clinical trials are currently underway in the United States, several are being planned.

# Selegiline (Eldepryl)

Researchers expressed a lot of interest in *selegiline,* brand name Eldepryl, in the mid 1990s in relation to its potential benefits for AD patients. The drug was introduced in 1981 as a treatment for Parkinson's Disease, and researchers looking at its method of action hypothesized that it might be beneficial for AD patients as well.

A well-controlled, randomized double-blind study conducted simultaneously at 23 Alzheimer's Disease Cooperative Study sites (and reported in the April 24, 1997, issue of the *New England Journal of Medicine*) compared the effects of vitamin E against those of selegiline in AD patients. Both vitamin E and selegiline delayed progression to severe dementia and institutionalization by approximately seven months. However, selegiline did cause more side effects, including insomnia, falls and fainting, and some incidents of significantly increased blood pressure. Because vitamin E provides the same benefits without the same risk of side effects, doctors now prefer it over selegiline. Vitamin E is also currently being investigated in a number of clinical trials to determine if any additional therapeutic benefits can be gained with larger doses or by using vitamin E in combination with other substances, such as selenium, a vital trace mineral that seems to play an active role in the prevention of a number of degenerative diseases. Vitamin E is also being tested to determine if can help patients with Mild Cognitive Impairment (MCI).

# Valproate (Depakote)

Valproate is an anti-seizure drug that's recently found some favor in the treatment of Alzheimer's Disease patients who suffer from agitation and psychosis. A two-year clinical trial is nearing completion. Investigators were trying to determine whether Valproate can help delay the onset of agitation and psychotic episodes, and also nail down whether it has any neuro-protective effects. We'll have to wait some time before the study results are known.

# IPA

*Indole-3-propionic acid* (IPA) is a potent, naturally occurring antioxidant that's been shown to interfere with the action of enzymes contributing to amyloid plaque formation in the brains of AD patients. A preliminary study looked at the safety and tolerability of IPA in patients with AD. The information from that study is currently being evaluated to see if conducting further clinical trials are warranted.

If you look up IPA on the Internet, about 90 percent of what you'll get back from the search engine pertains to the International Psychogeriatric Association, a group with members in more than 70 countries. Although the IPA does a good job of bringing the disparate groups that are studying AD together, the group has nothing to do with the IPA that stands for Indole-3-propionic acid. If you enter the full name of the antioxidant in your search engine, you'll get much better and more informative results.

## Certain B vitamins

The theory behind taking certain B vitamins to combat AD is that they help to lower the levels of the amino acid *homocysteine* in the body. High levels of homocysteine have been linked with an increased risk for developing AD. Although folate is thought to be the key factor in controlling homocysteine levels, vitamins B-6 and B-12 seem to work together to enhance its benefits.

The National Institutes of Health is currently conducting a large clinical trial to find out if lowering homocysteine with folic acid (vitamin B-9), pyridoxine (vitamin B-6), and cobalamin (vitamin B-12) will slow cognitive decline in patients with AD. Results from this study are several years away.

Wondering how much folate, B-6, and B-12 you should add to your diet? Look for a good multivitamin that supplies 400 mcg of folate, 2 mg of B-6, and 6 mcg of B-12. Modern diets rarely provide enough folate, so taking a daily multivitamin that provides all the B vitamins, along with other vitamins and minerals essential for good health, is a good strategy.

## Non-steroidal anti-inflammatory drugs (NSAIDS)

News about non-steroidal anti-inflammatory drugs (NSAIDS) is contradictory. Last year, in the September 24, 2002, issue of *Neurology,* researchers reported results of a study of a group of 5,000 people who were monitored for several years after being asked about their use of aspirin and other NSAIDS. The incidence of AD was 45 percent lower among people who reported regularly taking aspirin or some other NSAID for two years or more. Even low doses, such as the 81 milligrams, taken daily for aspirin therapy were associated with reduced risk. No protective benefit was reported among people who took NSAIDS infrequently or sporadically, nor did people who took non-NSAIDS painkillers, such as acetaminophen, appear to gain any protection.

However, a study published in the June 4, 2003, issue of the *Journal of the American Medical Association* reported that two NSAIDS, COX-2 and naproxen, did not slow the rate of cognitive decline in people with mild to moderate AD.

But the National Institute on Aging still believes that while NSAIDS may not be able to slow AD once it gets started, they may still play a role in preventing the disease.

Not all NSAIDS appear to have the same effect. Although the study published in *Neurology* looked at aspirin use, researchers believe that there's more at work than just aspirin's well-known anti-inflammatory action, although there are five or six competing theories as to exactly what that might be.

---

# A note about ginkgo biloba

There has recently been a flurry of interest and excitement about the Chinese herb ginkgo biloba and its potential to help people with AD retain memory. Although ginkgo has a solid reputation among herbalists, based upon thousands of years of use and experience for a number of conditions, results of a recent study conducted at Williams College in Massachusetts and published in the *Journal of the American Medical Association* didn't show that the herb has any measurable effect on Alzheimer's Disease. Critics of the study say that the problem was that doses given to study participants were too low. But the charge simply highlights the fact that getting a standardized dose of any herbal preparation is nearly impossible since their manufacture and quality standards aren't regulated. In contrast to what's available to consumers over the counter (that is, herbs that vary wildly in their quality, purity, and percentage of active ingredients), the ginkgo given to participants in the Williams College study was pure and standardized to insure that each study participant received the same dose of gingko's active ingredients.

A meta-analysis of 40 ginkgo biloba studies conducted by Dutch researchers in 2001 seemed to indicate that the herb did provide significant benefits to people suffering from what it called "cerebral insufficiency." Ginkgo's ability to improve blood flow to the brain is well documented and accepted within the scientific community, but how this may help people with AD is unknown at this time.

Ginkgo biloba is the subject of a number of additional ongoing studies. The National Institute on Aging is currently co-sponsoring a five-year study, using a 240 mg per day dose — twice what was given in the Williams College study. Results of this study aren't yet available.

None of the controversy has deterred people from buying ginkgo biloba, and many people swear that it's made a huge difference in their memory abilities. Unfortunately, anecdotal evidence isn't the same as evidence from a controlled scientific study.

Ginkgo biloba hasn't been shown to cause any significant side effects at recommended dosages. So if you really think that you'd like to try it or give it to your loved one, there's no reason not to (unless you or your loved one is taking blood-thinning medications or have a blood disorder that affects clotting; ginkgo biloba is not recommended under these circumstances). Keep in mind, however, that vitamin E (which is much less expensive than ginkgo) and cholinesterase inhibitors have been *proven* to help people with AD maintain a higher level of cognitive functioning for many additional months.

Don't start dosing yourself up with aspirin just yet. Aspirin is a powerful drug that can have devastating side effects in some people, including irreversible kidney damage and gastrointestinal bleeding. Just because you can get aspirin from your local pharmacist without a prescription doesn't mean you should suck it down like lemon drops. Only your doctor can decide if aspirin therapy is appropriate for you, and he or she will only prescribe it for use in cardiovascular problems, not for AD — at least, not yet.

Researchers have a lot more work to do regarding NSAIDS before they can comfortably recommend them as a treatment for AD. Scientists are currently working on the molecular structure of certain NSAIDS to see if they can design a drug that provides desirable protective properties without the toxic side effects normally associated with long-term NSAID use. But we're still years away from seeing something like that on the market.

# Testing Positive: Looking for the Definitive Diagnosis

No matter how many times doctors tell AD patients and their families that there's still no definitive test that can reveal a 100 percent positive diagnosis of Alzheimer's Disease, people keep asking for one. With this constant request in mind, some researchers are devoting their efforts to finding a test for Alzheimer's Disease, with decidedly mixed results so far. In Chapter 8, we discuss some self-administered home tests. Now, in this section, we take a look at a subject of some controversy — gene testing for Alzheimer's Disease.

## Genetic testing: Still not accurate

You may be asking yourself why genetic testing provokes such controversy. Well, the test is controversial because it's not definitive. Just because you have one of the genes associated with an increased risk of developing AD doesn't mean that you'll ever get the disease.

Doctors have a real ethics problem when deciding whether or not to administer genetic tests, especially to members of families that do seem to have the familial form of the disease. The reason is the level of stress that receiving a positive result can create in the life of the person tested. Can you imagine how you would feel if, at age 40 or so, you took a test that told you were doomed to get Alzheimer's? You'd probably go through the rest of your life scared and angry, always wondering when the axe is going to fall. Now, imagine how you'd feel if you spent all that time worrying and wondering only to never actually get AD.

You see why doctors are so reluctant to administer genetic testing for AD screening purposes. It simply isn't an accurate predictor of who is and who isn't going to get AD; it only tells you who has the gene that increases the risk of developing AD.

## New imaging tools for diagnosis

Researchers are trying to develop some sort of brain imaging protocol that would be 100 percent accurate for the diagnosis of Alzheimer's Disease. They're not even close yet, but two imaging modalities, PET and SPECT scans, are offering some intriguing research possibilities.

One of the things that most frustrates doctors about Alzheimer's Disease is their inability to "see" and definitively identify amyloid plaques and neurofibrillary tangles in the brain, which are the characteristic signs that prove that AD is present in a particular patient. In theory, doctors could simply drill into the skull, obtain a bit of brain tissue, prepare it, and slap it under the microscope to see what's going on.

But in actual practice, due to the high risks associated with brain biopsy, such procedures are reserved for only the gravest of illnesses where the likelihood of neurosurgery is high anyway. For example, brain biopsy and brain surgery are often part of one extended surgical process for patients with a suspected fast-spreading malignant brain tumor.

What's involved in a brain biopsy exactly? Well, the procedure requires that a patient be placed under general anesthesia. After the patient has gone under, surgeons drill a small hole in the skull and then skillfully guide a needle through that hole to a specific area of the brain, using CT or MRI scans obtained before the procedure as a guide, to obtain a tissue sample. Brain scarring following a biopsy has been known to trigger seizures, so it's not a procedure to be taken lightly.

Doctors believe that drilling into the skull of a patient who doesn't require brain surgery for any other reason, in order to satisfy a family's desire to know with 100 percent certainty that their loved one does have AD, is simply unethical. It's especially unnecessary when so many other tools available that are able to provide a reliable and accurate diagnosis with minimum risk.

Nonetheless, the desire to know the whole truth and nothing but the truth persists, so researchers are currently testing several different advanced imaging modalities to determine their potential usefulness in the diagnosis of AD. Up until now, the ability to image the brain and see amyloid plaques and neurofibrillary tangles (the Holy Grail of AD diagnosis, so to speak) has eluded researchers. Many scientists say that it'll never happen. New imaging techniques, however, such as PET and SPECT scanning, are giving doctors a glimpse into the overall structural and functional changes that occur in an AD brain. And that's helping them to understand what happens as patients progress through the course of the illness.

### PET scans

PET stands for *positron emission tomography.* Unlike CT (computerized tomography) scans and MRIs (magnetic resonance imaging) that make images of body structures or anatomy, PET scans are metabolically based. In other words, PET scans make images of the way the body works. Patients are injected with a radioactive pharmaceutical and then rest for about an hour to allow the injected materials to circulate throughout the body. When the materials have made their way through the body, the PET scan is performed. A PET scan can show the beating of a heart, the smallest of cancerous tumors, the human brain at work, and the faltering brain of an AD patient.

PET scanners have been around since the mid 1970s, but they required such a huge support team, including a licensed nuclear physicist, and were so heavily regulated by the federal government that it just wasn't practical for any facility other than the largest research centers to maintain one. In addition, the radioactive pharmaceuticals required for PET scans degraded very quickly and had to be produced in a giant machine known as a *cyclotron* just before injection into the patient's body. Because most hospitals don't have a place where they can park a cyclotron or the skilled personnel required to operate such a complex machine, keeping a PET scan on the premises was even more impractical. Now, the development of smaller cyclotrons and radioactive pharmaceuticals that degrade much more slowly has made it possible for one centrally located cyclotron to serve the needs of many medical facilities. This central location also relieves the facilities that have PET scans on the premises of the requirement to keep a nuclear physicist on staff and the responsibility of operating and maintaining the cyclotron, which, like any other equipment involving nuclear material, is still heavily monitored and regulated by the government.

What has most researchers so excited about the application of PET scan technology to the diagnosis of AD is that a PET scan may be able to detect the subtle changes in brain function that would predict AD years before the patient shows any symptoms at all. This ability raises intriguing possibilities for early intervention with drugs that can delay the onset of symptoms, especially as doctors are now finding that the earlier they start a cholinesterase inhibitor, such as Aricept, Exelon, or Reminyl, the longer and more effectively it works.

A *cyclotron* is not a fancy bicycle. It's a huge and rather complicated machine that uses alternating voltage to propel charged particles in a magnetic field. A cyclotron is crucial to the preparation of radioactive pharmaceuticals that supply gamma rays for detection by PET and SPECT imaging equipment.

# How PET scans work to diagnose AD

When a PET scan is performed, a glucose-based radioactive pharmaceutical material is injected into a patient's bloodstream prior to the scan and circulates freely through the blood, emitting gamma rays. As the patient lies on a table that moves slowly through the PET scan machine, cameras inside the machine record the gamma rays coming from the patient and turn them into electrical signals, which are processed by a high-speed computer to generate images.

When the patient is asked to perform a specific task, such as looking at a picture of a face, or trying to identify a smell, the area of the brain responsible for performing those activities becomes more active, thereby increasing blood flow to the part of the brain that's working. These active areas of the brain show up on PET scans as bright areas of contrast. As Alzheimer's Disease progresses, subsequent PET scans show that fewer and fewer areas of the brain are working correctly, plus a clear and ongoing loss of brain tissue is present.

The issue is how to determine who should undergo a PET scan screening for Alzheimer's Disease. A recent study conducted at UCLA found that routinely using PET scans to screen for Alzheimer's Disease correlates to a 65 percent decrease in avoidable months of nursing home care and a 48 percent drop in unnecessary drug treatment. But most insurance plans, including Medicare, don't reimburse for PET scans performed for AD screening. Medicare currently reimburses for clinical evaluation of cognitive impairment according to the practice parameters set out by the American Academy of Neurology in May 2001, including general cognitive screening instruments and a variety of medical tests, such as a complete blood count, depression screening, and liver and thyroid functions tests among others.

However, in April 2003, the Centers for Medicare and Medicaid Studies announced that is was designing a demonstration to evaluate the potential role of PET scans for patients with suspected dementia, as well as a multi-disciplinary expert meeting to fully explore the value of PET scan for Alzheimer's Disease. Medicare already covers PET scan tests for certain cancers and some types of cardiovascular disease. If Medicare decides to cover PET scans for AD screening, many private insurers are likely to follow suit.

Because the average cost of a PET scan currently ranges from $2,000 to $3,000, it's still much too expensive a procedure at this point to be used for routine screenings in the same way as mammogram ($65 to $125) or prostrate screening test (about $65), or many other routine annual health screenings.

If you're worried about radioactive material being injected into your loved one's body, don't be. Modern radioactive pharmaceuticals decay so quickly that the actual dose of radiation delivered is minimal and well within the guidelines established for other imaging equipment, such as traditional X ray machines.

## The significance of digital imaging technology

A long time ago, in a galaxy far, far away, all imaging modalities required the use of film to produce usable images. Now, doctors rely on pixels to give them the information they need to make a diagnosis. Digital imaging technology offers many advantages over traditional film technology. Here are just a few:

✔ Taking several digital shots is cheaper than making one film shot, so doctors feel free to order images from many different angles, increasing their odds of accurate diagnoses.

✔ Digital images can easily be sent via the Internet to a consulting doctor in another hospital or even in another state. With film images, expensive copies must be made if another doctor wants to review the case.

✔ Digital images are sharp and clear and can be manipulated to provide maximum information.

### SPECT Scans

SPECT stands for *single photon emission computed tomography.* It was developed about the same time as PET technology, and like PET, its reliance on fragile radioactive pharmaceuticals kept it confined to research centers for a long time. It also is a metabolically and not structurally based imaging system, so it shows things like blood flow and areas of infection.

Back in 1979, experts expressed a real interest in using SPECT scans to determine if patients with memory problems were likely to develop AD after a study by Harvard researchers reported that reviews of SPECT scans from 136 patients revealed reduced blood flow readings in four key areas of the brain, three of them related to memory.

Researchers hypothesize that those areas may be the first to be affected by AD. Today, SPECT scans are used primarily to provide information about blood flow to tissue, in cases like stress fractures, tumors, and infections. Some researchers initially speculated that SPECT imaging might be useful in the diagnosis of Alzheimer's Disease, but in its May 2001 practice parameters, the American Academy of Neurology specifically recommended against its use in routine evaluation of a patient with suspected AD.

## Comparing imaging procedures

Table 10-1 compares the benefits and disadvantages of currently available imaging procedures that may be used in the diagnosis of AD. Not all procedures are available at all facilities. Readers in large metropolitan areas may find their costs for these procedures are higher than the average listed.

| Table 10-1 | Comparison of Imaging Techniques Used in Alzheimer's Disease | | | |
|---|---|---|---|---|
| *Type of Scan* | *Average Cost* | *Average Length of Exam* | *Benefits* | *Disadvantages* |
| CAT Scan or CT Scan | with contrast $739; without $655 | 10 to 30 minutes; 30 minutes to 1 hour | Relatively inexpensive | Some patients may experience allergic reactions to injected contrast material. Difficulty in clearly seeing brain tissue may result in under estimation of brain atrophy. Higher radiation dose than tradi-tional X-ray limits total number of scans that may safely be given to one patient. |
| MRI | $1,155 | 30 to 90 minutes | Three-dimensional images, clearly distinguishes between cerebrospinal fluid and gray and white matter, no radiation | Noisy, not recom-mended for claustrophobics. Patient must lie still for a long time. More expensive than CAT scans. |
| PET Scan | $2,000 to $3,000 | 1 to 2 hours | Contrast mate-rial is non-toxic Shows both brain structure and function | Most expensive brain imaging technique. Slightly increased risk of cancer from radioactive tracers used in procedure. |
| SPECT Scan | $1,200 | 60 to 90 minutes | Shows both brain structure and function | Slightly increased risk of cancer from radioactive tracers used in procedure |

# Chapter 11

# Finding Alternative Therapies

. . . . . . . . . . . . . . . . . . . . . . . . . . . . . . . . . . . . . . . . .

*In This Chapter*

▶ Discovering ways to calm Alzheimer's Disease patients

▶ Planning structured social events

. . . . . . . . . . . . . . . . . . . . . . . . . . . . . . . . . . . . . . . . .

Although you may often feel powerless to help your loved one (and your-self) cope with the effects of Alzheimer's Disease (AD), some new programs are proving that you *can* effectively calm the agitation and address the self-imposed isolation that so often accompany AD by involving your loved one in various alternative therapies. Many of these alternative therapies can serve as valuable accompaniments to the drug therapies and family counseling offered by your healthcare team.

In this chapter, we use the term *alternative therapies* to describe a broad array of community support services that can help you manage your loved one's condition and provide a better quality of life for the both of you. We do *not* mean untested, unproven potions and devices like the sort we describe in Chapter 8.

Most communities do offer some support services for elderly patients, including patients with Alzheimer's Disease. Your community center should have information on programs and services that are available locally. You can also try contacting your local Council on Aging or area Agency on Aging (www.aoa.gov) for information. Even if you live in a rural area that offers few services, you should be able to find some sort of program available in a nearby urban center.

The therapies we discuss in this chapter have proven benefits, but remember that no one can predict how an individual will respond to a particular activity. For example, although most people find music to be soothing and comforting, music may, in fact, increase your loved one's agitation instead of calming it. When you start a new therapy for your loved one, monitor his or her reactions to it for the first few sessions to make sure that your loved one is actually enjoying the activity. You may have to do a bit of experimenting, but if you're persistent, you can find some beneficial activity that your loved one enjoys.

# Calming Alzheimer's Disease Patients

One of the most significant problems that families with AD patients often face is agitation. Agitated behaviors may include

- Asking the same question over and over again
- Pacing
- Hoarding
- Screaming
- Physical or verbal aggression

Several studies suggest that agitated behavior is twice as prevalent among patients with AD as it is among patients with other forms of dementia — although researchers aren't sure why.

*Agitation* in an AD patient is defined as any inappropriate verbal, physical, or motor activity that can't be explained by physical needs or pain.

Some experts believe that lashing out is a way for AD patients to attempt to communicate their fear and anxiety to the outside world, but this suggests that the behavior is purposeful. Regardless of the reason for the behavior, the key to dealing with agitation is to determine what triggers the episodes in your loved one and then figure out effective strategies that can either prevent them from happening or limit their duration and intensity.

Agitation is a major source of distress for caregivers. (For more detailed information on handling agitation, please see Chapter 16.) Repetitive episodes of agitated behavior increase the risk that a caregiver may lose control and exhibit anger and aggression — or perhaps even become physically abusive with his or her loved one. It is also a predictor of nursing home placement. That's why programs that help to calm patients and give caregivers a bit of a break are so important.

Effective programs and management strategies distract the AD patient, engage his or her attention (however briefly), and redirect the patient's focus toward the pleasant activity being offered. In this section, we discuss a few programs that have been proven beneficial for AD patients.

## Getting help from man's best friend: Pet visitation programs

One of the most difficult things for many people to give up when they must enter a residential care program is the love and companionship of their family pets. To address this need, many different groups and organizations have established visitation programs to bring pets to people confined to nursing homes or enrolled in adult daycare programs.

Many different groups have established pet visitation programs that bring well-trained, docile domestic pets to nursing homes on a monthly basis to give residents a chance to pet and interact with the animals. Call your local SPCA to see if they administer a local program.

Volunteers and staff members for the various organizations bring dogs, cats, rabbits, guinea pigs, and even birds to nursing homes, adult daycare centers, and other care facilities to visit with residents. All the animals are pre-screened to ensure that they have the proper temperament to be a visiting pet. After an animal passes the pre-screening, it must go through extensive training so that it will know how to behave when it starts to work in the visitation program.

The visiting animal is just half the team. The human volunteer who accompanies the animal also undergoes extensive training, so that he or she will know how to handle the animals properly and how to interact with the residents. The program gives volunteers the opportunity to share the love of their pets to comfort someone who, because of his or her living circumstances, has no other way to interact with animals.

### Benefiting from pet visitation programs

You may be wondering how much good a visit from a dog or cat can really do. Well, let us tell you that visits from animals do plenty of good. A number of studies show that interacting with animals lowers blood pressure, reduces stress and anxiety, encourages vocalization and social interaction, and even increases survival rates following a heart attack or major surgery. In addition, pet visitation programs may also do the following:

- ✔ Decrease aggressive or hyperactive behavior
- ✔ Increase physical and social activity
- ✔ Help patients deal positively with their feelings of loneliness and isolation
- ✔ Provide an opportunity for positive nonverbal communication
- ✔ Relieve depression and disorientation
- ✔ Improve morale, self-esteem, self-confidence, and self-respect
- ✔ Provide a nonthreatening environment for play and self-expression

Pet visitation programs may help AD patients interact more positively with those around them by allowing them to focus on something other than their own worries and problems. The programs give them an opportunity to engage in nurturing behavior in a safe environment and to receive immediate rewards in the form of tail-wags, licks, nuzzles, and purrs from the visiting animal companions. Animals allow AD patients to establish emotionally satisfying bonds that they perceive as safe and fulfilling, because therapy animals make no demands in return for their freely given affection. People who've been feeling isolated because of illness are able to feel a sense of connection with a therapy animal, and that connection may sometimes lead to improved socialization with caregivers, fellow patients, and family members. Even if the effect is only temporary, it's always welcome.

The simple act of physical contact and gentle touch can provide something that many of these patients may be lacking in their day-to-day lives. The playful interaction and exchange of affection, in turn, provides mental stimulation because the company and entertainment provided by the animals can help patients recall happy memories. Therapy animals help to liven things up, and they bring a spark of happiness to institutional settings that may otherwise seem depressing. You'll probably notice many additional benefits after your loved one starts participating in a pet visitation program.

Not every pet is suited for pet visitation programs. Some are too quick to snap; others have nervous temperaments. Remember, too, that you must do everything you can to protect therapy pets from inappropriate behavior by the patients they're visiting. Just like a child, an AD patient may accidentally squeeze a puppy too hard or drop it without meaning to. So make sure that the people administering the pet therapy program pay as good attention to the safety and happiness of the therapy pets as they pay to the safety and happiness of the human patients.

### Finding programs

Looking for a pet visitation program near you? A golden retriever enthusiast named Rochelle Lesser maintains an excellent nationwide group listing of pet visitation programs arranged by state. For more information, visit www.landofpuregold.com/rxb.htm and scroll down to your state.

Many other organizations in addition to the SPCA sponsor pet visitation programs with the goal to use domesticated animals to bring a little comfort and joy to patients whose lives are constrained by illness. If you need help finding a pet therapy program in your community, call your local humane society, animal shelter, or SPCA.

# And a one, and a two — music therapy

*Music has charms to soothe the savage breast,*
*To soften rocks, or bend a knotted oak.*

–William Congreve
The Mourning Bride – 1697
Act 1, Scene 1

We all respond to music: Sad music makes us blue, romantic music makes us feel all mushy, and happy music lifts our spirits. The philosopher Plato once declared that education is not complete unless it includes "music for the mind."

Music for the mind is the idea behind music therapy. The modern science of music as a healing therapy was born after World War II when doctors noticed that both the physical and emotional healing of the wounded soldiers they were treating got a measurable boost after musicians visited the hospitals and performed. Experts soon realized that a need existed for specialized training to develop musicians specifically interested in music as a therapy.

According to the World Federation of Music Therapy, *music therapy* is the use of music and/or its musical elements (sound, rhythm, melody, and harmony) by a qualified music therapist, with a client or group, in a process designed to facilitate and promote communication, relationships, learning, mobilization, expression, organization, and other relevant therapeutic objectives in order to meet physical, emotional, mental, social, and cognitive needs.

### What music therapists do

If you're thinking that a music therapist is just someone who pops a CD into a boom box and then stands there and claps his hands and smiles until the music is over, you couldn't be more wrong. Music therapy is an emerging specialty. According to the American Music Therapy Association, music therapists "assess emotional well-being, physical health, social functioning, communication abilities, and cognitive skills through musical responses; design music sessions for individuals and groups based on client needs using music improvisation, receptive music listening, song writing, lyric discussion, music and imagery, music performance, and learning through music; and participate in interdisciplinary treatment planning, ongoing evaluation, and follow-up."

One of the most appealing things about music therapy is that patients don't need any sort of musical talent or ability in order to participate in and enjoy a musical session.

Music therapy for individuals is prescribed by the patient's healthcare team in much the same way that counseling or a particular medication may be prescribed. For groups, a doctor responsible for monitoring the group writes what's known as a *standing order,* giving music therapists permission to come in on a regular basis and provide a specific program.

### How music therapy helps AD

Music therapy programs designed especially for AD patients primarily utilize sing-alongs and the playing of simple rhythm instruments, as well as movement to music if the patients' conditions allow it. The aim of these programs is to assist patients to reach nonmusical goals, including a decrease in episodes of inappropriate behavior, and to help with stress reduction and pain management.

In one study, soothing music played during mealtimes significantly increased food intake. This result is important because maintaining sufficient caloric intake in AD patients becomes more and more difficult as the disease progresses.

In another study, music therapy increased social interaction in AD patients and decreased agitated behaviors during the therapy session. Researchers noted that patients continued to respond favorably to music despite the ongoing progression of their disease.

As with any other therapy, individual responses to music therapy vary widely. The sort of music that's played does seem to make a difference. In the eating study, patients responded more favorably to soothing music than to pop music or familiar folk songs. Classical music also seems to be effective, especially in reducing *repetitive disruptive vocalizations* (RDV), which is an agitated behavior.

# Having Some Fun and Easing Isolation

As the disease progresses, AD patients have a tendency to become socially isolated. They may suffer from low self-esteem related to their loss of identity, or they may feel so frustrated that they begin to exhibit behavioral problems. These problems impact not only the patient but also the caregiver, because the caregiver has to shoulder the burden of "entertaining" his or her loved one.

Any number of planned therapeutic activities are appropriate for AD patients, including painting and ceramics classes, crafts, cooking, community gardening, and exercise groups. In addition to providing AD patients with some entertainment, these activities offer the caregiver a much-needed break and an opportunity for some personal time.

AD patients tend to get overwhelmed in large groups of unfamiliar people, so before you enroll your loved one in a program, check out the size of the classes. People with AD do much better in small-group activities where they can bond with the other members of the group and develop a sense of camaraderie as they enjoy the scheduled activity.

Some activities will be available only if you enroll your loved one in an adult daycare program. Many others, however, are offered by local senior centers, particularly for patients who are still in the mild stage of AD.

## Small-group activities

Small-group activities include arts and crafts, gardening, and cooking. They're structured to provide participants (usually six to ten people) with easy-to-accomplish goals. They give AD patients an opportunity to talk and socialize in a fun, safe, and nurturing environment. Successful completion of projects rewards group members with a feeling of satisfaction and accomplishment — emotions that are all too often absent from the lives of AD patients. In addition, structured small group activities help keep patients oriented to holidays and family dates of importance, such as birthdays and anniversaries.

## Recreational activities

Recreational activities include gentle exercise, sports and games, music therapy, and pet visitations. These types of activities can help to prevent physical or emotional decline that result from social isolation, immobility, and inactivity.

No matter what activity you plan for your loved one, remember to let him or her take it at a comfortable pace. It may take several attempts at participation before a person falls into a routine. If the program isn't in an AD center, your loved one may be more likely to participate if they go with someone else. The goal is to establish involvement in enjoyable, structured, regularly occurring activities that provide a feeling of community and accomplishment.

If your loved one doesn't want to participate on a particular day, honor that feeling and allow your loved one to withdraw if he or she chooses. Trying to force an AD patient to do something only leads to behavioral problems. Keep in mind that your loved one may be subject to fatigue and can be easily overwhelmed in new and unfamiliar situations.

# Part III
# Providing Care for the AD Patient

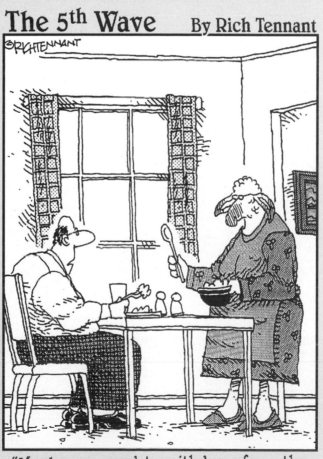

The 5th Wave    By Rich Tennant

"Maybe you need to withdraw from the clinical trial."

## In this part . . .

We offer valuable information regarding the myriad medical, legal, and financial issues you have to deal with as an Alzheimer caregiver. You discover how to find the best doctors and how to deal with attorneys and CPAs. You also find everything you ever wanted to know about Medicare regulations and evaluating the cost of care. In addition, you get some smart ideas about what to do if your family doesn't have adequate resources to provide care, and we evaluate the care options available so that you can choose what's best for your family.

# Chapter 12

# Making Medical Decisions

*In This Chapter*

▶ Understanding the importance of a good healthcare team

▶ Considering alternative therapies and clinical trials

▶ Looking at drug and treatment options

▶ Being aware of end-of-life care options

▶ Pondering brain donation

*A*lzheimer's Disease (AD) is a complex disease that isn't entirely under-stood — not even by doctors and scientists working on the forefront of AD research. It would be nice if, like treating a cold, your loved one could just throw some chicken soup at it, rest a few days, and feel better. But AD is a progressive condition, and the medical decisions that you and your loved one make become more and more critical with the passing of time.

The first and, perhaps, most important decision is choosing the healthcare providers who'll be your partners throughout the journey you're embarking upon. Having a sympathetic and knowledgeable healthcare team that's willing to take the time to listen to your concerns and dispense thoughtful advice will prove immensely helpful as you navigate the many twists and turns that AD may put in front of you and your loved one.

After you have your healthcare team in place, you'll have to make dozens of other decisions, including whether or not your loved one should participate in clinical trials, what sort of end-of-life care you want your loved one to have, and whether a *Do Not Resuscitate* (DNR) order is right for your family. You may even have to make decisions about what's going to happen after your loved one's death, such as whether to donate brain tissue for ongoing research projects that have already yielded valuable clues in the fight against AD (this decision usually needs to be made in advance of death).

In this chapter, you find practical advice and information to guide you as you try to make the best possible medical decisions for yourself and your loved one.

# *Finding the Right Healthcare Provider*

In order to illustrate the importance of finding the right healthcare provider (or team of providers), allow us to introduce you to two different families who each have a loved one with AD: Family A and Family B (pretty creative naming, huh?).

Family A suspects that something might be wrong with their elderly loved one. They've had the same primary care physician for 20 years, and, after an initial examination, he diagnoses the loved one with AD and refers him and the family to a nearby university medical center where the family encounters a warm and sympathetic core group of healthcare providers — medical doctors, nurses, psychologists, social workers, specialists in caregiving, and many others. These people, if they don't already know the answer to one of the family's questions, at least know where to get the answer and are willing to go the extra mile to get the answers the family needs.

Throughout the course of their loved one's AD, the family feels validated and listened to; they feel like they're an integral part of the team that's providing the best possible care for their loved one and that the healthcare team actually does care about the patient.

When their loved one passes away, the heartbreak of that event is eased by their experience with their medical team and the preparation they'd been given over the years. They're sad, but they're able to cope because they know that they and everyone else involved did their best for their loved one.

According to the Alzheimer's Association, a person with AD lives an average of 8 years from the onset of symptoms, but may live as long as 20 years. That's why finding healthcare providers whom you like and trust to serve as your partners during this journey is so very important.

Family B also suspects that something's wrong with their loved one and schedules a doctor's appointment. Their primary care physician is part of a huge practice group managed by an outside company. The doctor, who's never seen the patient before and doesn't know anything about her history other than what was on the form the family filled in just before the appointment, takes one look at the patient, pronounces her "depressed," and hands the family a prescription for some antidepressants and some sleeping pills because her nighttime restlessness has been disturbing other family members' rest.

The patient doesn't like the pills, and getting her to take them has become a real physical battle. The family finally resorts to crushing a couple of sleeping pills and stirring them into her iced tea. The next morning, she's groggy, and when she tries to get out of bed, she falls and fractures her pelvis. Suddenly, a patient who was showing signs of early dementia has become a patient who's bedridden with a potentially life-threatening injury. A patient who required about three to four hours of supervisory care each day now requires hospitalization and, after discharge, almost round-the clock maintenance and supervision from the family, plus a visiting nurse to monitor her medical condition.

What's the only difference here? The medical team. Surely all are competent healthcare providers, but one team is deeply experienced in treating AD patients, while the other team is relatively inexperienced. One team is familiar with the patient's history and personality and made an appropriate referral for a full work-up with a specialist, but the other team that "doesn't know the patient from Adam" looks only at the most obvious symptoms without looking any deeper.

Keep these fictional families in mind when you begin the process of selecting your medical team. Although insurance constraints may make it difficult to get the exact team you want, be persistent and keep pushing for your first choice of doctors. Even if you have to go out of your insurance network in order to visit a knowledgeable doctor or specialist, it may be worth it to pay a few extra dollars. The point is, if you're not satisfied with the outcome of your doctor visit, seek a second opinion.

Sometimes, if a doctor is especially experienced in or knowledgeable about one particular condition, such as Alzheimer's Disease, insurance companies will allow you to visit that doctor even if he or she isn't on the regular roster of providers. Check with your insurance provider to see whether you can do this. And be sure to get your permission to visit that specific out-of-network doctor in writing, so that there won't be any confusion about reimbursement later on.

# Building a Team

In Chapter 3, we talk about the different kinds of specialists who may see an AD patient. We also tell you that your family doctor is a good place to start, and in many cases, can provide the majority of the care your loved one requires. Your primary care physician can refer you to specialists, if needed, and other sorts of healthcare providers, such as visiting nurses, who may be available to help your family provide proper medical care for your loved one.

Keep in mind that not every person with AD absolutely needs to see a specialist. Many primary care physicians can do a fine job, particularly if they're very familiar with the patient and his or her family. In addition, finding and regularly visiting a specialist is unrealistic for many families because of finances or geography.

Other factors may influence your choice of physician and the number and type of people included in your loved one's medical team. For example, if your loved one has diabetes in addition to AD, your medical team might include a diabetes specialist, such as an endocrinologist, and probably a dietitian — experts who typically wouldn't be required for the day-to-day care of an AD patient but who can provide essential expertise when needed. If your loved one has cardiovascular disease, your team might include a cardiologist, and you may seek out a rheumatologist if your loved one has arthritis. In other words, the makeup of your particular medical care team is dictated by your loved one's medical needs. If AD is the only diagnosis and your loved one is healthy otherwise, you may do very well with a small team consisting of your family doctor, an AD expert, and someone such as a psychologist, visiting nurse, or social worker, to provide support and information about caregiving issues.

As the disease progresses, you should be alert for changes in his or her condition that may require the addition of a new doctor or other healthcare professional to your team. For example, if your loved one develops symptoms of depression, you may well want to add a psychiatrist to your team. If you worry that your loved one is becoming too sedentary, you may seek out someone who specializes in gentle, enjoyable, age-appropriate exercise activities to add a little movement to the daily routine.

In addition, you must also attend to routine maintenance issues, such as eye and dental exams, hearing tests, well woman or man exams, and so on. AD patients may not reliably attend to their own health issues and medical needs. Alternatively, a person may attribute symptoms of AD to a medical condition such as hearing loss and not pursue treatment for his or her cognitive problems.

Sometimes, families get so used to the day-to-day routines of caring for a loved one with AD that they're unsure how to react when a medical crisis not related to AD presents itself. If your loved one shows any signs of unusual pain, persistent heartburn and/or indigestion, dizziness or fainting, bleeding, or any other symptom that would indicate a significant medical problem, you should have him or her evaluated as quickly as possible by your family doctor. If the condition seems critical or life-threatening, call 9-1-1 or immediately transport your loved one to the nearest hospital emergency room for treatment.

# Keeping Good Records

Now is a good time to prepare a filing system to keep track of the many medical documents you'll receive over the course of your loved one's AD treatment. You don't need anything fancy to store your files; a simple cardboard filing box is fine. If you want to get a little more elaborate, purchase a metal filing cabinet. Whatever you choose, the important thing is that this place is where every single piece of paper relating to your loved one's AD will go. Try to get in the habit of filing the papers as soon as you get home from a doctor's appointment. If this isn't feasible, keep one manila folder in the front of the filing cabinet where you stick all the medical records until you have time to file them properly.

Keeping medical records straight will be much easier if you establish a good filing system to begin with. Get a box of manila folders and give each one a specific label, such as "Prescriptions," "Medicare Documents," "Hospital Bills," "Dr. John Doe," and so on. You'll be surprised how much time you save by keeping your loved one's medical records in one easy-to-access place. It beats digging frantically through piles of papers and junk mail any day.

If you don't have time to file the documents yourself, consider paying another family member (perhaps a teenage son or daughter who always seems to be asking you for money?) or a neighbor you know and trust to help you. All these little pieces of paper may not seem important now, but down the road, you may need to correlate information on two different medical records to make a more informed medical decision. If your loved one is seeing several different doctors, keeping them informed of what medications the other doctors are prescribing will help prevent an accidental conflict in prescriptions. By keeping all this information at hand, you'll always be ready to answer any questions your healthcare providers may have, and you'll also have exact times and dates available.

To keep track of medications more easily, make up a list of medications (including any vitamins or other supplements) your loved one takes and laminate it for your wallet, and make a copy for your loved one's wallet as well as copies for various healthcare providers. Be sure to update the card each time a medication is added or stopped, or the dosed is changed.

Before each appointment with a doctor, counselor, social worker, or other important member of your loved one's care team, make copies of the information you want to share and put them in a manila envelope to give to the doctor. Having the info with you can help you remember to discuss any questions you have or important issues that have come up since the last visit.

Always bring copies rather than your original documents. If you were to happen to lose the originals along the way, they'd be difficult to replace.

# Using Alternative Therapies

We live in an age where more information is available than ever before, and it's coming at us 24/7 from a dozen different directions. But trying to decipher whether the information is good or bogus is difficult, to say the least.

Nowhere is separating good info from bad more confusing than in the world of alternative therapies. If you believe half of what you read on the Internet, we've already cured Alzheimer's Disease. (But if that were really true, don't you think the mainstream press would have reported that breaking news by now?)

On the other hand, don't assume that just because a treatment isn't "mainstream medicine" it has no therapeutic value. Large doses of vitamin E used to be considered an alternative treatment for AD; now that its therapeutic value has been shown in a series of scientific studies, the therapy has entered the medical mainstream.

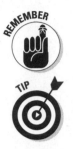

If you decide that you want to investigate alternative therapies for your loved one, just be sure that you don't use them in place of proven medical care. And please keep your doctor informed of everything you're doing, so that he or she can advise you of any potential conflicts or problem areas.

For more information on so-called therapies and cures that you should avoid, see Chapter 8. For more info on alternative therapies that really work, see Chapter 11.

# Evaluating Clinical Trials

One of the decisions a person with AD and their family may face is whether to enroll in a clinical trial. The advantages of being enrolled in a trial of a treatment that may provide unforeseen benefits can be tremendous, but you must also keep in mind the potential for side effects from an experimental treatment, some of which may be serious or even life-threatening.

Unless you happen to have a working crystal ball, you have no way of knowing in advance what the outcome of a particular clinical trial will be. So does this lack of certainty mean that you shouldn't run the risk of participating? Maybe yes, maybe no. It's a difficult decision and a lot depends on the personalities of the people involved. If your loved one likes the idea of participating in something that may help him, that may well be historic, that could lead to vastly improved treatments for AD, he just might be the sort of person who'd jump at the chance to participate in a clinical trial. However, if your loved one is primarily concerned about potential side effects or has other worries, enrolling him in a clinical trial may not be a good idea.

At the very least, you need to discuss the clinical trial with your loved one and provide an explanation of the rationale for the study, the risks and benefits, and other factors in language that your loved one can understand. The study coordinator can help with this discussion when he or she reviews the consent to participate.

Enrollment in a clinical trial requires some dedication on the part of the caregiver to make sure that appointments are kept, log books and journals are filled out in a timely fashion, and medications are administered as directed. And don't forget that you may be putting yourself and your loved one through all this hassle only to discover that you've been given a placebo. Although control groups that receive placebos are vitally important to validate the integrity of clinical trials, finding out that your loved one isn't actually receiving the investigational new drug can still be disappointing.

You can take some comfort in the fact that clinical trials are well controlled, and researchers make every effort to ensure the safety of trial participants.

# Understanding the Importance of Cholinesterase Inhibitors

Despite the terrific advancements made in the diagnosis and treatment of Alzheimer's Disease in recent years, the sad fact is that only one in four AD patients ever receive *cholinesterase inhibitors* (see Chapter 7 for more info), and of those that do, most stay on the drugs only three to six months. Considering that ongoing clinical observations — in other words, reports coming from doctors who are using these drugs in current patient populations — suggest that cholinesterase inhibitors provide significant benefits for greater periods of time than previously thought possible, the fact that so many patients are not receiving these drugs is a tragedy

Cholinesterase inhibitors are the very best treatment currently available for AD and have injected a note of hope into what used to be a rather bleak outlook. If your doctor is reluctant to prescribe them or tries to take your loved one off the medication after a few months without a clear reason for doing so, you should switch to a doctor who understands the vital role these drugs now play in maintaining AD patients in a higher level of functioning for long periods of time.

The original clinical trials of the cholinesterase inhibitors lasted from three to six months, and for reasons unknown, there's a persistent belief among some members of the medical community that the drugs lose their effectiveness and shouldn't be taken for any longer period of time. In actual practice, however, patients who start cholinesterase inhibitors soon after diagnosis and stay on them for extended periods receive the most therapeutic benefit. Considering that these drugs delay admission to nursing homes by an average of seven months and may preserve a higher level of functioning for many patients, you should push your doctor to prescribe one of the currently approved cholinesterase inhibitors for your loved one. With very few exceptions, everyone deserves the chance to try an approved AD medication, regardless of the severity of his or her disease.

AD patients who are fortunate enough to have a doctor who understands the importance of early diagnosis and treatment, and who understands the necessity of reaching a therapeutic dosage, do better than patients who haven't been treated with these drugs or who've been treated for a short time and then taken off or unjustifiably switched.

When AD patients remain on cholinesterase inhibitors, some families report that their loved one remembers family members' names, remembers how to perform basic household tasks and personal hygiene routines, and retains more of his or her unique personality. The drugs may reduce agitation and have even been shown to reverse some psychotic tendencies in patients with more advanced AD. These gains can be significant for both the patient and the family.

# Deciding on End-of-Life Care Options

Talking about end-of-life care options may seem a bit disheartening, especially if the end still many years away. But now, as soon as possible after diagnosis, is the right time to discuss your loved one's wishes for his or her end-of-life care. You're going to have to make more decisions than you might think, so you want to start early.

If a patient is in the early stages of AD, she should make these decisions for herself, and her caregivers should then carry out her wishes. Making these decisions soon after diagnosis allows your loved one to participate in the decision-making process in a meaningful way, and gives you time to consult an attorney to have any necessary documents drawn up.

To make sure that the patient's choices for end-of-life care are carried out according to his or her wishes, you should prepare one or more documents called *advanced directives* and contact your attorney for help in drawing up the necessary documents. (For more information on advanced directives and how they work, see Chapter 13.) When a patient hasn't prepared an advanced directive and is no longer capable of making such choices, the caregiver and the family must make these decisions for the patient.

Some AD patients succumb to physical ailments other than AD, such as heart attack, stroke, or complications of diabetes. In fact, most people with AD don't die from the disease but rather from a complication of the disease, such as aspiration pneumonia. Although good care enables many people with AD to experience a good quality of life following diagnosis, no matter how excellent their care, near the end of life, most AD patients aren't able to make any decisions for themselves. That's why you should discuss these issues and make these decisions now while your loved one can still make his or her wishes known.

When your loved one is in the final stages of AD, he or she may experience a life-threatening medical crisis, such as pneumonia, and you must decide what sort of care will be provided. In this sort of situation, you have three major choices available: letting nature take its course, palliative care, or aggressive care. Read on for a better explanation of each option.

## *Letting nature take its course*

When you've lived with an AD patient for many years, by the time you approach the end of the road, you may decide that you'll just ride out whatever happens and let nature prevail. If you choose this course, you absolutely must make these wishes known to your healthcare provider by signing a *DNR* (Do Not Resuscitate) order. All this order means is that when your loved one is dying, the medical care facility and its staff will allow that natural process to proceed without interfering.

Only doctors can order DNR forms, but only families and competent patients can request them. If you do ask for a DNR, the doctor will sign and ask the patient or whoever is legally empowered to represent the patient to sign the document as well. The DNR, which is a binding, legal document, is then put into the patient's medical record so that anyone who provides care knows what to do if the patient experiences a life-threatening crisis.

If you feel squeamish about taking the responsibility for signing a DNR, your loved one may wish to consider creating a document called a living will soon after diagnosis. Living wills specify the exact types of medical treatment and interventions that patients do and do not want performed if they're in a crisis situation. For more information on living wills and where to find forms for your state, see Chapter 13.

You may be thinking, "Well, of course if an AD patient is dying, they're just going to let them go." That's not always the case, though. Even when a patient's quality of life isn't good, some healthcare providers are determined to prolong his or her life no matter what. They may aggressively resuscitate a dying patient, inserting ventilator tubes and performing other invasive procedures to restore life. But if you and your loved one have had the foresight to sign a DNR, both the attending doctors and the medical facility must honor that request.

## *Palliative care*

*Palliative care* means that your loved one will be fed and kept comfortable and free from pain. It also means that appropriate care and medications will be given to alleviate any distressing symptoms the patient may display. For example, if an AD patient is running a fever and is uncomfortable, the doctor may administer acetaminophen. But no aggressive or invasive measures will be taken to artificially extend the patient's life.

The verb *palliate* derives from the Latin, palliatus, which means "to conceal." Palliative care does just that; it "conceals" the intensity of an illness through moderation of its effects with appropriate care and medications. However, it does not change the course of the illness.

## To feed or not to feed?

A lot of discussion is occurring among both medical professionals and families about the use of a feeding tube in a dying patient. Many years ago, some religious organizations insisted that as long as a patient was alive, he or she had to be given food and water. It seemed the ethical and humane thing to do. But recent studies show that feeding tubes can cause infections and increase the patient's discomfort. Other studies have shown that at the end of life, the lack of food or water doesn't cause pain or discomfort. So don't be surprised if, near the end of your loved one's life, no food or water is offered, because study data doesn't support the contention that placing a feeding tube improves or maintains the patient's quality of life.

Palliative care often goes hand in hand with a DNR order. It's a way for a family to let healthcare providers know that they want to ensure their loved one's comfort and safety, without taking any extraordinary or aggressive steps to save that person's life if he or she experiences a potentially fatal health crisis.

## *Aggressive care*

Some families just can't accept the idea of letting go of a beloved family member, no matter how far advanced his or her illness. These families may chose to opt for aggressive end-of-life care, authorizing their physicians to employ whatever means necessary to prolong their loved one's life, including the use of ventilation equipment to maintain breathing and oxygenation and defibrillators to restart the heart.

Although end-of-life care is an extremely personal choice and no one else can tell you what to do, choose carefully if you're considering an aggressive approach. Aggressive care is appropriate and understandable in situations where someone has suffered a traumatic injury or is in a critical stage of an illness. If these patients can be helped through their crises, they may recover fully and go on to enjoy many more years of a good quality of life.

The situation is different with people who lack quality of life, however. Even if you "save" your loved one, ask yourself: "What am I saving him for?" You have to determine to what degree your loved one has quality of life. You and your loved one have already been through a lot simply dealing with AD. If there is no quality of life, there's absolutely nothing wrong with choosing to let life end naturally.

# Considering Brain Donation

Many advances in our understanding of Alzheimer's Disease and its effects upon the brain have come from the study of brains donated by the families of deceased Alzheimer's patients. In addition, some families find closure when they choose to donate their loved one's brain, because a post-mortem brain autopsy is still the only way to confirm a diagnosis of Alzheimer's Disease with absolute certainty.

If you do decide to donate your loved one's brain after his or her death, you need to start the process now. Most institutions only accept brains from individuals who've been enrolled in their study programs, so that any information gathered can be understood within the context of that patient's medical history. In some cases, you must also go through an interview and screening process in order to be accepted as a candidate for brain donation. Please read on for a list of organizations that are currently accepting brains for the study of Alzheimer's Disease.

Researchers study not only the brains of AD patients, but also brain tissue donated by elderly people who've died from causes unrelated to AD. They need brain tissue from normal elderly people to compare to brain tissue from AD patients, so that they can document the changes that AD causes in the brain. The hope is that this sort of research may eventually lead to a cure for AD and more drugs that will help to delay or prevent the onset of AD symptoms in susceptible people.

## Deciding whether brain donation is right for your family

Many factors come into play when a patient or a family is thinking about donating their loved one's brain for research purposes. Your family may have religious issues that must be taken into consideration, and some family members may consider the procedure to be distasteful.

If you have concerns that brain donation may somehow violate the ethical or moral standards of your religion, the best thing to do is consult your spiritual advisor or whoever you feel is the most qualified person to assist you in making such an important decision.

If you're struggling with whether or not to donate your loved one's brain for research, you may be comforted to know that none of the major religions prohibit a brain autopsy or tissue donation.

## Brain donation and autopsy

Some families get confused when they receive a bill for a brain autopsy following the death of their loved one. Although brain donation generally doesn't cost the family anything, some institutions do charge families for autopsies that are performed to provide important information to the family.

*Brain donation* means that you're giving your loved one's entire brain to a research facility for use in their Alzheimer's Disease research projects. *Autopsy* means that a pathologist examines portions of your loved one's brain tissue to look for the neurofibrillary plaques and tangles that are characteristic of AD. When you sign the papers stating that you intend to donate your loved one's brain for research, you'll be asked about autopsy at that point. Some institutions, particularly those affiliated with medical schools, provide autopsy services for their patients as a courtesy for families who are donating brains; others charge for the autopsy (the average cost is $1,750 to $2,000). When you meet with your brain donation counselor, be sure to ask how that particular facility handles this issue.

Your loved one's wishes must be taken into consideration as well. Many AD patients are happy to donate their brains in the hope that doing so can help to advance the fight against AD; others are absolutely against it. If they're given the opportunity to consider this topic soon after their diagnosis, many AD patients opt to participate in brain donation programs.

If you have family members who are vigorously opposed to the idea of brain donation, you'll have to decide how much weight to give their objections. Reaching a decision that makes everyone happy may not be possible. The important thing is to do what makes your loved one happy and to try to honor his or her wishes as best you can.

## Understanding the donation procedure

After you agree to donate your loved one's brain, the facility you've selected will inform you of its donation procedures. You'll be asked to fill out several forms and assigned a donation coordinator with a 24-hour phone number to call in order to alert program coordinators when your loved one is about to pass away. You'll also be asked to sign a legal consent giving the facility permission to collect your loved one's brain for research purposes. Before the autopsy can proceed, you must also provide a death certificate signed by the attending physician who verified your loved one's death. The facility will generally coordinate transportation of the body directly with the funeral home you've selected, or you may be told to arrange this yourself. It's helpful and can save a lot of time if you select a funeral home in advance and discuss your intent to have an autopsy performed.

What if you agreed to donate your loved one's brain, but you change your mind later and decide against the procedure? No problem. Simply contact the agency that made arrangements for the brain donation and let them know that you've changed your mind, and they'll note your loved one's medical records accordingly so that the donation procedure isn't performed.

Some people are reluctant to agree to brain donation because they fear that it'll somehow disfigure their loved one or make having an open-casket funeral impossible. This is simply not the case. They may also worry that brain donation will delay the funeral, but the procedure requires just a few hours. As soon as it's completed, your loved one's body is transported back to the funeral home so that it can be prepared for burial.

Ideally, brain tissue is harvested within 6 hours of death; in fact, the sooner the better for research purposes. However, if the procedure can't be performed within this time frame, you should instruct the funeral home to embalm your loved one's body. An autopsy can still be performed on embalmed tissue. The pathologist removes the brain in such a way that the donor's normal appearance is maintained.

Even if your loved one has already indicated on her driver's license that she's agreed to be a potential organ donor, that's different from specifically donating one's brain for research. Most donor registries that are tied into state drivers' license programs only provide for the removal of transplantable organs and tissue, such as the heart, lung, kidneys, and corneas at the time of death. If your loved one wants to donate her brain for Alzheimer's research, she must enroll in a specific brain donation program.

After the brain's been obtained, individual sections may be removed and mounted on slides for microscopic examination. If the family has requested autopsy results, the pathologist will prepare a report for release to the family. The rest of the brain is either placed in a preservative solution or is frozen. Most research institutions make samples of brain tissue available to other qualified researchers, along with pathological documentation.

## Finding research facilities that accept donated brains

Various research facilities across the United States accept brains for donation. Most of these facilities are not only in need of brains from AD patients, but also brains from older people with normal cognitive functioning for purposes of comparison.

Even if you think you're 100 percent prepared for your loved one's death, it'll still be a difficult, emotional time. Take the time now to prepare a folder with the name and address of your funeral director and any specific requests your loved one may have made for his or her funeral and give this information to the coordinator of the brain donation program your family has chosen. Keep a copy of the information for yourself, along with the location and number of your loved one's cemetery plot and the title to the property.

If you're unsure whether your city has a brain donation program, you can call either the local chapter of the Alzheimer's Association or a nearby medical school or teaching hospital to find out if a program is available to you.

Here are a few representative brain donation programs to give you an idea of what's out there. Call the local chapter of the Alzheimer's Association for guidance on what's nearest to your home.

- Baylor College of Medicine (www.bcm.tmc.edu/neurol/struct/adrc/adrc5f2.html): The Baylor College of Medicine Alzheimer's Disease Center runs a brain donation program in the Houston metropolitan area to collect brain tissue for use in ongoing Alzheimer's Disease research. However, the program only accepts donations from patients who have been enrolled in the Center.

- Boston University (www.bu.edu/alzresearch/btd.html): The Alzheimer's Disease Center at Boston University maintains a brain donation program.

- Northwestern University (www.brain.nwu.edu/mdad/generalprocedures.html): The Northwestern Alzheimer's Disease Center in Chicago runs a brain donation program.

- Oregon Brain Bank (www.ohsu.edu/som-alzheimers/br-bank.html): Established with the assistance of the Alzheimer Research Alliance of Oregon in 1991, the Oregon Brain Bank program provides support for families of AD patients by supplying accurate post-mortem confirmation of AD diagnosis through autopsy, and by providing brain tissue samples for study by interested researchers.

# Chapter 13

# Understanding Legal Issues for Alzheimer's Patients

· · · · · · · · · · · · · · · · · · · · · · · · · · · · · · · · · · · · · · · · · · · · · · ·

· · · · · · · · · · · · · · · · · · · · · · · · · · · · · · · · · · · · · · · · · · · · · · ·

*O*ne of the most difficult issues for both Alzheimer's Disease (AD) patients and their families is figuring out how to handle legal decisions or decisions that affect their own or a loved one's legal status. Laws about determining competency and the granting of guardianships and powers of attorney vary so widely from state-to-state that something that's legal and entirely appropriate in one state may raise eyebrows in another. How can you figure out what to do?

Legal decisions can be emotionally wrenching; in many states, you must first have your loved one declared mentally incompetent before you can put a guardianship in place. Families may be understandably reluctant to do this, and if you're an AD patient, you certainly won't like the idea of being labeled incompetent. But in order to protect your assets and get your family through the next few years in the best possible shape, everyone involved must sit down together as soon as possible and make these important decisions.

In this chapter, we explain the ins and outs of the many legal issues that can affect AD patients and their families, and we also tell you why getting your legal ducks in a row as soon as possible after your own or your loved one's diagnosis is so essential. Legally, many of these decisions can only be made by the person with AD. If you wait too long to make them and become incompetent in the eyes of the law, your family will have to go to the trouble and expense of seeking a guardianship in order to manage your affairs.

You must decide how to handle many issues. You have to determine whether you want to try to preserve assets or transfer them to a responsible party for administration. You have to figure out how to provide for your own care (if you're the AD patient) or your loved one's care (if you're the caregiver) without impoverishing remaining family members. You must deal with Social Security and insurance issues and take steps to protect yourself or your loved one from fraud or abuse. These decisions certainly aren't small ones.

The information provided in this chapter is in no way intended as a substitute for professional legal advice. If you have a specific legal question, your best bet is to consult an attorney who understands your local statutes and the laws that apply to your particular situation.

# Getting Started

Before you pick up the phone and call an attorney, take the time to do a bit of organizing. You'll save yourself a lot of time and money down the road.

First, get a sturdy manila folding file or any other type of spacious file you prefer to hold documents in an organized fashion. Because you're going to be dealing with a lot of paper over the years, you may want to invest in a hanging folder system that helps keep your files straight and your paperwork in good condition.

If space is tight in your home and you don't want a giant, ugly metal filing cabinet cluttering things up, consider using a cardboard banker's box to store your loved one's documents. They come in packs of three or six and are ideal for storing either letter- or legal-size documents. You can even fit them with a small rack to accommodate hanging files. Use one box for medical records, one for legal records, and a third for financial records.

Get a packet of manila file folders and label them. For example, in a folder marked "Will," you might have a copy of your loved one's will and written documentation stating where the original, legally binding copy of the will is stored. If you have more than one attorney, as in the case where one attorney is dealing with elder law issues and another attorney is dealing with financial issues, make a separate folder for each one. Proceed in this fashion until you have folders for every legal issue you're dealing with.

Although all this labeling and preparation may seem like a lot of work, doing so saves you so much time in the long run that you'll be happy you took the time to prepare your filing system properly to begin with. And don't make the mistake of thinking that you have to do all this work by yourself. Your loved one or your children and grandchildren may be happy to help you with this important paperwork.

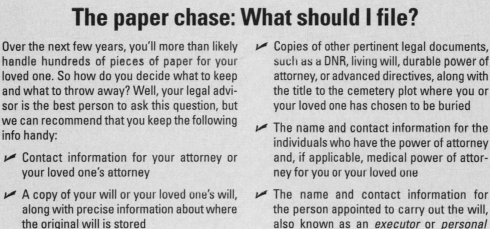

## The paper chase: What should I file?

Over the next few years, you'll more than likely handle hundreds of pieces of paper for your loved one. So how do you decide what to keep and what to throw away? Well, your legal advisor is the best person to ask this question, but we can recommend that you keep the following info handy:

✔ Contact information for your attorney or your loved one's attorney

✔ A copy of your will or your loved one's will, along with precise information about where the original will is stored

✔ A list of any trusts that have been executed

✔ Copies of other pertinent legal documents, such as a DNR, living will, durable power of attorney, or advanced directives, along with the title to the cemetery plot where you or your loved one has chosen to be buried

✔ The name and contact information for the individuals who have the power of attorney and, if applicable, medical power of attorney for you or your loved one

✔ The name and contact information for the person appointed to carry out the will, also known as an *executor* or *personal representative*

If you feel like you're just too overwhelmed to tackle this chore and don't have anyone who can help you, consider hiring a professional organizer who can come in for a day or an afternoon. Pros can whip through all your paperwork so fast that your head will spin. Yes, you may have to shell out a few hundred bucks, but consider it an investment in your own mental health. And the good news is that after the filing system is set up, maintaining it on your own will be relatively easy.

## Evaluating Your Legal Options

After your loved one receives a diagnosis of AD, you have many different ways to handle his legal affairs. The three most common legal options are

✔ Durable power of attorney

✔ Legal conservatorship, or, as it's known in some jurisdictions, a guardianship

✔ Trusts

Each option has distinct advantages. In this section, we discuss these three choices, so that when you consult your attorney, you have a basic knowledge of what's involved in the decisions you're about to make.

Sort out your loved one's legal affairs as soon as possible. We can list many reasons why, but one of the most important is that after your loved one reaches the stage where the law would consider him incapable of making informed decisions, giving you or another family member a power of attorney to handle legal business is no longer possible. You would then have to go through the process of getting a guardianship to obtain the right to handle your loved one's affairs, a process that is both expensive and pretty traumatic for all involved.

# Durable Power of Attorney

You probably take your ability to make your own decisions for granted, so you may find it tough to face up to the fact that the day may come when your loved one might truly be incapable of making informed decisions in her own best interests. Or perhaps you're an AD patient in the early stages of the disease and you want to specify who will handle your affairs after you can no longer do so. That's where powers of attorney come in.

A regular or *nondurable power of attorney* covers the transfer of legal authority for one or more specific events for a specific period of time. To protect you and your interests, this type of authority ends automatically if you become incapacitated, because it is assumed that you would no longer be able to give informed consent or make any proper legal decisions.

A *durable power of attorney* is a legal document that authorizes a person to make caregiving, financial, and/or medical treatment decisions on behalf of a patient who's become incapable of making her own decisions. The person who receives the AD patient's legal authority is called an *attorney in fact,* but you may also hear this person called an *agent* or a *proxy.* The person granting the power of attorney is called the *principal.* A durable power of attorney can be granted only if the patient transferring the authority is still considered mentally competent.

When dealing with a health situation where a person may become increasingly incapacitated, you need a durable power of attorney. This instrument that transfers broad legal decision-making authority to the caregiver or another designated person for an indefinite period of time was designed specifically to provide care for future unknown circumstances. A power of attorney allows AD patients to exercise their authority and choose someone trustworthy to handle future decisions while they're still able to make informed decisions. After the power of attorney is designated, the person with AD should discuss her future wishes with that person to make sure she's understood.

Take care of the legal planning as quickly as possible after diagnosis. If you don't, you're essentially handing your family's legal decision-making power over to a disinterested, overburdened court that will make its decisions with little regard to your family's wishes or situation. Once the person with AD is no longer considered to be legally competent, the court will require the appointment of a conservator or guardian to manage her affairs, and that will cost more money.

If you're diagnosed with AD and are already holding a power of attorney for another family member such as your spouse or child, you should arrange to transfer that authority as soon as possible. Discuss the situation with the person who gave you the power of attorney and decide together who can best handle the power of attorney for her.

## *How many agents are needed?*

The number of agents you appoint depends on your particular situation and the abilities of the individual agents. The only person who can make these appointments is the person who anticipates becoming incapacitated, whose assets and legal and business affairs must be tended in an uninterrupted fashion despite that incapacitation. For example, if your father has AD and doesn't appoint an agent before becoming incompetent, you can't appoint an agent for him.

Each family can tailor its power of attorney to fit its needs. For example, if a woman has two children, one a nurse and the other an accountant, she might choose to draw up two powers of attorney, giving the nurse the right to make medical decisions and the accountant the right to make financial and legal decisions for her when she can no longer make these decisions for herself. When appointing more than one agent, to avoid conflict, you should appoint people who get along well together and who'll work together to protect your interests.

Another consideration is proximity. Typically, a family must deal with Alzheimer's Disease over a long period of time, so the agent must live relatively close by. Even if you have the best relationship with your daughter who lives in Juno, Alaska, and trust her the most out of all your children, consider how very difficult it will be for her to be onsite, sometimes for weeks at a time, in order to handle your affairs. This would be especially difficult if she has small children or a busy career.

When selecting an agent, try to find someone you love and trust who could be forceful if required. If no one in the immediate family is able to take on this responsibility, it's possible to transfer power of attorney to a close friend or significant other. But you and your loved one must be sure that person is willing to accept the responsibility before proceeding, and you must also make sure the person is someone you both trust implicitly to do the job because that person is about to get an awful lot of power.

The principal can grant his agent as much or as little power as he wishes. Most durable power of attorney forms actually have checklists of powers that may be granted; for example, real estate transactions and banking. If your loved one wishes the agent to have a particular power, he leaves it on the list, but if your loved one wants a specific power to be excluded from the agent's authority, he crosses that off the power of attorney document.

Appoint several alternate agents in your order of preference if, for some reason, your first choice of agent is unable to carry out his responsibilities.

You may well be happy with just one agent, but even if you are, most attorneys will tell you that it's a good idea to appoint an independent third party to review your agent's accounting after you become unable to review the accounting yourself. It's just an extra layer of protection to help keep everything on the up and up.

Handling the legal, financial, and medical affairs of another person is a lot of work, so don't beat yourself up if it's something you'd rather not do. Perhaps the responsibility can be split between several members of the family, so that the entire burden of care doesn't fall on one person.

## Should power of attorney be given to my lawyer?

If you're a person with AD and don't have any relatives or anyone you feel you can trust to handle your affairs, or if you're a caregiver and you feel like you can't handle being your loved one's agent and no one else in your family can either, you may transfer legal authority to your lawyer so that she may serve as your or your loved one's advocate. But check your local statutes to make sure that this is allowed where you live. Some jurisdictions may consider it a conflict of interest.

An agent is required by the court to take her role in safeguarding the principal's property and assets very seriously. The agent should keep the principal's property and assets separate from her own, maintaining separate bank accounts and other accounts as necessary, and also provide regular, accurate accountings supported by receipts of all transactions conducted on behalf of the principal.

If your jurisdiction allows the person with AD to transfer power of attorney to her lawyer, the patient and two witnesses will be asked to sign a legal document giving proxy to the attorney. Naturally, you should make sure that the attorney you choose is held in high regard, both in the community and among her peers. Also, check with your state Bar Association and the local Better Business Bureau to make sure that no complaints have been filed against the attorney. If you have any doubts at all, keep looking until you find someone you trust and feel comfortable with. Local Senior

Centers or the Council on Aging or the local chapter of The Alzheimer's Association might have names of reputable lawyers experienced in handling elder law issues.

How you handle your family's legal issues depends in large part on the laws where you live. The advice of an attorney can be invaluable because she can steer you to take advantage of those laws to create the best possible legal plan for your family.

## Choosing the correct type of power of attorney

You can handle a durable power of attorney in two ways. If you're worried that your health is deteriorating rapidly, you may request that it take effect immediately upon the signing of the legal documents. That means that from the moment you walk out of the attorney's office, your designated proxy (agent) will be handling most or all of your affairs. If you're still able to manage your affairs and prefer to do so for as long as possible, you may sign what's known as a *springing durable power of attorney.*

This type of power of attorney automatically "springs" into effect after you meet the definition of incapacitation set out in the document, and that incapacitation has been certified by your attending physician. In other words, with a springing durable power of attorney, you won't give up your legal authority until and unless you become incapacitated.

You can use a standard definition of incapacitation or tailor one to suit your circumstances. Your attorney can advise the best course for your particular situation.

While springing power of attorneys may seem like an attractive alternative, in actual practice they can be problematic because there is nothing concrete on the face of the document that states the document is now in effect. As a result, third parties such as banks and insurance companies are frequently reluctant to honor them, even after the necessary certifications have been obtained. Consult your attorney to see what power of attorney is right for you.

In all states, a patient must still be demonstrably competent and capable of making informed decisions when he signs a durable power of attorney. That's why executing a durable power of attorney as soon as possible after a diagnosis of AD is so essential. If you wait until after your loved one has lost significant mental capacity, the courts will no longer allow you to obtain your loved one's power of attorney because he's no longer capable of giving informed consent to the arrangement.

## What kind of "powers" does power of attorney bestow?

You may feel confused about what a person can or can't do with a power of attorney. Though specific authority varies from state to state, generally speaking, agents acting on behalf of an incapacitated individual (also known as a principal) may

- ✔ Collect by whatever means are necessary any monies or valuables that are owed to the principal

- ✔ Save, invest, or disburse monies, or use them on behalf of the principal for the purposes intended

- ✔ Sign new contracts or modify existing contracts on behalf of the principal, on terms agreeable to the attorney of record

- ✔ Buy, sell, or lease property on behalf of the principal

- ✔ Settle claims or court cases in favor of or against the principal

- ✔ Hire and fire attorneys, accountants, or any other personnel necessary to attend to the principal's business and legal affairs

And that list is just the short one. In plain English, an agent may be handling real estate and personal property transactions, stocks and bonds, commodities and bonds, banking, business operations, insurance, annuities, estates, trusts, claims and litigation, personal and family issues, Social Security, Medicare, Medicaid, pensions from private corporations or from civil or military service, retirement plan transactions and income, and personal and property taxes.

In addition to the things an agent *may* do, there are also some things that she *must* do to satisfy the requirements of the law. Agents must

- ✔ Always act in the best interests of the principal and not engage in any act that furthers their own interests

- ✔ Keep appropriate records of each transaction, including a complete accounting of receipts for expenditures and disbursements

- ✔ Manage the principal's legal and financial affairs in an honest and competent manner

## Can someone use power of attorney to steal assets?

To be brutally honest, yes. When you or your loved one gives power of attorney to another individual, that person has the authority to make legal decisions. The agent has the power to handle all the banking, property, and investments for the principal and has access to all related information. That's why you and your loved one must choose someone of the highest moral character, who you trust completely, as your agent. If the person you choose has a questionable character, the temptation of having free access to your family's money and property may be more than he can handle.

Putting as many layers of protection in place as possible when drawing up a power of attorney is a good idea. Doing so creates a system of checks and balances to ensure that the people entrusted with your assets or your loved one's assets execute their responsibilities honestly.

A power of attorney gives the proxy an enormous amount of authority. Some unscrupulous people will try to force someone to sign a power of attorney in order to gain legal authority over that person's assets. If someone in your family, a friend, or an acquaintance is trying to force you or your loved one to sign a power of attorney, don't let it happen! Contact the police or your local elder abuse hotline immediately for guidance and information about how to handle the situation. In some states, trying to force someone to sign a power of attorney through threats and abuse is considered extortion, so if you feel that you or your loved one is unsafe, don't hesitate to call the authorities for help in removing and dealing with the person who's threatening you or your loved one.

## Changing your mind

If you or your loved one is unhappy with the appointed agent's conduct, the power of attorney can be revoked at any time, as long as the person who granted the authority in the first place is still considered competent to make decisions. You or your loved one must inform the agent in writing that the power of attorney is revoked and must also inform the lawyer, bank, and other financial institutions that the agent no longer has the authority to manage your affairs.

Once your loved one becomes incompetent, you should keep watch over his affairs even if you're not the agent to make sure the person granted the power of attorney is behaving responsibly. If you're not the primary caregiver and you feel like the agent is abusing the power of attorney, you should file a complaint with local law enforcement authorities or pursue guardianship. Because the person with AD is no longer competent to make his own decisions, the court must intervene to investigate any instances of misconduct. Only the court has the authority to dissolve a power of attorney in situations where the principal is no longer competent and the existing agent is not performing his duties responsibly. But the court does not have the authority to grant a new power of attorney; that's why it's a good idea to appoint several agents at the time the power of attorney is granted. If one doesn't work out, another can step up and take over the job. If the principal names only one agent and his authority is revoked, then the family must apply for a guardianship to gain legal authority to manage the affairs of the person with AD.

If your jurisdiction required the power of attorney to be filed with the local clerk of court, the lawyer must file a copy of the revocation with the clerk to make things official. At the same time, you and your loved one will probably want to consult with your attorney about the appointment of a new agent and the creation of a new durable power of attorney. If you put this off and don't select a new agent in a timely fashion, your family may be required to go to the expense of getting a conservatorship or guardianship.

## *How much does it cost?*

A power of attorney is a relatively inexpensive legal procedure. You can spend $50 on legal software that contains the necessary forms and simple instructions. Or you may download a power of attorney legal form for free from your state's Council on Aging Web site and fill it out yourself if your situation is straightforward. Filing fees vary from town to town, but most jurisdictions charge in the neighborhood of $10 to $20 dollars to file a power of attorney with the clerk of court.

However, your best bet is probably to hire an attorney who's experienced in elder law to help you, especially if your legal, financial, and/or family situation is complex and requires sorting out.

To find an elder law specialist in your area, call the state Bar Association or the local Alzheimer's Association or Administration on Aging for suggestions. You can also talk to other families dealing with AD to see if they can suggest a good lawyer, or just look in the phone book. If you want to use an Internet search engine, enter the phrase "elder law" and then the name of your town or city. The results should give you contact information for any attorneys specializing in elder law in your area.

In addition to the filing fee and attorneys' fees, your loved one should be aware that it's reasonable for an agent to ask for a monthly stipend to cover the expenses that she may incur while managing the affairs of the person with AD. The agent may have to give up her job to care for you or your loved one, or change from full-time to part-time work, so she might suffer a real loss of income as a result of agreeing to be the agent. Even if the agent keeps working full time or already doesn't work at all, she will still incur considerable expenses, such as gas, postage, phone, legal bills, and other professional fees. The amount of this stipend can vary dramatically, depending on the number and value of the assets to be managed, the relationship between the agent and the principal, and prevailing rates in your area. Ask your attorney what amount is customary.

Families tend to prefer durable powers of attorney because they transfer broad authority to manage their loved one's assets without the hassle and expense of constant court interference. However, if your loved one's diagnosis of AD is made well after she has become incompetent, you'll be required to seek a conservatorship or guardianship in order to make legal decisions for her. We discuss other valid reasons why some people choose to seek a guardianship instead of a durable power of attorney in the next section. So read on if you aren't sure which route to take.

# Guardianships or Conservatorships

Depending on where you're located, the next level of legal oversight and decision-making authority may be called either a *guardianship* or a *conservatorship*. Simply put, a *guardian* or *conservator* is charged with "guarding" the assets and interests of his ward and making decisions based solely upon the principal's best interests. The court oversees and supervises all decisions that the guardian makes.

For the purposes of a guardianship, a *ward* is defined as a person who, by reason of incapacity, is under the protection of a court either directly or through a guardian appointed by the court. A ward may also be called a *protected person*.

When an AD patient has already passed the point of being able to make competent decisions in his own best interest, guardianships can be used to give the family the ability to manage the affairs of the person with AD. Guardianships are also a good idea if there are disagreements between the patient and family members or among various family members about how the situation should be handled and who should get the power of attorney. In the case of family squabbles, a guardianship with court oversight is a good way to guarantee that the best interests of the person with AD are maintained.

If your loved one set up the guardianship while he was still considered to be competent, then your loved one would've been able to set out the exact terms and conditions he wanted, including selecting his own guardian. If the guardianship was set up by the court after your loved one was already considered incapacitated, the court appoints the guardian, and a family may not have as much say-so in that appointment as they'd like. There may be disagreement among family members who are vying for the appointment and if the judge so chooses, he may appoint a guardian that is not even a member of the family. (Yet another argument for settling legal matters long before your loved one loses his legal status as a competent person.)

## What does a guardian do?

When a guardian's appointed, the first thing that she must do is deposit a court-determined amount of money called a *bond* to ensure that she will honestly manage the protected person's assets. Sometimes, however, the court won't require this bond, especially if the assets of the estate are limited.

---

# Who determines competency?

You may feel confused or indifferent about the whole issue of competency, but the courts take it very seriously. Competency is a legal, and not a medical, decision. However, an attorney or the court may rely, in part or in whole, upon the medical expertise and opinion of a doctor or other healthcare provider who is familiar with the case and who can provide the results of neurological testing to give the court a legal basis for making a determination of incompetency.

---

A guardian must provide for the basic needs of

- ✔ Food
- ✔ Shelter
- ✔ Medical care

In addition, the guardian must manage the ward's assets in a skillful and prudent manner and pay the wards' bills in a timely fashion, using the ward's assets whenever possible. Finally, the guardian must prepare an annual report for the court describing all transactions made on behalf of the ward.

## *How are guardianships awarded?*

If your loved one has set up a guardianship in advance, its provisions will kick in as soon as you've satisfied the court that your loved one has reached a point of incapacitation. If your family hasn't made any legal plans in advance and your loved one is now incapable of caring for himself, you may now determine that a guardianship is right for your family (at this point, a durable power of attorney is no longer an option). In either case, the first thing you must do is petition the court:

- ✔ If the guardianship has been set up in advance, you simply have to prove that your loved one is no longer capable of caring for himself. In this case, courts usually accept a written report from the attending doctor as proof, but in some instances, they may require the doctor to appear and testify in person.

- ✔ If your family hasn't planned for a guardianship in advance, you (or whoever's up to the task) must ask the court for the right to be named your loved one's guardian. Before the court appoints you, you must prove that your loved one is incapacitated by providing valid medical documentation. Sometimes, when the presiding judge isn't happy with the way the family's conducting itself, she may decide to appoint the court itself or a court representative as the guardian. This may also happen when the ward doesn't have any immediate family members available to act as guardian. To ensure the best outcome, hiring an attorney to represent you at these proceedings is imperative.

# Why choose a guardianship?

Sometimes, people who are still competent choose a guardianship over a durable power of attorney. In the following situations, this is a wise move:

- ✔ **The individual has no one to look after her.** If an individual doesn't have anyone to look after her, setting up a guardianship while she's still competent allows her to choose how her assets are managed and also have a say in her medical care, living arrangements, and end-of-life care options. Because the guardianship is managed by the court, your loved one has a way of making sure that her wishes are carried out.

- ✔ **The individual's family members don't get along.** When family members either don't get along or actually engage in out-and-out warfare, a guardianship outlines what must be done on behalf of an AD patient. Even though the family members may still fight, they must follow the guidelines of the guardianship exactly and have no authority to change them or go against the wishes the principal or the court have set out in the guardianship documents.

Guardians must operate within very narrow parameters set out by statute in their jurisdictions. If they mismanage an estate or commit acts not in the best interest of the protected person or engage in outright fraud, they may face severe civil and criminal penalties, including fines or even a jail sentence.

Court supervision of all transactions under guardianships makes it almost impossible for a guardian to pull any kind of stunts with the principal's assets. So if your loved one is worried that certain family members might not be trustworthy when handling her assets, she can sidestep the entire issue by setting up a guardianship.

On the downside, guardianships make it much more difficult for family members to conduct business or make decisions for their loved one because every single thing they do has to be approved by the court prior to doing it. And each time the family's involved with the court, fees must be paid; papers must be signed, notarized, and filed, and a dozen other little details must be dealt with in order to satisfy the dictates of the court. So overall, guardianships are more expensive to set up and manage than durable powers of attorney.

Your loved one's lawyer can review the relative benefits and drawbacks of both types of asset management and help her decide which is best for your loved one. We offer a quick comparison of the two in Table 13-1.

| Table 13-1 | Durable Power of Attorney Versus Guardianship | |
|---|---|---|
| *Type of Instrument* | *Advantages* | *Disadvantages* |
| Durable Power of Attorney or Springing Durable Power of Attorney | Gives an AD patient the ability to plan his own future and make sure that his wishes are carried out by someone he trusts | Gives broad powers to the appointed agent; lack of monitoring makes it possible for an unscrupulous agent to steal assets |
| | Can be tailored to meet the family's situation; authority may be split between several people | May make AD patient feel left out or overlooked unless "springing" form is used |
| | Provides for broad range of authority along with thefreedom and flexibility to make decisions for the principal without court oversight | |
| | Relatively inexpensive | |
| Guardianship or Conservatorship | Has the built-in safeguard of court supervision of the agent's activities on the person's behalf, which helps to prevent fraud and abuse | Relatively expensive com pared to a durable power of attorney, generally costing at least $1,000 to set up |
| | Can serve to settle arguments when family members don't get along or disagree on how the principal's assets should be managed | More difficult to make deci sions because everything must first be approved by the court. Crowded court dockets in most areas mean that months or even years may pass before a court renders its decision |
| | | Cuts AD patient out of the decision-making process and deprives him or her of many rights |
| | | Principal must be declared incompetent in an open court before guardian can be appointed |

## Another possible legal option: Personal custodians

Some states allow for the appointment of a *personal custodian* to handle business and legal affairs for an impaired person. Under this type of law, the impaired person transfers some or all of her property to the custodian for management. The individual retains ownership, but the custodian manages and invests the individual's property according to her wishes. If the impaired person is transferring real property, such as homes, raw land, or investment buildings, she must sign and execute a deed trans-ferring the property to the selected custodian, always being sure to include language that makes it clear that this transfer is for purposes of management only and is being done under the authority of local personal custodian statutes.

Check with your loved one's attorney to see if personal custodianship is available in your juris-diction and for advice as to whether a durable power of attorney or a personal custodianship would best meet your loved one's needs.

# Living Trusts

Living trusts take effect as soon as they're executed and can be an excellent tool to manage assets during the grantor's life. Trusts can be either revocable, which means that you can change the terms of the trust or cancel it entirely even after you've put it in place, or irrevocable, which means that the trust can't be changed or revoked.

Don't be confused if you see the terms grantor trusts, inter vivos trusts, and living trusts all used together, because they all mean the same thing. Uncle Sam and the IRS use the term grantor trusts, lawyers use inter vivos trusts, and the rest of us just call them plain old living trusts.

The person who creates and funds a trust is called the grantor. The person who manages the trust is called the trustee. In most cases, the grantor and the trustee are the same person. Property and assets are placed in the trust and managed by the trustee for the benefit of the grantor in accordance with the terms of the trust. However, a successor trustee is usually designated. This successor trustee assumes his responsibilities upon the death or dis-ability of the trustee. These documents provide an extraordinary amount of flexibility in the management of assets.

Trusts transfer property from you to the trust, and then after you die, the trust transfers the property to the people you selected, effectively avoiding probate. Probate is the process a court goes through to establish the validity of a will and to distribute your assets. Probate can take anywhere from 12 to

18 months or longer, playing havoc with a family's finances. Because living trusts don't require court validation, they save a huge amount of time and trouble for families.

## The advantages of a living trust

Living trusts bypass the probate courts, so they save more of your assets for distribution to your heirs because they won't have to pay court costs, attorneys' fees, and executor's commissions. They also help to reduce estate taxes. In addition, living trusts can help shield a family's privacy because your family's business isn't being aired out in open court.

## Transferring property into a living trust

How your loved one transfers property into a living trust depends on the kind of property and whether or not she has an ownership document, such as a deed, for the property. For things that have deeds, like cars, boats, and houses, your loved one must actually transfer ownership of the property to her trust by re-registering the property in the name of the trust. This action effectively makes the trust the legal owner of the property. If your loved one doesn't take this step, the person she appoints as her trustee won't be able to transfer this sort of property after your loved one dies.

Even though your loved one transfers ownership of her property and possessions to her trust, she still retains full control and use of the property during her lifetime.

Property that doesn't have an ownership document, such as household furnishings and personal possessions, can be transferred easily to your loved one's trust by simply listing them on what's known as the *trust schedule,* which is just an inventory of the property that's owned by the trust.

## Exploring Miller trusts

*Miller trusts* are a legal instrument that help people who have too much income to apply for Medicaid assistance meet the income requirements. They are also called *income cap trusts* or *income assignment trusts.* A person with AD can create a Miller trust to receive his Social Security and pension checks. In the eyes of Medicaid, if a trust is receiving a person's income, then the person is not receiving that income, even though he may still have the benefit of the money.

The Social Security administration always complies with requests to transfer monthly checks to a Miller trust, but some private pension plans will not cooperate or make it unnecessarily difficult.

A Miller trust can be set up either by the person with AD or his agent. A bank account must be created in the name of the trust, but it must have a zero opening balance. Some banks will not accommodate this requirement, so shop around until you find a bank that will. When the bank account is open, write the Social Security administration and the company that manages your pension and ask them to deposit the monthly checks directly into the trust account. Attorneys are very helpful to make sure the trust is set up and administered correctly. Once the trust is operating, the trustee uses the funds to pay for the personal needs of the person with AD and administrative fees associated with the trust.

# Making Choices for Medical Care

To make sure that your choices or your loved one's choices for medical care and end-of-life care are carried out as desired, you can prepare a legal document called an *advance directive*. Advance directives provide precise instructions as to the type of medical care you or your loved one wish to receive. *Living wills* specify the end-of-life care you wish to receive, and *healthcare proxies* allow a pre-selected agent to make medical decisions for the person with AD after she becomes incapacitated.

## Advance directives and living wills

Advance directives allow you or your loved one not only to select end-of-life care options but also to exclude procedures that are specifically not wanted. For example, if the person with AD doesn't want to be put on a ventilator to assist his breathing, this request would be stated in an advance directive.

The Partnership for Caring provides free, downloadable advance directives, living wills, and healthcare proxies along with instructions for every state on its Web site. Just fill out a short form, click on your state, and the correct form will be downloaded to your computer. With another click, you can download the accompanying instructions. Visit www.partnershipforcaring.org/HomePage/ and then click on "Advance Directives" and follow the instructions.

Other things your loved one might consider for his advance directive may include the following:

- Feeding tubes
- Pain medication
- Surgical procedures
- Defibrillation to restart his heart
- DNR (Do Not Resuscitate) orders

Although it's possible for the person with AD to create an advance directive that doesn't include DNR instructions, if he does want to specify a DNR order, the request must include it as part of the advance directive in order to make it legally binding.

A *living will* is a type of advance directive intended to reduce unnecessary suffering when a patient is terminally ill. A living will protects patients from prolonged pain and ensures that his wishes for end-of-life care are respected by the attending doctors and nurses.

## Healthcare proxies

In some jurisdictions, a durable power of attorney can't be used to make healthcare decisions for a principal. Your loved one must execute a separate document called a *healthcare proxy* or a *medical power of attorney* that grants agents the authority to make medical decisions for their loved one.

Your loved one should *not* give her healthcare proxy to a healthcare provider. In some jurisdictions, lawmakers have protected patients' interests by making it illegal to do so. Doctors and hospitals frequently have different agendas from patients and their families. They may be caring and competent, but healthcare providers won't necessarily have your best interests in mind or be routinely diligent about carrying out a DNR order.

The sad fact is that the quality and consistency of end-of-life care isn't very dependable in the United States, nor do many healthcare providers or facilities maintain a strong, clear policy for handling DNRs and advance directives. That's why it's so important for your loved one to have a strong family member insist that your loved one's wishes are carried out when the time comes.

If you want more information on the current status of end-of-life care in your state, visit www.lastacts.org/scripts/la_tsk01.exe?FNC= BetterEndHome__Ala_newtsk_laxlike_html and click to download the "Means to a Better End" report. This comprehensive 108-page document is a report card that grades the various states according to how well local health-care facilities respected and carried out the last wishes of their dying patients. You may be surprised at how poorly some of the states fared.

In many jurisdictions, giving a healthcare proxy to a healthcare provider is illegal. Although legislators have enacted these laws to protect consumers from overzealous healthcare providers, this can thwart your wishes if the relative you want to appoint as your agent is also an employee of your preferred healthcare provider. Check with your attorney to see what the statutes in your area require.

# Drawing Up a Will

Generally speaking, anyone who's an adult over the age of 18 and sound of mind and body is legally able to make a will. A person who makes a will is called a *testator*.

As with all other legal issues, making a will is much easier to do while your loved one is still considered competent and capable of making informed decisions. If you wait until after she's incapacitated, the courts will oversee the writing of the will and the distribution of the estate, and it'll be a lot harder on your family and cost a lot more money than if you take care of it now.

Never throw an original will haphazardly into a drawer or file box or bury it in a stack of unrelated papers. A will is a valuable legal document that helps an executor or the courts settle your loved one's estate according to her wishes. The original copy of the will should be stored in a fireproof box, and notarized copies should be kept with the attorney who drew up the will. By taking these precautions, in the unlikely event of a fire, flood, or natural disaster, your loved one's wishes can still be carried out. Please note that a safety deposit box in a bank is not a good place to store a will. In many states it may be necessary to open the estate before anyone can gain access to the safe deposit box of the person who has died.

## Understanding the benefits of a will

Wills allow people to control how they want their assets to be distributed after death. They help people transfer their assets to their surviving spouse, children, friends, or charitable organizations in a way that eases the tax burden and also satisfies the desires of the person making the will as to how those assets will be divided among the heirs. A will also serves as a road map for the court that lets the court clearly understand the wishes of the person who's died.

A will does many things besides the obvious. Along with allocating your estate in the way you want, a will can also do the following:

- Leave more assets for your heirs by minimizing estate taxes and other expenses that would be incurred in a court-managed distribution of your estate

- Provide for the most economical distribution of your assets

- Ensure that your assets are distributed to your heirs without undue delay

The property a person leaves behind after he dies is called his *estate*. An estate includes all property and cash assets owned at the time of death, including bank accounts, the family home, other real estate and buildings, land, furniture, cars, jewelry, royalty income, stocks and bonds, and proceeds from investments, along with proceeds from life insurance policies and pension plan policies that are payable to the estate.

## Deciding if you need an attorney to make a will

Like any other legal documents, wills can be simple and straightforward, or they can be complex and hard to understand. If your loved one has a small estate and just one or two heirs, you and your loved one can certainly write out the will yourselves, have it witnessed and notarized, and file it with the court. Doing so is fast, and it's economical.

A handwritten will is called a *holographic will*. In order to be valid, it must be written entirely in the hand of the person creating it, and it must be signed and dated. About half the states in the U.S. accept a handwritten will. Some require that it be witnessed and notarized; others do not. For a list of states that allow holographic wills, visit www.sphinxlegal.com/sphinx/freeresources/handwrittenwills.asp.

If your loved one has a larger or complex estate and a number of heirs, trying to write the will yourself can be a mistake that costs your family thousands of dollars in unnecessary taxes, not to mention court and attorneys' fees. Lawyers can often make money-saving suggestions that more than cover the cost of their fees.

When making a will, your loved one needs to take several things into consideration. For instance:

- ✔ Is the bulk of her property owned jointly with her spouse?
- ✔ Does your state have forced heir laws that require a certain percentage of her assets go to her children?
- ✔ Does she want to leave a bequest to a favorite charitable organization or research institute, or make sure that her son with the 12 nose rings and orange hair gets nothing until he reaches a certain age?

Attorneys experienced in probate, estate planning, and the laws of your state can help your loved one make her way through the conflicting information and also help her make good decisions about how to distribute her estate.

## Dying without a will

Dying without a will is called dying *intestate*.

If you or your loved one dies without a will, your family may be thrown into a maelstrom of trouble. Heirs may fight over the distribution of the assets; the spouse can be left destitute. All sorts of undesirable things can happen. And worst of all, the state will step in and tell your family how they have to distribute the assets, and they'll take a bigger chunk of your loved one's property as taxes than they would've if an attorney experienced in estate planning and probate had been hired to draw up a will.

According to the National Committee on Planned Giving, as many as 70 percent of Americans don't have a will. The legislature of your state has already determined how to distribute the assets of people who die intestate and you may not like some of their ideas very much. For example, if your wife dies without a will in the State of Louisiana, all her estate automatically goes to your surviving children, leaving you, the spouse, high and dry. So if your wife wants to be the one who decides how her estate is divided and who gets what, she needs to make her will now.

## Making a will for an incompetent person

In order to write a legal will for a person who's been declared incompetent, you must be appointed as his guardian. Along with the other powers granted by the court, you have the power to write a will for your loved one and determine, with the court's guidance, how his assets should be distributed following death.

Writing a will can get tricky because guardians aren't supposed to do anything in furtherance of their own self-interests, but if you're appointed guardian for one of your parents, it's reasonable to expect to inherit a portion of the assets remaining after their medical and burial expenses have been paid. You should consult an attorney to familiarize yourself with the statutes that govern the making of a will for an incapacitated person because they vary widely from state to state.

If family members disagree as to how assets should be distributed or who should be named as your loved one's guardian, consider visiting a mediator to work through your disagreement and reach an equitable compromise. Your family is going through a difficult time and everyone is going to have his own opinions about how things should be handled. Try not to let this be the cause of a permanent rift.

Despite what you may believe after watching too much late-night television or seeing too many bad movies, videotaped wills are not acceptable because all wills must be in a written form in order to be valid and legally binding.

# Chapter 14

# Working through Financial Issues for Alzheimer's Patients

Although no illness is cheap, taking care of a loved one who has Alzheimer's Disease (AD) for an extended period of time can leave a family financially devastated. You must figure out not only how to pay for your loved one's normal expenses, such as food, clothing, and shelter, but also how to cover all his medical expenses — without bankrupting either yourself or your loved one. It can be a daunting task to say the least.

A long bout with AD can wreck even the most careful financial planning. Insurance coverage may run out, and money put aside to pay for a carefree retirement must be diverted to pay for long-term care. Families without health insurance face even more dire circumstances, sometimes falling into poverty in order to maintain a good standard of care for their loved one.

If your loved one is still gainfully employed, you must help him determine when to stop working and how to deal with the loss of his job and his income. When it becomes apparent that he can no longer manage his own finances, you have to decide who in the family can step in and take over or find a trustworthy professional to handle financial issues. You have to evaluate your loved one's insurance coverage and formulate a plan to cover shortfalls and gaps in coverage. Finally, your family may be one of the many that eventually run out of resources after caring for a loved one with AD for many years.

In this chapter, we guide you through the complexities of the many financial issues that families and AD patients may face. We offer some savvy tips for making the most of what resources you do have and point you in the direction of community resources and local organizations that can help you cope with your situation.

# Reviewing Financial Needs and Resources

Yes, Alzheimer's Disease is an 800-pound gorilla, and you have to wrestle with it whether you want to or not. But don't be afraid to face your financial situation head-on. Having accurate financial information can actually empower you to make better choices.

You should have only one unknown variable in your financial equation: how long you'll have to provide care for your loved one. That's the one thing you can't be sure about. However, a good bet is to plan for costs that will rise as your loved one's disease progresses and additional care is required.

Before you worry yourself into a tizzy, take some time to sit down with your loved one and review her current and projected financial needs, and also take a look at her resources. Doing so gives you a reasonable idea about whether your loved one's available resources are sufficient to cover her needs. If they're not, you at least have an idea of how much the projected shortfall may be. After you have this information in hand, you can use it to chart your financial course and figure out if you need to develop additional resources to cover the cost of care.

## Comparing resources to needs

Make two columns on a sheet of paper and label one "Resources" and the other "Needs." Under "Resources" list the following:

✔ Your loved one's cash on hand and in savings and checking accounts

✔ Any recurring monies due from:

- Salaries
- Rents
- Trusts, including Miller trusts
- Royalties

- Stock dividends
- Outstanding loans
- Any other source of steady, recurring income

✔ Any payments due your loved one from:

- Insurance settlements
- Retirement packages
- Any other type of investment

✔ Real property assets, such as the family home, car, jewelry, land, artwork, collections, and so on

Under "Needs" list current monthly bills and a projected amount that will be required to maintain your loved one as her AD progresses. Depending upon whether you provide care in the home by a family member, or in-home care by an outside caregiver, or place your loved one in a care facility, your medical costs can range anywhere from about $1,000 a month to more than $6,000 a month. Most families find that costs increase as needs change and more hands-on care is required.

## Projecting future costs

Although not every AD patient ends up in a nursing home or other residential setting, those who do experience an average stay of two and a half years. Sometimes, families transfer AD patients to a hospice for their last few months of care, particularly if the patient has other serious health problems, such as diabetes, cancer, or heart disease. If you anticipate needing hospice care, be sure to include your share of those costs in your estimates. Medicare pays for the majority of hospice costs; call 800-MEDICARE for complete information or download a free hospice care booklet at www.hospiceinfo.org/public/articles/index.cfm?cat=7.

Nursing home and hospice costs vary widely from region to region, so call local care facilities and get an average cost for residential care in your area. Then determine the average number of doctor visits per year, the cost of prescriptions, and so on, and add this to your estimated costs for providing care, and you have a reasonable estimate of how much you'll have to pay each month to care for your loved one.

In July 2002, the Alzheimer's Association reported that the average lifetime cost of caring for an AD patient is $174,000. The vast majority of that amount (an estimated $139,000) is expended after the patient is admitted to a nursing home or other residential care facility.

Compare your resources with your needs to see whether you have sufficient resources available. Knowing what you have helps you determine how to manage your situation and whether or not you should liquidate some investments to generate additional cash. Be sure to have a contingency plan in place if your planning indicates that your loved one's needs outstrip his ability to pay for his care.

You may find that your loved one does have enough resources to cover his care, but those resources are in the wrong form. For example, your loved one might have stocks or bonds that must be liquidated to provide cash to pay bills. Or he may be holding some property for investment in the hope that it would appreciate. Even if you don't net as much as you may want, selling the property and investing the money in a liquid fund may be a good idea so that it'll be available to pay bills as needed.

Before you make any financial decisions that you may regret later, consult an expert for advice. Many banks offer financial counseling services to their customers; you may also seek financial advice from an accountant, attorney, broker, or an independent financial advisor such as a Certified Financial Planner (CFP).

What if the worst happens, and you find out that your loved one doesn't have a penny saved and can't contribute to his own care at all? Although this news may not be exactly what you wanted to hear, finding it out now so that you can figure out what to do about it is far better than finding out when it's too late to do anything. We give you some tips for dealing with this situation later in this chapter.

## Managing paperwork

When you do take over your loved one's finances, you must establish a well-organized filing system right from the get-go, not only for tax purposes but also for legal and insurance reasons.

Consider buying a small, inexpensive filing cabinet or even a set of banker's boxes so that you can store your loved one's paperwork separately from your own. If you don't keep up with the paperwork, you may have to pay dearly. Sometimes, insurance companies will send you affidavits that you have to sign and return within a certain period of time, and if you don't do so, you lose benefits.

Although filing may just seem like extra work in an already overburdened schedule, it'll save you lots of time and energy in the long run when you realize that you can always put your hands on whatever papers you need simply by pulling open a drawer or lifting the lid from a box.

## Reviewing your own financial needs and resources

In the midst of taking care of all your loved one's business, don't let yourself lose sight of your own finances. You absolutely must review your own resources and needs, just as you did for your loved one's finances (see "Comparing resources to needs" earlier in this chapter), and come up with a financial plan for yourself — particularly if you're going to be at least partially responsible for some of your loved one's expenses. If handling both sets of "books" is too big a job for you, ask your spouse or an adult child to help out. Or consider hiring a financial professional to do it for you.

Letting your own bills slide is all too easy when you're caring for a loved one with AD, but you don't want to wreck your own credit while protecting your loved one's interests. Try to achieve a balance by setting aside an hour or so each week to review your own finances and pay any bills that are due. Then set aside a separate hour to deal with your loved one's finances. After you get organized and get into a rhythm, you'll probably find that you can manage on your own without too much difficulty.

# Taking Over the Financial Reins

As the fog of Alzheimer's begins to cloud your loved one's mind, her ability to handle even the most simple financial transactions becomes impaired. Early on, the person with AD may be having problems calculating tips, writing checks, and making correct change. She may also lose money, forget to pay bills or pay the same bill twice, and hide money and then accuse someone else of stealing it after she forgets where she hid it. In other words, she's doing things that should indicate that she's no longer capable of handling her money independently. You don't want health insurance or long-term care insurance policies to be canceled for nonpayment of premiums, especially because your loved one can't get long-term insurance back after being diagnosed with AD.

Begin discussing financial issues with the person who has AD at the time of diagnosis. Perhaps one family member can serve as a financial manager to take this pressure off the caregiver. You can establish a power of attorney early while gradually transferring the day-to-day management of money to this financial manager. For example, the patient can sit with the financial manager and open bills. The financial manager writes out the check to pay the bill, and the patient signs the check.

If you dealt with this issue soon after your loved one's diagnosis, all you have to do when you reach this point is have your family doctor declare your loved one incapable of handling her own affairs, and the power of attorney you put in place then springs into effect, giving you the authority to manage your loved one's finances with very little hassle. We discuss obtaining a power of attorney, as well as other AD-related legal issues, in Chapter 13.

If you wait until a crisis occurs to figure out how to manage your loved one's finances, it may be too late. After your loved one is incapacitated, your options are much more limited and much more costly than if you'd planned ahead and put a power of attorney in place while your loved one was still mentally competent. Planning ahead gives you the chance to protect your loved one's assets from fraud or mismanagement by others and also minimizes the bite that court costs, attorneys' fees, and taxes will take.

## Protecting your loved one from fraud

Congress estimates that telemarketing fraud involving sweepstakes and cheap prizes costs Americans about $40 billion a year. According to the American Association of Retired Persons, more than half those victims are 50 years of age or older. The sad but true fact is that millions of elderly Americans become victims of fraud every year. This is particularly true for people who have AD. Older people are vulnerable to scams for lots of reasons, including the simple fact that they were raised in a time when it was considered rude to hang up on a caller, even a dishonest one. Con artists know this and play on it to help their schemes succeed.

Discuss a plan for a checks and balances system to monitor your loved one's finances for signs of fraudulent activity that might indicate that she has fallen prey to a dishonest scheme. If you do suspect fraud, try to gather as much evidence as you can and contact the appropriate authorities. Then change your loved one's phone number immediately to get her out of the clutches of the con artists because they don't stop until they've wrung every possible penny out of their victims. Some con artists have even

convinced some of their older victims to sell their homes and send them all the proceeds.

You should also report the problem to the fraud divisions of your loved one's bank and credit card companies. Ask them for guidance in canceling existing accounts; they'll probably flag the accounts to monitor them for fraudulent activity. In the meantime, you will have taken your loved one out of harm's way. You may have to spend some time and effort recovering lost assets and seeking reimbursement. Attach doctors' statements of diagnosis to the letters you write when attempting to have charges waived.

In 1995, the National Consumer's League launched a project to help determine those factors that make older people more vulnerable to fraud. They produced a free booklet called "They Can't Hang Up," that includes tips to help seniors recognize and avoid fraudulent schemes. It can be downloaded at www.fraud.org/elderfraud/theycan'thangup.htm. If you don't have the capability to download a PDF file, you may read the brochure at www.fraud.org/elderfraud/hangup.htm.

If you didn't put a power of attorney in place, you may have a fight on your hands. One of the characteristics of Alzheimer's Disease is episodes of suspicion, in which the AD patient believes that family members are stealing from him. This atmosphere isn't exactly conducive to finding a way to transfer control of your loved one's finances into your hands. That scenario plays right into an AD patient's suspicions that everyone is out to rob him blind.

Remember that as the disease progresses, you may have problems obtaining a power of attorney. As we explain in Chapter 13, the person granting the power of attorney must be of sound mind when granting it. If your loved one's condition is advanced, you'll have to seek a guardianship in order to gain authority to manage your loved one's finances. And with today's crowded court dockets, getting this guardianship can take some time.

In the meantime, meet with your loved one to see if you can work out a plan to make sure that bills are paid on time and that enough cash is on hand to buy groceries, gas, and other everyday necessities.

If you don't get control of your loved one's finances as quickly as possible, after he becomes incapable of managing his money on his own, you're setting him up as a potential victim for scamsters and con artists. (See the upcoming sidebar for details.) And even if the person with AD doesn't fall victim to a fraud, multiple subscriptions to the same magazine and series of books can still be damaging and costly.

# Understanding Changes in Tax Status

Along with all the other changes AD brings to your life, it also changes your loved one's tax status and gives you another chore that you must manage — handling their taxes as well as your own — all while trying to figure out which deductions you can take to compensate for the cost of your loved one's care.

If you're going to take even one deduction, take them all, or at least take as many as you qualify for because many of the following benefits can only be claimed by someone who's filing a return that itemizes deductions. Generally speaking, a caregiver can only deduct his loved one's medical expenses if they total more than 7.5 percent of adjusted gross income. If you're filing as a head of household and are claiming your loved one as a dependent, the amount to be deducted can include the total medical expenses for you and all the members of your immediate family as well as all the medical expenses for the AD patient. This helps you reach the 7.5 percent figure.

Where you deduct the expenses depends on your situation. If your loved one is living with you and you're claiming him as a dependent, you'd make the deduction on your 1040. If your loved one is still living independently, you may deduct qualified medical expenses on your loved one's tax return. You can also deduct the cost of making any necessary improvements to your home in order to better care for your loved one.

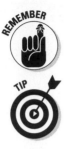

If you're claiming your loved one as a chronically ill individual, that fact must be certified annually by a licensed healthcare professional.

For a complete overview of the tax implications for AD patients and their families, visit the Alzheimer's Association Web site at `www.alz.org/ResourceCenter/ByTopic/Planning.htm` and click on "Taxes and Alzheimer's Disease" to download an excellent booklet on the topic. If you need additional guidance, consult a tax attorney or a financial advisor.

# Deciding Whether You Need a Financial Advisor

If you have a trusted financial advisor who can help you and your loved one look at your resources and formulate a plan to pay for ongoing expenses, you're ahead of the game. But you don't absolutely have to have a financial advisor to survive, particularly if you're fairly knowledgeable about how money works and feel confident making financial decisions. But like legal issues, financial management can be complex. Unless you have a very thorough understanding of money and long-term financial planning, for your own peace of mind, you should consult an accountant, attorney, financial advisor, or other expert.

People with the early onset form of AD must be especially thoughtful about their financial planning because their young age may mean that they don't qualify for some programs and benefits available to older adults. Also, 20 to 30 percent of people with AD live alone. They should ask a friend to go with them to the appointments when seeking financial counseling.

Before you can start managing your loved one's finances, you must first have written legal authorization to do so, either from a power of attorney or a guardianship. See Chapter 13 for complete information.

Fees vary widely, so be sure to get a quote in writing. Check out the person's credentials and find out whether she has any complaints against her on file with the Better Business Bureau (BBB), the Certified Financial Planner Board (CFP), National Association of Securities Dealers (NASD), or the Securities and Exchange Commission (SEC). A good financial advisor can save you the cost of her fees many times over, but a bad one can cost you money, or worse yet, engage in dishonest, commission-producing practices that eventually drain your entire account.

## Types of financial advisors

Just because someone's in your Sunday School class doesn't mean that you should automatically make him your financial advisor. You should take several steps to ensure that the person you select to help you with your finances is honest, knowledgeable, and doesn't have any potential conflicts of interest.

What kind of conflicts of interest? Well, for example, if your financial advisor is encouraging you to buy a particular security over another, more highly rated security, you may ask yourself why until you discover that he receives a commission on sales of the less desirable product. When advisors recommend products that they also earn commissions on, that represents a potential conflict of interest. However, just because the potential for a conflict exists doesn't automatically mean that your advisor is up to something. As long as he fully explains his relationship to the recommended product and that he earns commissions from its sale, he's satisfied the requirements of full disclosure and given you everything you need to make an informed investment decision.

Sometimes, if you give your advisor too much autonomy in handling your money, he may be tempted to churn your account to make extra money. Always maintain a hands-on involvement in your loved one's finances to provide an extra measure of security and oversight.

*Churning* has a very different meaning in the world of finance than it does in the world of dairies and cows. In financial circles, it means that your advisor is turning your money over again and again, investing in first one stock or bond and then in another, in order to earn more commissions. Before this type of fraud came to light, many people had their entire investment accounts drained by unscrupulous investors who churned their way right down to the bottom of their clients' capital, producing not butter, but gravy.

There are many different types of financial advisors, but they all must be licensed, which means that you are able to check their backgrounds and performance histories. Although honesty is certainly an important characteristic to look for, you also want someone who's compassionate and caring, who understands your needs and your goals, and who can assess your resources and advise you on the best way to make those resources stretch to cover the cost of your loved one's care.

In recent years, *Certified Financial Planners* (CFPs) have emerged as leaders in the field of financial advice because they have a broad range of knowledge and experience and are able to help people put together comprehensive financial plans tailored to their individual requirements and tastes. But several other types of financial advisors may meet your needs just as well. Check out your options in the following list:

- **Certified Financial Planner (CFP):** A Certified Financial Planner is someone who's studied and passed a rigorous examination administered by the Certified Financial Planner Board of Standards. A CFP commits to uphold high ethical standards and voluntarily submits to the regulatory authority of the CFP Board. CFPs must stay current in their skills by passing a new certification test every other year.

- **Chartered Financial Consultant (ChFC):** A ChFC is a financial professional who's completed an eight-course certification program, meets experience requirements, and agrees to uphold a code of ethics.

- **Chartered Financial Analyst (CFA):** A CFA is a financial professional who meets the Association for Investment Management and Research's (AIMR) requirements for education, experience, and ethics. A CFA must also pass a test administered by AIMR. CFAs focus on the analysis of investments.

- **Certified Public Accountant (CPA):** A CPA has completed extensive education and supervised work experience before taking a difficult national examination to receive certification. Although the majority of accountants are concerned with tax returns, financial statements, and audits, in recent years, many CPAs have expanded into the area of financial planning.

- **Attorney:** An attorney who specializes in estate planning may sometimes diversify into financial planning as well, particularly when her practice concentrates on elder law and the preparation of documents, such as wills and trusts, that enable families to take over the management of their loved one's assets.

- **Stockbrokers:** A stockbroker is a licensed individual who's certified and regulated by the National Association of Securities Dealers (NASD). A stockbroker recommends securities, such as stocks and bonds, for investment purposes and earns commissions on those transactions that her clients actually execute.

   All financial planners who are paid by clients to execute, buy, or sell orders for mutual funds, stocks, bonds, commodities, or other securities must be registered with the NASD and licensed by the appropriate securities agency for their state.

- **Investment advisors:** An investment advisor provides advice regarding the purchase of securities in exchange for a fee. Depending upon the size of the person's business and the breadth of her practice, anyone who performs this service must either register with the Securities and Exchange Commission (SEC) or the local state securities agency.

✔ **Money or asset managers or portfolio managers:** A money manager manages her client's portfolio of investments. Depending on training and experience, a money manager may either design the investment portfolio herself or use a design provided by a CFP or some other sort of financial advisor. The manager's fees are usually a percentage of the value of the portfolio.

Okay, so you never knew that so many different kinds of financial advisors existed, and now you're more confused than ever. Don't despair. Ask your friends for the names of financial advisors they've worked with and trust and then go through the checking and interviewing process described earlier in this chapter before you make your selection. The local chapter of your Alzheimer's Association may also have names of financial planners who are familiar with the specific needs of people with AD.

Shop around, get recommendations from your friends, check credentials and references, and then interview your top two or three financial advisors. Only then should you make a selection.

## Cost issues

How much a financial advisor costs you depends on how his charges are structured. For starters, you should know how the advisor gets paid, whether by commission or by fee. This seemingly small fact can make a world of difference in how much you're charged and in whether the recommendations you're given are unbiased or based upon the advisor's desire to sell financial and investment products he represents in order to earn additional commissions.

Never hire a financial advisor who won't fully disclose, in writing, how he's paid or how much he's going to charge you.

Financial advisors usually base their charges on one of the following five models:

✔ **Fee only:** Your advisor charges you a fee for each service he renders. In the case of attorneys or accountants, you may pay an hourly fee.

✔ **Fee based:** Your advisor charges fees plus commissions. The fees are for assessing your financial situation, and the commissions are earned on the sale of investment products he recommends.

✔ **Percentage fee:** The fee is based on a percentage, typically 1 to 2 percent, of the value of the assets the advisor's managing for you.

✔ **Commission only:** Your advisor's earnings come strictly from commissions on investment products he sells; insurance agents and stockbrokers generally use a commission-only fee structure.

✔ **Salary:** Employees of banks and credit unions who provide financial advice generally are paid a salary, but they may receive performance bonuses.

Ask what sort of records the advisor keeps and what access you have to those records. Check to find out whether the advisor's records are regularly audited and by whom.

In addition, try to find out if your potential financial advisor has any conflicts of interest, has been prohibited from taking part in the management of a company for reasons of fraud, has had any criminal convictions within the past five years, and has declared bankruptcy.

# Quitting Work

By the time most people are diagnosed with AD, they've already retired from their careers. However, improvements in the diagnostic procedure mean that doctors are diagnosing the disease earlier in the course of the illness. Consequently, a greater percentage of people receiving an AD diagnosis are still employed. These people and that small percentage of people who experience an earlier onset must decide when to quit their jobs and when and how to tell their bosses and co-workers about their diagnosis.

Your loved one's decisions in this regard depend upon the type of work he does and how much on-the-job authority he has. Obviously, the lead designer for a revolutionary new fighter jet has a lot more riding on the accuracy of his work than a person who performs a less challenging job or who works in a support position. Even if they don't specifically know that they have AD, people often understand very early that something is profoundly wrong because they can no longer easily perform even the most basic tasks required by their jobs.

According to the General Accounting Office (GAO), by the year 2050, between 8 and 13 million people will be living with AD in the United States. The difference in the figures represents projections if there is a significant breakthrough in prevention and treatment (8 million potential patients) and if there's no significant breakthrough (13 million potential patients).

## Properly timing the departure

Sometimes, AD patients deny that anything's wrong, and a boss or compassionate co-worker must tell them that their performance is lagging. If your loved one hasn't yet been diagnosed and the co-worker is unaware that cognitive impairment is the cause of the problems, this confrontation can be particularly difficult. The drop-off in performance produced by early AD can baffle fellow workers, particularly if it comes from a valued long-term employee who's always been a reliable producer in the past.

---

# Top five signs your financial advisor may be getting ready to move to Acapulco

Okay, so maybe we didn't really mean the Acapulco thing, but there are distinct ways to tell whether a financial advisor has your best interests at heart or is working toward her own financial goals. Think about switching to another advisor if the one you're working with exhibits any of the following behaviors:

✔ Starts recommending various financial products within minutes of meeting you, long before she knows anything about your personal financial situation or your financial goals or problems

✔ Baffles you with a rapid-fire presentation of dense technical lingo and then tells you not to worry; he'll take care of everything

✔ Asks you for permission to manage your funds independently and make trades and purchases without first getting your permission for each transaction

✔ Fails to disclose that she's been disciplined for dishonest practices in the past

✔ Fails to deliver promised documentation or contracts

---

When your loved one can no longer perform his job effectively and/or without undue stress, the time's come for him to quit working. If you wait too long to talk to your loved one about quitting, you may have to deal with him being let go or laid off, which may negatively affect insurance coverage. Talk to the benefits counselor in the Human Resources Department to determine the best way to quit.

Your loved one may be able to take a medical leave of absence, which will cover some medical expenses for a fairly extended period of time. Or perhaps he should accept a disability package that will pay him a portion of his salary for a period of time, as well as allow him to keep insurance coverage. Finally, allowing the company to terminate your loved one so that he's eligible for COBRA Insurance coverage may work out best. Other companies, particularly smaller ones, may not have such a variety of options available. Find out from your loved one's employer what your best options are.

COBRA stands for the *Consolidated Omnibus Budget Reconciliation Act* of 1985 that requires employers who offer group health plans to give their employees the opportunity to continue their group health coverage for a period of time even if they're terminated, laid off, or experience some other change in employment status. Individual companies handle COBRA insurance in different ways, so be sure to consult with your loved one's Human Resources benefits counselor to determine the best way to handle leaving.

If your loved one is forced to stop working and is too young to receive Social Security benefits, and his company has no real plan in place to cover a long-term disability like AD, see if he's eligible to apply for a state-run disability program. He may also get *supplemental security income* (SSI) if his income level is low enough. Patients with early onset can really suffer financially because income, retirement, and insurance benefits may be lost or reduced because of early termination of employment — all at a time when the cost of medications and treatment are increasing.

## Sharing the diagnosis

Whether or not to tell the boss or any co-workers is a personal decision that your loved one must make. Of course, human resources must know the truth about your loved one's condition in order to help him plan his departure, but by law, they cannot share any of your loved one's private medical information with anyone else, not even with his boss.

The most important consideration is making sure that your loved one doesn't try to hang on too long at work. Even though it's great to keep getting that paycheck, staying at work past the point where your loved one can truly be effective can create more problems than it solves.

## Not everyone understands

If your loved one does decide to share the AD diagnosis with co-workers, be aware that although many will be supportive, a few may not be. Most people will handle the news well, but a few may not respond as favorably. Some people may have a built-in prejudice against anyone with any sort of disability; others are afraid of anyone who has a condition of any sort. If a trusted co-worker turns cold after hearing that your loved one has AD, encourage your loved one to not make it her problem. That co-worker must deal with that issue on her own, so don't let yourself or your loved one get drawn into the drama.

Personality issues or other conflicts in your loved one's workplace may make her feel that she shouldn't make her AD diagnosis common knowledge. Or perhaps your loved one is a private person who'd prefer not to share medical problems with anyone other than close family members. That's fine, too. Just be aware that if your loved one works closely with others, they may already know that something is going on. Telling them about the diagnosis allows your loved one to talk about it openly, seek support, and educate others about the disease. Your loved one may also find that other co-workers are struggling with AD issues at home, and this situation provides an opportunity for sharing and education.

# Evaluating Insurance Coverage

Insurance coverage regulations can be complex and confusing. Trying to figure out what's covered by a particular policy and what isn't and who covers what practically requires a PhD in handling paperwork and reading hundreds of lines of tiny type. But if you're tempted to just throw in the towel, don't: Buried somewhere in that type that you can barely see may be a sentence that has profound implications for your loved one's financial situation.

Insurance companies can either be one of your biggest allies in the fight to provide good care for your loved one, or they can be the biggest thorn in your side. In this section, we review some of the most common forms of insurance coverage and tell you how to deal with your insurance providers effectively and, if necessary, fight them to get the coverage you've paid for.

## Medicare

Medicare is a federally sponsored healthcare insurance intended to help provide medical services for people aged 65 and over. It's also available to some disabled people and some people with advanced kidney disease.

Medicare is divided into two parts: Part A and Part B. You can also choose something called *M + C,* which means "Medicare plus Choice," which allows you to choose your own insurer to provide coverage for items like long-term disability coverage and prescription medications that Medicare doesn't cover. This type of coverage is popularly known as *Medigap* insurance because it helps to fill in the gaps in current Medicare coverage.

---

### Who really pays?

According to the AARP, the cost of medical care for seniors is divided among a number of payers:

| Source | Percentage Paid |
|---|---|
| Medicare | 50% |
| Medicaid | 15% |
| Patient | 20% |
| Private Insurance | 10% |
| Other Sources, includ ing Charitable Groups | 5% |

---

### Part A coverage

Part A is available for all people ages 65 or older or anyone who's receiving Social Security benefits. If you receive these benefits, you automatically receive a Medicare card. Part A covers inpatient hospital stays, skilled nursing facility and hospice care, and some home healthcare services. (Assisted living and AD units are not considered skilled nursing units.) This part, funded by a 1.45 percent payroll tax collected from both employees and employers, is provided free of charge. It covered an estimated 41 million recipients in 2002 (35 million seniors and 6 million permanently disabled young adults).

In the past, many Medicare carriers programmed their computers to automatically reject claims for certain services from AD patients. In April 2002, the administrator of the Centers for Medicare and Medicaid Services issued a press release stating: "Medicare may pay doctors and other healthcare providers for neuro-diagnostic testing, medication management, and psychological therapy when provided to patients with Alzheimer's Disease." This ruling was a big victory for AD patients and their families who routinely had to fight to get their Medicare claims paid.

### Part B coverage

Part B Medicare is optional coverage. You have seven months to sign up for this coverage, beginning three months before your 65th birthday and ending four months after your birthday. You can enroll simply by calling the Social Security Administration's toll free number: 800-772-1213. If you don't enroll during this initial period, the cost of the coverage goes up 10 percent for each 12-month period that you wait.

The monthly premium of $58.70 is taken out of your Social Security check each month before it's mailed to you. It covers doctors' fees, tests, outpatient hospital care, and some other outpatient services such as physical and occupational therapy. Low-income seniors may be able to get their states to pay part of their monthly Part B premium and may also be eligible for assistance with medications.

### Cost issues

Part A Medicare beneficiaries pay part of the cost of the medical services they receive through co-insurance payments and deductibles. For example, in the year 2003, Medicare inpatient hospital services are subject to an $840 deductible for the first day of a hospital stay and a $203 per day co-insurance charge for each day thereafter up to 90 days. Medicare will reimburse the hospital for the balance of the bill for up to 90 days of hospitalization. Medigap insurance can help pay for some of the deductibles and co-insurance charges.

Part B beneficiaries pay a $100 annual deductible; thereafter, Medicare pays 80 percent, and you're responsible for a co-insurance payment to cover the 20 percent balance.

In response to many inquiries and complaints about Medicare from the families of people with AD, the Alzheimer's Association in conjunction with the American Bar Association launched a Medicare Advocacy Project to identify problems, gather information related to the problems, and develop effective strategies to help solve the problems. They're focusing on a pattern of denials of coverage and reductions in services for people with AD that's emerged in recent years. They're working to get more effective coverage for Alzheimer's Disease incorporated into Medicare regulations.

### What's covered and what's not

Medicare doesn't cover long-term, non-acute care like that required by AD patients. Nor does it cover prescription medications, which is a sore point with a lot of seniors because the number of prescriptions written has jumped to an average of 28.5 prescriptions per senior per year in 1999, up from 19.6 in 1992. The average cost of a prescription has risen from $28.50 in 1992 to $42.30 in 1999 (the last year for which such statistics are available). Although seniors represent 13 percent of the general population, 34 percent of all prescriptions are dispensed to seniors, and they account for a disproportionate 42 percent of all prescription drug spending. There's currently a movement backed by several Congressmen, the AARP, and other senior advocacy groups to change Medicare regulations to cover long-term, non-acute care and prescriptions.

Even though most prescriptions aren't covered by Medicare, several state programs do provide assistance for seniors struggling to pay for their prescription medications. Medicare maintains a search engine at www.medicare.gov/Prescription/Home.asp that can help you determine if such a program is available in your area. Enter your zip code for the best results, or you can search by state.

In the current healthcare climate, drug prices are rising much faster than inflation, and pharmaceutical companies, despite their claims to the contrary, have the healthiest profit margins of any Fortune 500 companies — an average 16.5 percent net profit from 1993 through 1999 compared to an average 5 percent profit for all other Fortune 500 companies combined. This price hike puts many seniors in a tremendous financial crunch and often forces them to choose between paying their rent and buying food, or buying their prescriptions. Government agencies are being asked to address this issue as well.

If you have questions about your Medicare coverage and what services are available, visit www.medicare.gov/Coverage/Home.asp. Scroll down to the box entitled "Select Search Criteria" and select your state and the subject you're interested in, and click "View Results."

### The rules, paperwork, and hassle

Although Medicare was a good idea on paper, in reality, it's grown into a dense tangle of sometimes conflicting rules and regulations — as many as 100,000 pages of them at last count — that doctors and hospitals must adhere to in order to get reimbursed by the government for the services they render to patients. Many doctors and hospitals complain because they aren't reimbursed in a timely fashion or never get reimbursed at all for the services they provide because Medicare denies the claims. They then have to try to collect the entire balance owed from their patients who are often seriously ill and unable to satisfy their 20 percent co-pay, much less the entire bill.

A high profile 1999 conviction of two officers of the Hospital Corporation of America for alleged Medicare fraud was recently thrown out in April 2002 by a federal appeals court judge who found that the officers' interpretation of the convoluted and contradictory Medicare regulations was at least as reasonable as the government's, meaning that no fraud had occurred, only an honest disagreement as to what the regulations actually specified as acceptable Medicare billing practices.

As a result of this bureaucratic nightmare, many doctors today refuse to accept new Medicare patients, making it increasingly difficult for senior citizens to find good healthcare at an affordable price. In addition, many of the companies that used to underwrite Medicare Part B coverage have pulled out of that business, citing their inability to make a profit due to slow pay and continually reduced reimbursements by the federal government. To make matters worse, Congress keeps adding new Medicare regulations, price controls, and coverage limits, clouding an already murky picture.

Want more bad news? Medicare reimbursements are based upon regional *Fee For Service* (FFS) norms, which can vary wildly from one city, county, or state to the next. So if you live in Miami, Florida, local regulations may allow you to get coverage for prescription drugs, which isn't available to Medicare recipients in Houston, Texas. HMOs that provide Medicare services in Miami are reimbursed at nearly twice the rate for the same services as HMOs in Minneapolis-St. Paul, Minnesota. No one can offer a credible explanation for these variables; they just exist. And in order to make good financial decisions for your loved one, you have to be aware of them.

Congress is discussing what to do about the impending epidemic of Alzheimer's Disease cases. Some Congressmen are arguing that people with AD should be classified as disabled so that they can receive disability benefits both from government and private insurance resources. Others are trying to rewrite Medicare regulations so that long-term disabilities, such as AD, are covered.

So how do you thread your way through all the paperwork? For starters, you can visit the Medicare Web site at www.medicare.gov/default.asp and click on "Medicare Personal Plan Finder." After you enter your zip code, this specialized search engine asks you a few questions and quickly help you search out the best Medicare plans for your situation.

If you need more assistance, contact the State Health Insurance Assistance Program for one-on-one counseling and assistance with Medicare problems. The people there can help you select the right coverage for your situation, solve billing and claim problems, and provide referrals for low-income seniors to receive assistance from a variety of community organizations. To find the nearest local chapter, call 800-MEDICARE and ask for health insurance counseling or visit www.medicare.gov/Contacts/Related/Ships.asp.

## Medicaid

Medicaid is an insurance program that's jointly sponsored by the federal government and individual states that provides medical services for low-income individuals. Although the program is funded by the federal government, it's administered by the states, which each establish their own eligibility standards and determine the type, amount, duration, and scope of services. They also set the rate of payment for services.

Most Medicaid services are delivered to families with children, but they're also available to certain older people who meet their state's guidelines for assistance. To qualify, a person must

✔ Be 65 years of age or older, or blind, or disabled

✔ Be a U.S. citizen with a Social Security number and be a legal resident of the state where the application is made

✔ Have total gross assets, income, and personal property that meet certain standards; to look up federal poverty level guidelines for your state, visit www.elderweb.com and click on the "Regions" tab

✔ Fill out and sign an application and undergo an interview with a Medicaid specialist

Because Medicaid eligibility may change from month to month because of changes in income or resources, Medicaid cards originally were supposed to be valid for one month only and had to be renewed every month. However, as a practical matter, eligibility is re-determined on an annual basis. If you have questions, seek out an attorney that specializes in Medicaid qualifications.

## Medigap

Medigap, also known as Medicare plus Choice, is private insurance intended to help people cover the cost of the "gaps" in Medicare coverage. Medigap covers co-insurance payments and deductibles and, in some cases, may even cover medical supplies and prescription drugs. Consult your insurance agent to see what coverage is available in your location.

Be aware that if you purchase a Medigap plan, it must cover at least the same benefits offered under Part A and Part B Medicare. Depending on the type of coverage you select, you may have additional benefits, such as prescription drugs or extra days in the hospital.

You should also know that many insurance carriers have dropped their Medigap policies because they claim that getting reimbursements from the government in a timely fashion is too difficult.

If you're having trouble locating a Medigap plan provider, fill out the form available at www.medicare.gov/Coverage/Home.asp. This is Medicare's Personal Plan Finder, which can help you locate suitable insurance carriers in your state.

## Private insurance

Private insurance can include your regular health insurance as well as long- or short-term disability coverage. Talk to the human resources benefits counselor at your loved one's place of employment to see what sort of coverage your loved one has in place.

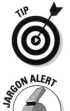

Get copies of your loved one's policies and read them through from the first page to the last, paying particular attention to information about coverage of chronic illness and long-term disability.

*Disability insurance* is different from health insurance in that it provides a cash payment to help people cover their basic living expenses in the event that they become ill and are unable to work for an extended period of time. *Extended* or *long-term care policies* are used to help pay for home or residential or adult daycare for your loved one as his AD progresses and care requirements increase.

According to the American Association of Retired Persons (AARP), about 50 percent of seniors over the age of 65 will ultimately require long-term care, either in the home or in a care facility. Long-term care policies range from $500 to several thousand dollars per year, depending on age, the benefits selected, and location. But you have to plan ahead; after your loved one is diagnosed with AD, they're no longer eligible to purchase long-term coverage.

Insurance experts recommend long-term care coverage for families with extensive assets they want to protect. Because it's expensive, it's not something that every family will choose.

## Long-term care insurance

Long-term care insurance is meant to help families cover costs of providing for a loved one who has a degenerative condition or a chronic illness like AD. Some people are under the impression that the government pays for long-term care through Medicare or Medicaid, but it doesn't. Medicare only covers skilled nursing care for a short period of time following surgery, an accident, or a period of acute illness. Regular health insurance policies and Medigap insurance policies make no provision for long-term care either, so if it's something you think your family needs, you should get it right away. After a diagnosis of AD or any other chronic, incurable illness is made official, you or your loved one are no longer eligible to purchase a long-term care policy.

Depending on which options are selected when the policy is purchased, services can be provided in a variety of settings, including your home, assisted living centers, or nursing homes. Long-term care policies take effect when the insured is unable to perform basic self-care tasks for a period of 90 days or longer. Although exact coverage varies from company to company, long-term care usually provides a daily benefit to help cover the cost of hiring someone to provide assistance with the activities of daily living such as bathing, toileting, dressing, and eating.

Before you purchase a policy, visit www.longtermcareinsurance.org. The site, sponsored by The Long Term Care National Advisory Council, features lots of information to help you make the best decision when purchasing a long-term care policy.

## Help for veterans

Individuals who served in the military are eligible for a variety of benefits, including excellent healthcare and prescription benefits, along with some limited nursing home benefits. More than 50 percent of men over age 65 are veterans, and with today's coed military, that figure will someday include a high number of women as well.

For complete information about veterans' eligibility, visit www.va.gov/elig.

# Running Out of Resources: What Next?

No matter how well you plan, you may one day have to face the fact that your loved one is running out of money to cover his monthly expenses. Perhaps your loved one didn't have enough resources to begin with or maybe he's outlived your best projections and has started to chip away at his capital. You can try several strategies to buy yourself a few extra months or years of solvency.

## *Using permanent assets*

The most likely place to turn when looking for additional funds is your loved one's family home, particularly if it's paid off. You can get an equity loan that gives you a line of credit based upon the value of the house. The advantage of this type of credit line is that it's flexible to meet your needs and available for you to use whenever you need it without having to go back to the bank to reapply for another loan.

If the house isn't completely paid off, refinancing the mortgage may be a good idea if interest rates are low. Lower monthly house payments can put an additional hundred dollars or more back into your monthly budget. Call around to find the best rate and ask for a loan analysis to make sure that refinancing is a smart move for your situation.

Taking out a second mortgage on the home is also something to consider. A second mortgage allows you to consolidate your loved one's debts at a lower rate of interest. Depending upon how much equity has built up in the home over the years and how much you want to take out, you may be able to collect a substantial sum of money to help cover monthly bills.

If none of these ideas is practicable for you and your loved one has reached the point where he can no longer live on his own, you may want to consider selling the home. It might be the best way for you to access the cash you need to pay your loved one's bills.

While you're thinking about ways to raise money, take a look at your loved one's unused household possessions. You might raise a few thousand selling furniture and appliances, or even more if cars, collectibles, artwork, or jewelry are available to be sold. But even if you have a power of attorney giving you full authority over your loved one's possessions, if your loved one is capable of participating in decision-making, include him and, if he's married, his spouse to make sure that neither of them objects to your selling those particular items.

If neither you nor your loved one has any resources left to cover the cost of care, community organizations can help you. Call the nearest chapter of the Alzheimer's Organization for a list of local volunteer groups and charitable organizations available to assist people with AD and their families.

If you're unable to continue providing care, either for reasons of your own health or for lack of funds, it's possible to surrender your loved one to the custody of your state or local authorities. After your loved one becomes a ward of the state, he will be eligible for care in state facilities. Obviously, before you do this, you should check out the facility where your loved one will be housed to make sure that it meets your standards for cleanliness, safety, and compassionate personnel.

No matter what, give yourself credit for doing the best you could do over a long period of years and for stretching the available resources as far as they could go.

## Getting help from other family members

Don't wait until you've completely exhausted your financial resources to ask other family members to contribute money to your loved one's care. Just because you're the primary caregiver doesn't mean that you should have to shoulder the entire cost of providing that care. If you need help paying for sitters, daycare, or medical expenses, say so. Your other family members don't know what you need unless you tell them.

Make copies of your caregiving budget and send one to each family member who is in a position to offer financial assistance. Be specific about what you need. Don't demand that your sister pay $200 a month and your brother $400; you may not know their true financial situation. Tell them what you need and ask how much they can comfortably contribute on a regular basis. Even if it's just $50 a month, that's $50 less that you have to come up with.

Discussions about financial matters go more smoothly when the participants feel like they have the full picture, so be open and honest; don't hold anything back or overstate the problem.

## Getting help from your community

If you've run out of resources to provide care for your loved one, you may be able to get help from a variety of local resources. Call your local center of government, whether it's a city hall or county courthouse, and ask for the number of the local Council on Aging or any other organization that deals with the concerns of the elderly. Then call the organization to see what resources are available to help families in your situation.

You may be able to find an adult daycare center that offers either free care or rates that are based on a sliding scale according to your income. Some churches in your community may offer free respite care or help you find low-cost or volunteer sitters, drivers, and other types of helpers as needed.

Your state or local community may offer free or reduced-cost home health aides or free placement in a state-run nursing home if your family meets local income guidelines.

# Chapter 15

# Evaluating Care Options

· · · · · · · · · · · · · · · · · · · · · · · · · · · · · · · · · · · · · · · · · · · ·

· · · · · · · · · · · · · · · · · · · · · · · · · · · · · · · · · · · · · · · · · · · ·

As the number of families dealing with *Alzheimer's Disease* (AD) has continued to grow, the availability of good care options has blossomed as well. Your chance of finding a good adult daycare program and a decent selection of residential care options and qualified in-home care assistants has increased over the past several years. In fact, the range of options has grown to the point that trying to sort out what kind of care would be most suited to your family's situation can get pretty confusing.

When you're considering care options for your loved one, you have to face the fact that, at some point, you're going to need somebody's help. Even if you think that you can do it all by yourself, the time will come when you realize that you do need assistance, even if it's just in the form of a three-hour break a few afternoons a week.

In this chapter, we look at the various care options and discuss the pros and cons of each type of care. We define the standard of care for AD patients, so that you'll know what to look for and be able to determine whether the care being provided for your loved one is adequate.

You also discover good resources for caregivers, including organizations that can give you information on local services, advice and help with problems, as well as a link to other caregivers who are going through similar problems and who can lend a sympathetic ear.

# Identifying Your Options

When you sit down to start planning what sort of care would be most appropriate for your loved one, the first thing you and your loved one must do is discuss your goals and identify your options. If you have financial concerns, your local Council on Aging and Alzheimer's Association can point you to some community resources that may be able to help.

First, establish your goals. When making a plan for care, consider immediate, short term, and long term needs. Decisions about care may be influenced by many factors, including

- ✔ Patient safety
- ✔ Your health
- ✔ Your loved one's health
- ✔ The presence of certain behavioral symptoms
- ✔ The level of care needed on a daily basis
- ✔ Various practical issues such as financial considerations

Here are some questions to consider:

- ✔ Do you want to help your loved one maintain her independence for as long as possible, or would you prefer to get her into a more controlled environment right away?
- ✔ Do you want to keep your loved one in her own house, bring her to yours, or place her in a residential care facility?
- ✔ Will you be shouldering the bulk of the care, or will you hire someone else to come in and provide care?

You should make every effort, insofar as is practical and possible, to honor your love one's wishes. However, there may be times that you will have to be the "bad guy" and make an unpopular decision. This may be the case if your loved one wanted to continue living alone and driving despite evidence that it was no longer safe for him to do so.

Keep in mind that your loved one won't require as much care in the early stages of AD as he or she will in the later stages. For someone with very mild AD, perhaps all you will need is someone to ensure that medications are taken as prescribed. The care plan you start out with will change and become more comprehensive as your love one's condition progresses. Tables 15-1 and 15-2 present the various care options that are available for AD patients.

### Table 15-1    Respite Care Choices for Alzheimer's Disease Patients

| Respite Care Choice | Care Provider | Location | Cost |
|---|---|---|---|
| Informal unpaidcare | You or another family member, or neighbor | Your home or your loved one's home | No out-of-pocket cost other than medical bills, but you may have to adjust your work hours, take FMLA, or give up your job to provide care, depending on your loved one's level of need |
| Paid caregiver or companion service | You may contract with an individual or hire a paid caregiver from an agency | Your home or your loved one's home or elsewhere depending on need (e.g. acute illness requiring hospital stay — hire a sitter to stay with patient overnight in the hospital | U.S. Department of Labor reports average is $8.17 per hour Agency referred $12 to $25 per hour |
| Visiting nurse or home health aide for patient with co-existing medical needs | Home health aide, LVN, RN licensed to provide med-ical services | Same as paid caregiver | $25 to $50 per hour depending on cer-tification often covered my Medi-care or private insurance |
| Adult daycare | Paid staff and volunteers | Free-standing center for adults with dementia or affiliated with a hospital, church, or care facility | $35 per day and up; may include trans portation or provide it for a nominal fee; services such as bathing cost extra |
| Day healthcare for patients with AD and co-existing medical illness that requires nursing services | Paid staff | Free-standing facility or hospital-based | $50 per day and up; services such as bathing cost extra |

# Fast facts

Here are a few tidbits of info on elder care:

✔ According to the American Association of Retired Persons (AARP), in 2001, 22 percent of 45- to 55-year-olds were caring for or helping to financially support an older family member.

✔ The Kaiser Family Foundation reported in 2002 that an estimated 45 million family

caregivers provided 80 percent of the long-term care required in the United States.

✔ A 1997 survey by the National Alliance for Caregiving said that the typical caregiver is female, married, 46 years of age, and employed outside the home. One in five caregivers reported caring for a person who suffers from some sort of mental confusion or dementia, including Alzheimer's Disease.

| Table 15-2 | Residential Care Choices for Alzheimer's Disease Patients | | |
|---|---|---|---|
| *Residential Care Choice* | *Care Provider* | *Location* | *Cost* |
| Assisted living | Paid staff | Assisted-living center | $27,000 a year and up |
| Licensed residential care home (also called a personal care home) | On-site non-medical staff | Neighborhood home licensed to provide care for a certain number of people on site | $850 to $4,000 per month, depending upon location and client need |
| Dedicated Alzheimer's care center or memory support unit | On-site medical and non-medical staff, visiting medical staff | Alzheimer's care center; maybe free-standing or be part of a continuing care retirement community that offers all levels of care from independent living to assisted living to AD care | $44,000 to $54,000 a year on average |
| Nursing home | On-site medical and and non-medical staff, visiting medical staff | Nursing home | $36,000 to $100,000 annually, depending upon location |

A common misconception exists that after someone reaches the age of 65, the government pays for all that person's medical needs, including long-term care. Unfortunately, that's simply not true. See Chapter 14 for more info on how much the government covers.

# Respite Care Options

Early on, the vast majority of patients with AD live in their own homes with minimal support from others. While 20–30 percent of patients with AD live alone, many live at home with spouses or relocate to live with a relative, usually an adult child. As cognitive abilities decline and the need for supervision or assistance with day-to-day activities of living increase, more time is required of the caregiver. In addition to the financial impact of paid care (Medicare doesn't pay for someone to come to your home and provide companion care), providing care at home can exact a profound psychological cost from the caregiver. What is important to remember is that you do not have to provide all the help that may be needed. A variety of options are available to you, and your care plan may include a combination of the in-home unpaid care you provide plus enrollment of your loved one in a daycare program and a few afternoons or days a week of paid companion care.

 In 1997, the National Alliance for Caregiving reported that 29 percent of caregivers acknowledged they'd deliberately passed up a promotion or the opportunity to receive additional job training in order to keep taking care of their loved one. Twenty-five percent reported passing up the chance to transfer to another location.

## Caring for your loved one at home

Many families feel that they don't have any other choice but to care for their loved ones at home without assistance. According to the Alzheimer's Association, 28 percent of caregivers have annual incomes of less than $20,000. Financial constraints force them to personally shoulder the burden of providing care for their loved ones. Families that have higher incomes and even two-income families may find themselves caught in that proverbial "sandwich" between the financial needs of their elderly parents and the financial needs of their college-age children. When money's tight, providing in-home care rather than spending thousands for care outside the home seems like the best choice. In fact, two-thirds of families caring for an AD patient choose in-home care for their initial care option.

### The benefits

Providing in-home care in your loved one's home or in your own home has some concrete benefits:

- ✔ You may worry less because you believe you can better keep an eye on your loved one.

- ✔ You have the opportunity to spend more quality time together.

- ✔ Your loved one may feel more independent.

- ✔ You know that your loved one is being well cared for and treated with love and compassion.

- ✔ Other family members may be able to help provide care as needed.

- ✔ You may feel a unique, deep sense of pride and accomplishment in your role as caregiver.

- ✔ You may learn things about yourself that you might have overlooked had you not become a caregiver. For example, you may find that you are more caring, supportive, nurturing than you knew, or perhaps you learn that you are an effective problem-solver who possesses great organizational skills.

- ✔ You get in touch with your ability to advocate for yourself and your loved one.

- ✔ You may learn that you are a resilient person.

### The drawbacks

Now for the cons:

- ✔ You may have to invest some money in refitting the house to accommodate your loved one's needs if the disease is severely advanced or if they have a co-existing medical illness. For example, you may have to install a grab bar in the bathtub and a toilet seat booster. However, funds may be available from the state or federal programs to offset the cost of these modifications.

- ✔ The strain of providing round-the-clock care by yourself and or overseeing paid caregivers can create a tremendous amount of physical and psychological stress and lead to health problems for the caregiver.

- ✔ Serving as a primary caregiver can negatively impact your marriage and your family relations.

- ✔ Serving as a primary caregiver can adversely affect your career.

- ✔ Creating space for your loved one in your home can lead to crowding for other family members. For example, siblings who previously had their own rooms may have to share a room, which can lead to problems.

- ✔ You may have to prepare a special menu to address your loved one's nutritional needs.

- ✔ You'll have very little free time for yourself and your family.

- ✔ The additional costs associated with caring for your loved one may impose a financial strain on your family.

- ✔ No matter how diligent you are, your loved one may still wander away or have an accident, which can lead to feelings of guilt for the caregiver.

Although it may sound like a lot of negatives are associated with providing in-home care, you can do many things to make it a more positive experience for the whole family. See Chapter 16 for a complete overview of what's involved in in-home caregiving, and how you can make it as stress-free and rewarding as possible.

### Cost issues

A 2002 study conducted by UCLA found that while direct costs (including prescriptions and doctor visits) of caring for an AD patient in the home average about $3,100 for a six-month period, the actual costs, including unpaid caregiver hours and time lost from work, brings the average cost to $30,000 for six months. For patients with milder symptoms still in the earlier stages of AD, the six-month figure was much lower, about $20,000.

## Paid in-home care

Perhaps you want to keep your loved one in his own home for as long as you can, but you're unable to directly provide any of the care yourself. In that case, you can hire a home companion, also known as a paid caregiver to provide the care.

Your loved one's condition and social needs determine the number of hours required for the outside help. If your loved one's in the early stages of AD and lives alone, she can probably handle most if not all of her day-to-day responsibilities. You should let her know you're going to monitor how effectively she' is handling these responsibilities, and discuss the possibility of eventually hiring a paid caregiver to come a few hours in the morning to make sure that she gets dressed and eats properly and takes her medications as directed, You and your loved one can define a paid caregiver's role according to current needs. Perhaps she needs or would enjoy having someone come in to cook or do laundry and other household chores. If your loved has been told to stop driving, a paid companion can serve as a driver/chauffeur.

It doesn't make sense to ask a person with memory problems to remember to take their medication.

Although home companions can perform a variety of tasks, they aren't licensed to provide skilled nursing care. Their primary responsibilities will be to help your loved one with his or her more complex and basic *activities of daily living* (ADLs) — shopping, food preparation, household chores, driving, errands, personal hygiene, exercise coach, and medication oversight, and so on. If your loved one needs something like a daily insulin shot, a service that provides home health aides rather than home companion/homemaker/paid caregiving services is required.

The types of services provided by paid caregivers vary from agency to agency, and also depend upon what your loved one needs and how much you're willing to pay. Generally speaking, the more services an aide provides, the higher the hourly rate.

- **Personal care or ADLs:** Assistance with personal hygiene, such as bathing, dressing, and toileting. Some may be willing to supervise light exercise and get your loved one in and out of bed.

- **Household chores:** Light cleaning, shopping, laundry, dishes, meeting and supervising repairmen, and so on.

- **Nutrition:** Meal preparation and cleanup, supervision of meals and snacks, shopping or ordering of meals from outside sources like Meals on Wheels.

- **Supervisory:** Transportation to doctor's appointments, daycare and senior centers, and so on.

- **Social services:** Companionship and activity planning.

- **Safety:** Ensuring that medication is taken appropriately. Inspection of premises for safety hazards, establishment of routine to ensure the safety of the AD patient. Making sure that the patient doesn't get injured, lost, or disoriented.

### The benefits

The pros of hiring a home health aide:

- Relieves you of the responsibility of providing care all by yourself

- Can help maintain your loved one in a familiar and comforting environment

- Can establish a daily routine for your loved one, which may include in home and outside activities (that is, going to museums, the park, shopping, visiting friends, eating out for lunch, and so on)

- Can help broaden your loved one's social network

- Can help safeguard your loved one

- Can help ensure that your loved one doesn't become exclusively dependent on you for care

- Companion may become like a member of your family after a long period of employment

### The drawbacks

The cons of hiring a home health aide:

- ✔ An aide can't provide medical services. You'll have to hire a visiting nurse if you want this type of service

- ✔ The cost of service — Medicare doesn't pay for the cost of a home companion

- ✔ Even with careful screening, occasionally, a home health aide turns out to be unsuited to the job, either by reason of dishonesty, neglect, roughness or abusiveness, or failure to perform the job adequately, or just a bad personality match with your loved one,

Although aides that you hire yourself can cost much less to employ, you do run a higher risk of encountering problems than you would with an aide from an agency because all reputable agencies have rigorous screening protocols to ensure a consistent quality of service.

### Finding a home health aide

You can start by checking the bulletin board in your local senior center or community center. People looking for work as aides often post their credentials there. If you can't locate any potential candidates that way, place an ad in the local paper or post a notice at the senior center. If you're a member of your church, ask around to see if anyone is interested in the job or has used such a service. Talk to co-workers, call assisted living or other care facilities to see if someone is seeking additional part time work, or call the Alzheimer's Association for information on local agencies.

The Family Caregiver Alliance has an excellent fact sheet entitled "Hiring In-Home Help" located at www.caregiver.org/factsheets/hiring_help.html. This guide can help you assess your needs, write a job description, rehearse a sample interview, and determine whether to use an agency or privately hire a home health aide. It also helps you locate resources within your own community that may be able to assist you in your search. Or look at New Lifestyles: The Source for Seniors at www.NewLifeStyles.com for an area guide to senior care options for more than 45 metropolitan areas across the United States.

You and your loved one should interview several candidates. Allow your loved one time to ask questions of the candidate and interact with him to assess whether they could be compatible. Also be sure to do the following:

- ✔ Ask for a work history and references, and actually call them, even if the person is someone you know.

- ✔ Discuss salary requirements.

- ✔ Ask whether the candidate has dependable transportation.

✔ Ask what services the aide will provide and what hours he or she is available to work.

✔ Clearly outline what the aide's responsibilities will be and invite him or her to ask any questions about the job and about your expectations and requirements.

✔ Describe a difficult scenario and ask them how they would handle it.

✔ Ask them if they know what AD is and what it means to them. This will give you a sense of their knowledge and experience of the disease, as well as their personal perception of those afflicted by it.

✔ Ask them why they chose to go into this line of work, particularly their desire to work with patients with AD.

✔ If a free training program for caregivers of patients with AD is available through your local Alzheimer's association, would they be willing to attend?

✔ Would they be willing to read literature suggesting ways to care for patients with AD?

For a different approach to finding a home health aide or companion, careguide.com maintains a great site to at `www.careguide.com/Careguide/educationcontentview.jsp?ContentKey=890`. The guide is chock full of sensible information that can walk you through the entire process from interviewing to checking references to hiring.

Tell the aide about your loved one's condition, but don't make the mistake of talking about your loved one as if he wasn't right there in the room with you — this dehumanizes the person with AD and can make him or her very angry or unhappy! Also tell the potential employee about any special needs your loved one has, such as requiring assistance with toileting or dressing.

Check with your insurance agent to see whether you need to adjust your policy to cover an in-home employee. When you do hire someone, make the job offer in writing, specifying hours, duties, and salary. Tell the aide how often you'll pay him or her, and on what days. Make a copy of the aide's Social Security card and driver's license. You'll need the card for tax purposes and the driver's license copy as a security measure. These steps can avoid a lot of confusion later on.

If, for whatever reason, the aide you hired doesn't prove to be a satisfactory choice and you find it necessary to replace the aide, give him or her written notice and a couple of weeks' severance pay to tide the aide over until he or she can find another job. Although you're not strictly required by law to offer notice and severance pay, it's a generous gesture that can go a long way toward smoothing out any difficulties that the firing may bring up.

If you pay the aide more than $1,400 a year, you must deduct Social Security and Medicare taxes from his or her wages. Once a year, you're required to report the income to the Internal Revenue Service and pay the taxes you've deducted. By law, you must provide your employee with copies B and C of IRS form W-2 by January 31 of the year following the year the wages were paid. You have until the last day of February to send Copy A to the Social Security Administration.

After you do hire someone, make sure that you pay the Social Security and Medicare taxes that are due on the wages you pay them, or else Uncle Sam may pay you a visit. Consult your financial advisor or visit the Social Security Web site at www.ssa.gov/pubs/10021.html for information about the financial responsibilities of people who employ household workers. If you don't pay the taxes on time, you'll have to pay the overdue taxes plus a penalty.

### Considering a live-in

You may prefer to have someone live in the house with your loved one, especially if your loved one is living alone. Providing room and board should allow you to negotiate a better hourly rate for services.

Follow the same procedures to find a live-in aide as you would for one who comes into your home to work. After you've made your selection, you need to figure out where you're going to house the person you've chosen.

Hiring someone to live in your or your loved one's home and then trying to cram that person into a broom closet is unfair. The aide should have his or her own private, clean, furnished room with adequate space to store personal belongings. Get your junk out of there before he or she moves in. The aide should either have his or her own bathroom or access to a nearby bath. You should discuss your expectations for use of the kitchen and other common areas of the house.

---

# What to look for in a caregiver

Everyone's personality is different, but you should look for a few key personality characteristics when seeking a caregiver for your loved one. The candidate should be

✔ Cheerful, upbeat, positive

✔ Patient and understanding

✔ Even-tempered

✔ Mature, sensible, cool-headed

✔ Caring, compassionate, empathetic

Just because someone is living in your home doesn't mean that he or she is available to work around the clock seven days a week. The aide is an employee, not a slave. Agree on his or her duties and draw up a written schedule before the aide starts work, and then stick to it. If, you require the aide to work more than 40 hours in one week, you should be prepared to pay him or her overtime, which is generally one and a half times his or her regular hourly rate.

Keep in mind, your live in will need a certain amount of time off per week, and may have an emergency that requires immediate attention. When you rely on others to provide care, you have to be ready to fill in or have a contingency plan in place to cover their responsibilities. See the following for options.

### Finding a home health agency

If you don't want the hassle of screening candidates and have neither the time nor the inclination to deal with tax forms and Social Security, you should probably hire your aide through an agency. Home health agencies take most of the work out of finding an aide because they've pre-screened all their candidates and send out only the people who meet their standards to interview for jobs. Best of all, you pay the agency, and they pay their aides, so you don't ever have to worry about collecting Social Security taxes and dealing with the IRS — at least not on your aide's account.

But using an agency does have a downside: Agencies frequently use a rotation of personnel to provide care, so the person sent to look after your loved one on Monday may be different from the person sent on Tuesday. This lack of consistency can be very upsetting and confusing for AD patients.

On the other hand, if one aide is sick, a qualified substitute is automatically sent, which means that you don't have to scramble trying to arrange last-minute care the way you would if you'd hired an aide privately.

You need to give the agency a complete overview of your loved one's physical and mental status, so that the staff can assign someone who's qualified to handle your needs. Review the information we provide under "Finding a home health aide" earlier in this chapter and use it to discuss terms of employment with your agency aide. Let the aide know your loved one's schedule and preferences, preferably in writing, and the duties you expect him or her to perform.

You can find a listing of home health agencies in the yellow pages, but of course, that doesn't give you much information about an agency's track record. Ask your loved one's doctor for a referral to an agency that he or she trusts, and ask friends who've used an agency and if they were satisfied with the care provided.

If, for whatever reason, the first companion the agency sends over doesn't work out, you can simply call the agency and ask for new candidates for the position. Of course you will want to make it clear from the beginning that you will be expecting the same companion to be coming each time.

### *Knowing when you need a visiting nurse*

Sometimes, your loved one needs more care than a home health aide can provide. If your loved one has multiple health issues, such as AD and diabetes or AD and heart disease, he or she will also require a visiting nurse. A visiting nurse can provide medical services that a home health aide can't, such as changing dressings, giving injections, monitoring vital signs, and so on. Visiting nurses provide services ranging from highly skilled nursing care to physical and occupational therapy, as well as hospice care for terminally ill patients.

Members of the Visiting Nurse Associations of America have a mission to provide compassionate, high-quality, cost-effective home health and hospice care in their respective communities through skilled nursing and therapy services and home health aides. To find a Visiting Nurse Association near you, enter your zip code in the search box at www.vnaa.org/vnaa/GeneralContentPages/ GeneralContentPage1.aspx?theHTML=HTML/Home.html&theCurrentChoice= Home.

Some nurse visits are covered by Medicare, especially if your loved one has just been discharged from a hospital. But generally speaking, hiring a visiting nurse is an expense that you'll have to cover.

## *Adult daycare*

If your loved one isn't yet ready for a nursing home but you don't feel that your situation is conducive to providing in-home care, adult daycare is for you. Adult daycare for people with dementia and its newer cousin, adult day healthcare, can be a real godsend for a two-career family that simply can't provide in-home care and doesn't particularly like the idea of leaving their loved one alone all day with an aide. Adult daycare provides some real benefits for AD patients as well, giving them the chance to socialize and participate in enjoyable activities with their peers in a safe and controlled professional environment.

Adult daycare evolved from the child daycare model; but should never be confused with child care. These programs are geared toward adults, with adult activities tailored to meet the capabilities of the participants, and an atmosphere designed for adults. Adult daycares are usually open five days a week during traditional business hours. These programs are designed to meet the needs of both functionally and cognitively impaired older adults, though programs can vary depending on the population they are targeting. In other words, some daycare programs are designed for patients with mild-moderate AD, while others cater to the needs of those with more advanced AD. Some adult daycare facilities provide transportation. All provide hot meals on the premises as well as some health monitoring and support services such as medication reminders and blood pressure screening. In addition to providing respite for the caregiver, these programs provide enjoyable and appropriate social activities and engagement for those with AD. Having AD does not mean that you no longer have a need to feel meaningful or socially connected to others. We all need a reason to get up in the morning and attendance at a day program can provide a sense of purpose.

AD patients are often leery of change, so you may encounter some resistance when you first pose the idea to your loved one. This is to be expected. Acknowledge that they have some "healthy skepticism," and reassure them that you will preview the program together. If you ask whether they want to go, you are almost certain to get a no. You would be wiser to ask if they would prefer to preview the "wellness center, senior center, or activity center" on Monday or Wednesday, thereby giving them a choice and sense of control but not the final decision about whether to go. Keep in mind that it may not be necessary for your loved one to know that they are formally enrolled in the program. You can tell them that they are attending on a volunteer basis. The staff of the day center is probably very familiar with this approach and will be most willing to acknowledge him as a helper or volunteer rather than a paid subscriber. Once you initiate enrollment, try to stick with it for a few weeks before quitting. After your loved one settles in, makes a few friends, and starts participating in the activities, he or she may begin bugging you to go to daycare even on the weekends.

Adult day healthcare offers more comprehensive care for patients who require specific medical or psychiatric supervision. It provides services, such as on-site nurses, social workers, physical therapists, and other medical and caregiving professionals, in addition to the social activities, meals, and transportation services offered by regular adult daycare.

The nice thing about these programs is that they don't use a "one size fits all" approach. Activities are tailored to your loved one's interests, needs, and abilities. One AD patient who has mobility problems may meet with a counselor while other patients who are more mobile participate in a light exercise class. Another patient may visit with a nurse and then join his fellow patients for a snack or musical entertainment. But the most important function adult daycare serves is that it eliminates the problem of social isolation that can overwhelm an AD patient who stays at home all the time. These places offer so many enjoyable planned activities, from crafts to music to board games, that your loved one is sure to find something to enjoy.

### Finding a daycare center

Adult daycare centers are licensed and regulated by the states where they're located, so you can be assured of a fairly consistent quality of care. But you still visit several centers with your loved one in advance, and once you narrow the field, check out the program and facilities and interview the personnel. This way, you'll be able to select a center that best fits your loved one's interests and personality, which gives you a better chance of a successful experience.

The following sources can help you find a good adult daycare center:

- ✔ The Administration on Aging maintains a comprehensive Web site with information about adult daycare at `www.aoa.gov/NAIC/Notes/adultday.html`.

- ✔ The National Adult Day Services Association maintains a searchable directory at `https://host.softworks.ca/AGate3/directory/?f=NADSA%2E0002`.

- ✔ You can visit the federally sponsored Eldercare Locator at `www.eldercare.gov/search.asp` and enter your state and zip code to obtain a list of organizations in your area that can help you locate appropriate care for your loved one.

### Knowing what to look for in a center

Look for a pleasant, secure, comfortable atmosphere that has plenty of space and good lighting. The facility shouldn't be cluttered or crowded, because that can lead to falls or other accidents. Patients should be attended to and well supervised involvement and ensure safety. The staff should be courteous, compassionate and caring, and experienced in dealing with the needs of older adults with dementia.

For more information on what to look for in a daycare center, a terrific checklist is available at `www.gltc.jhancock.com/facts/daycare_checklist.cfm`.

If the center provides transportation, inspect the vehicle the staff uses to make sure that it has an adequate number of seat belts and that the driver takes the time to belt each passenger. If your loved one uses a walker, wheelchair, or scooter, does the center have a way to transport the mobility equipment back and forth? Watch the driver for a few minutes to satisfy yourself that safety considerations are being observed.

Here are some other questions you should ask:

- ✔ What's the ratio of paid staff to attendees?
- ✔ Are the activities provided stimulating, enjoyable, age and cognitively appropriate?
- ✔ Are activities available for both large and small groups?
- ✔ Is the dining area clean? Are the meals nutritious and appealing?
- ✔ If your loved one has special nutritional concerns, such as a diabetic diet, can the center accommodate that?
- ✔ Can the center provide emergency medical care if your loved one needs it?

Don't forget to ask your loved one for input. If you're considering two or more centers, ask your loved one for his or her preference. If your loved one has had a hand in the choice, he or she will make a more successful transition to adult daycare.

# Making the Transition to Residential Care

No matter what sort of care approach you ultimately decide on, the first few weeks right after you start the new care arrangements may be difficult because it represents a change for both you and your loved one. Some older people are happy to get out from under the burden of caring for their home and into a more protected and supportive environment, but others will fight you tooth and nail if you so much as bring up the topic for discussion. You may encounter anger, bitterness, tears, grief, and accusations that you don't really care for your loved one and are just trying to shuffle her off into a corner somewhere to get her out of the way. Just knowing that these problems may crop up and having a plan in place to deal with them is half the battle.

Don't beat yourself up if the biggest feeling you experience after placing your loved one in a residential care facility is a huge blast of relief. Caregiving places profound burdens on the caregiver; if you've provided care for a number of years or even months, feeling relief at such a time is perfectly natural. Now, your relationship with your loved one will evolve into something new. You aren't finished caring for your loved one, but the nature of your work changes as you go from being a direct, hands-on caregiver to a care manager overseeing those providing the direct care.

Don't be surprised if you find yourself battling some difficult feelings of your own. Even if the thinking part of your brain knows that changing care settings is the best thing for your loved one, the emotional part of your brain may be weighing you down with guilt and an overwhelming sense of loss. You may feel like you've abandoned your loved one. Nothing could be further from the truth. Keep in mind that what's changing the caregiving situation is Alzheimer's Disease, not you.

Making sure that your loved one feels included in the decision-making and preparation process can help the transition. Take a tour of your loved one's new home and encourage her to ask any questions she may have. Give your loved one the opportunity to meet other residents and staff members and socialize. Visit at lunchtime so you can enjoy a meal together. Understand how very difficult it might be for someone who's lived in the same house for years, surrounded by family keepsakes and treasured possessions, to have to give up most of what she owns in order to move into a care facility. Help your loved one choose a few truly meaningful things to bring to her new home. Reassure her that her things will be kept safe and allow her to grieve the loss of a way of life she may have cherished. Offer support and hope for a "new chapter" in her life and reassure her that you will be a constant part of that chapter. Some caregivers make a scrapbook with favorite family photographs and include pictures of the family home, inside and out, to remind your loved one of the happy memories associated with the house. However, don't be disappointed if the person with AD shows little interest in this, or if reviewing it together sparks a negative reaction or no reaction at all. If you do use it, use it to reminisce and story tell, and not to quiz your loved one on his or her recall of their previous residence.

Another good idea is to move the furniture and other belongings in before your loved one arrives. This way, when your loved one arrives at his new living quarters, the room will be well organized and inviting. Arranging two or three pieces of furniture in a familiar setting with some of the same decorative objects that your loved one had at home is a good way to bring a little piece of his former surroundings with him into his new life. This gesture can be very comforting and help to cut down on the feeling of strangeness your loved one may experience when he first moves into his new place.

Patience and understanding can go a long way toward helping your loved one make a smooth transition to his new home. But if either one of you still has difficulty coping with your emotions after a few weeks, seek the advice of a professional to help you over the rough patch.

## How will I know when it's time for full time residential care?

The goal of effective management of Alzheimer's Disease is to keep the patient independent and living in a familiar environment for as long as possible. But you can watch for some signs that signal the time to place your loved one in a residential facility.

- ✔ You can no longer control your loved one's wandering.

- ✔ His or her nighttime restlessness is keeping the rest of the family from getting a good night's sleep.

- ✔ Your loved one's behavior is becoming increasingly unmanageable.

- ✔ He or she is frequently incontinent.

- ✔ Your loved one's had a fall or some other sort of accident.

- ✔ The strain of providing round-the-clock in-home care is threatening your family's stability.

# Residential Care Options

No matter how wonderful the care you give and your willingness to use respite services, the day may come when you simply can no longer provide the kind of care your loved one requires, in your home. Full-time residential care is a necessary consideration for many, many families caring for someone with AD. For many, it becomes a necessary step to keep their loved one safe and healthy. It is also a step that caregivers take when the level of care required becomes overwhelming. In the next section we discuss the various kinds of residential care available for AD patients. Even if you never intend to use this, it's wise to know about residential care and explore the options for placement in your community. It's better to be prepared to make a decision and do so before a crisis precipitates one.

Don't let anyone fool you: Making the decision to place your loved in a full-time residential care facility is probably one of the most difficult a caregiver can experience. It becomes even more difficult if you promised your loved one to never put them in a home. You may encounter some stiff resistance from your loved one when you first broach the subject of residential care, but don't let that sway you. You must make the decision based upon what's best for your loved one and for your family.

In all residential care situations you'll have some basic questions. For example:

- ✔ Will your loved one have a private bath or have to share a bath?
- ✔ Will you be able to install a private phone line in his or her room, or will your loved one have to use a community phone?
- ✔ Are the doors of individual rooms or suites equipped with locks?
- ✔ How often are housekeeping and laundry services provided?
- ✔ What social and entertainment activities are provided?

These questions are just the beginning. You can locate good checklists online at the following locations:

- ✔ Assisted Living Checklist: www.alfa.org/public/articles/details.cfm?id=75
- ✔ Nursing Home Checklist: www.medicare.gov/Nursing/Checklist.pdf

After you've made the decision to place your loved one in a residential care facility, you need to decide what kind of facility is right for his or her needs and your financial situation. The following sections describe the various types of facilities that are available for AD patients.

# Assisted living centers

Some people are confused by the idea of assisted living, thinking it means that someone comes into your home to assist your loved one. Actually, assisted living centers are full-time residential care facilities where the residents have their own apartments but are assisted with the activities of daily living. Your loved one's privacy and some sense of independence are maintained, but he or she has an added level of security and access to services needed to stay healthy and independent, yet supervised and safe.

The *Assisted Living Federation of America* (ALFA) defines assisted living as the following: "A special combination of housing, personalized supportive services, and healthcare designed to meet the needs — both scheduled and unscheduled — of those who need help with activities of daily living."

## What they offer

Placing your loved one in an assisted living center has many advantages. Perhaps the best, at least from your loved one's point of view, is that your loved one will still be living in a private home-like setting surrounded by familiar and comforting furniture and many of his or her "treasures," such as family photographs and keepsakes.

From your point of view, the best news is that assisted living is surprisingly affordable, even cheaper than keeping your loved one in his or her own home with a home health aide. How can this be? Well, after your loved one moves into an assisted living center, all the expenses associated with maintaining his or her residence — mortgage payments, taxes, upkeep, repairs, and so on — all just go away. In addition, if you've been paying a home health aide to watch your loved one, that expense disappears as well.

Assisted living centers are able to offer a high level of comprehensive services through economy of scale. Whereas it might be prohibitively expensive for 25 families to each hire a visiting nurse, when a 25-unit assisted living facility hires a full-time nurse to monitor the health needs of its residents, it makes good economic sense. Not every resident needs to see the nurse every day, but the nurse is there and quickly available when residents do need medical attention. According to ALFA, about one million residents are currently living in approximately 20,000 assisted living residences throughout the United States.

What should you look for in an assisted living residence? The Assisted Living Federation of America says that the following services are required for a balanced and effective assisted living program:

- ✔ Three meals a day, served in a common dining area
- ✔ Housekeeping services
- ✔ Transportation

✔ Assistance with eating, bathing, dressing, toileting, and walking

✔ Access to health and medical services

✔ 24-hour security and staff availability

✔ Emergency call systems in each resident's unit

✔ Health promotion and exercise programs

✔ Medication management

✔ Personal laundry services

✔ Social and recreational activities

Assisted Living is not a good choice for patients who require around-the-clock nursing care or extensive medical care and monitoring.

### What they cost

Depending on your location, assisted living facilities cost between $1,500 to $6,000 per month. Except for medical services and the cost of prescriptions, all your loved one's basic needs, including food, social activities, household services, and basic medical monitoring, are covered by the monthly stipend. Assisted living isn't covered by Medicare, but in some states, Medicaid patients may qualify for help in covering assisted living expenses. Consult a caseworker at your local senior center for information regarding your state's regulations.

### Where to look

A number of search engines provide help in locating an assisted living facility near your home. ALFA's search engine at www.alfa.org/directory/ is confusing to use, but if you ignore its requests for Last Name, Company Name, and so on and simply enter your state, you get back an extensive list of providers. The problem is that they're arranged alphabetically, not by locale, so you'll have to scroll through the entire list to find a nearby facility.

Another good search engine, maintained by Total Living Choices, is located at www.tlchoices.com/finder/showwizardprocess.asp. You have to go through a free sign-up process, but the information you get is targeted to specific types of care facilities within 10 miles or less of your current home.

Some states have what's called *licensed residential care homes* or *board and care homes,* where patients are cared for in a small, private home setting. We discuss this form of care in the next section.

## Licensed residential care homes

Licensed residential care homes are known by many names — board and care homes, adult family homes, adult foster homes, or adult group home —

but they all provide similar services, such as room and board, assistance with daily activities, and, in some cases, minimal nursing services. Unlike nursing homes and assisted living facilities, board and care homes don't have to be licensed in all states. According to the American Health Care Association, as of December 2002, 1,455,571 patients were living in 16,454 nursing homes throughout the United States.

In smaller communities, board and care homes may well be the only nearby choice available to families looking to place a loved one in a full-time residential setting. Care is frequently provided in single-family residences that have been modified to accommodate the needs of elderly residents. Generally, such homes care for no more than six patients at a time.

Although many such homes provide excellent care for their residents, instances of abuse have been reported, particularly in unlicensed homes. Before you decide to place your loved one in a board and care home, visit the facility several times. Note whether the other residents seem clean, content, and well cared for. Ask to see the room your loved one will be occupying, and if you'll be allowed to bring some of his or her furnishings into the room. Ask for a written list of the services provided and a list of references and then talk to other families that have had loved ones in the facility to see if they were satisfied with the care their family member received.

Finally, if you do decide to place your loved one in a board and care home, make sure that the fees and all the services your loved one will receive are laid out in writing in a formal contract, so that there's no confusion about what you expect. Most of these homes offer different levels of services for varying fees; make sure that you don't sign up thinking you're getting one level of service only to find out that the facility charges additional fees to provide the services, such as laundry, that you thought your loved one would be getting.

## Dedicated Alzheimer Care Centers

If your loved one's AD is advanced or he or she has developed additional health problems, you must put him or her in either a dedicated Alzheimer's Care Center or a nursing home where he or she can get the medical care they need. Dedicated Alzheimer's Care Centers are facilities designed specifically to meet the needs of AD patients, with special services aimed at creating personal satisfaction, preserving self-esteem and dignity, and creating a sense of independence — all in a secure and nurturing environment. Although some Alzheimer's Care Centers provide adult daycare only, most are residential facilities that also provide some level of medical services. Frequently, dedicated Alzheimer's units are part of a larger facility, such as a nursing home, that provides full-time care for patients with a number of physical conditions.

# Nursing homes

Just like hospitals, nursing homes are staffed 24 hours a day by healthcare professionals and support personnel who provide medical and personal care services for residents. Generally speaking, at least three different levels of care are available: basic care, skilled nursing care, and sub-acute care, as well as dedicated Alzheimer's units in some locations. According to the 1999 Nursing Home Survey, the average length of stay in a nursing home is about two and a half years.

Residents in nursing homes or *skilled nursing facilities* as they're sometimes called, get a furnished room, meals and snacks, housekeeping and laundry services, and basic medical services such as monitoring and the administration of medications. They also receive supervision and help with their daily activities, usually from *licensed practical nurses* (LPNs). Additional services, such as transportation, physical and occupational therapy, and doctor visits may incur additional charges over the basic monthly rate.

Patients who require more medical care usually live in *skilled nursing units* where *registered nurses* (RNs), therapists, and rehabilitation specialists can provide for their special medical needs. Skilled nursing services are more expensive than basic care services.

Someone who's recovering from surgery or a serious illness requires placement in a *sub-acute unit,* which means that they're not as sick as they were while they were in the hospital, but they're still much frailer and require much more care than the other residents of the nursing home.

Finally, people with AD are frequently assigned to *dedicated Alzheimer's units,* where, in addition to the basic, skilled nursing or sub-acute services that their condition requires, they also receive services and activities designed to enhance their quality of life.

Medicaid and Medicare may pay for some portion of nursing home care, but only if the home is Medicare certified and only under certain qualifying circumstances. Medicare only covers care in a skilled nursing facility that follows a qualifying hospital stay, not custodial care, which is how most nursing home care is classified. Generally speaking, families that don't have long-term disability coverage must pay for nursing home care out of their own pockets.

Nursing homes are the most expensive type of care, costing anywhere from $2,000 to $10,000 a month, depending upon the level of services your loved one requires, your location, and how nice the nursing home is.

In order to achieve a successful nursing home placement, you and your loved one should visit several facilities to see which one you both like best. Try to schedule at least one visit at night and one on the weekend, so that you can see how the nursing home performs when staff members aren't expecting visits from potential residents and their families. Eat a meal or two to test the quality of the food. Check to see if the residents are clean and properly dressed and if they seem content or agitated. Does the staff treat residents with courtesy and compassion, or are they short-tempered? When working with residents, do staff members seem patient or impatient? Are sufficient activities available for residents, or do most of them just seem to be parked in wheelchairs and staring off into space? Are residents offered appropriate assistance with activities like eating and toileting?

Assess your loved one's needs and select a nursing home that seems best suited to fulfill those needs. Give the placement at least a month to see whether it's working out, but if your loved one doesn't like the facility and isn't making a good transition, don't be afraid to change facilities.

In many ways, placing your loved one in a permanent residential setting can be very difficult to deal with. You may realize that your loved one is nearing the end of his or her fight with AD, and you may be disappointed in yourself that you're not able to provide all the care he or she needs right up to the end. That's just one of the many stresses that caregivers must face.

---

# AARP's signs of a bad nursing home

Not every nursing home is a great place. The American Association of Retired Persons published the following list of warning signs of a bad nursing home. If you encounter one or more of these negative indications, run, don't walk, out of there and definitely *do not* place your loved one in that facility.

✔ **Odors:** A strong smell of urine and feces indicates a shortage of staff to help residents to the bathroom or to keep residents and the facility clean.

✔ **Restraints:** Vests and other devices that tie or otherwise hold people down in their beds and wheelchairs are dangerous and humiliating. Good nursing homes seek safe and respectful ways to protect residents from falls and wandering.

✔ **Lack of privacy:** Residents should not be undressed or partly dressed in rooms or hallways in view of guests and other residents. Staff should knock before entering rooms.

✔ **Lack of dignity:** No resident should be spoken to disrespectfully.

✔ **Unanswered calls for help:** Every call bell or cry for help should be attended to promptly.

✔ **Loneliness and inactivity:** People-watching is fun, but residents shouldn't spend hours on end sitting at the nurses' station, front door, or in front of a TV.

✔ **Lack of help with eating:** Residents who can't feed themselves shouldn't spend the mealtime with full trays in front of them.

Information on more than 17,000 Medicare- and Medicaid-certified nursing homes is available for comparison on Medicare's Web site at www.medicare. gov/Nursing/Overview.asp. Scroll down the left side of the page and click on "Nursing Home Compare." On the next page, click on "Begin Nursing Home Search" to begin.

# Chapter 16

# Caring for the Alzheimer's Patient

· · · · · · · · · · · · · · · · · · · · · · · · · · · · · · · · · · · · · · · · · · · · · · ·

## In This Chapter

▶ Creating a care plan

▶ Explaining some key concepts in healthcare

▶ Understanding Alzheimer's Disease care standards

▶ Managing personal hygiene and nutrition

▶ Creating an exercise and activity plan

▶ Making a safe place for your patient

▶ Handling depression and other emotional problems

· · · · · · · · · · · · · · · · · · · · · · · · · · · · · · · · · · · · · · · · · · · · · · ·

*N*o matter what sort of approach you eventually choose to care for your loved one, throughout his illness you will be providing at least some of his care, and you will certainly be interacting with him on a regular basis whether you're serving as a direct, "hands-on" caregiver or as a "case manager." So it's important to familiarize yourself with the sort of behaviors you may encounter, and the type of assistance your loved one may need over the course of a typical day.

If we could recommend one word for you to remember around your loved one, we'd pick "patience." It can be mightily frustrating when AD patients repeat the same questions or stories over and over, lose things, then rummage through the house constantly looking for "lost" items, and accuse you or someone else of taking their things. As frustrating as these behaviors are, caregivers may ultimately face even more distressing behaviors including sleep disturbances, incontinence, irritability, agitation, restlessness, wandering, and verbal or physical aggression. But these behaviors are all part of the process, and getting mad at the person with AD won't make things any easier.

Make no mistake; having a family member diagnosed with Alzheimer's Disease presents one of the greatest challenges you may ever have to face. You're dealing not only with the gradual loss of the person as you once knew him, but also with having to provide thoughtful and compassionate care as this person slowly slips away and becomes more difficult to manage and less responsive to your care and compassion. As functional and cognitive skills decline, needs increase, and this escalating burden can be very difficult for caregivers to handle. Many caregivers experience feelings of grief and loss as their loved one is less able to respond to their needs and understand the demands of caregiving.

In this chapter, we go over the major issues you may have to deal with as an Alzheimer's caregiver, everything from choosing who in your family is going to serve as caregiver to a complete overview of the physical, emotional, and psychological challenges you and your loved ones could face together. Yes, you have a difficult task ahead, but if you stay focused, you can manage to take good care of your loved one, yourself, and your family, all at the same time.

# Making a Care Plan

Before you can provide care for your loved one, you must first determine what her needs are. If she's still able to prepare meals and perform household chores, then her needs are different from those of a person who can no longer operate a stove or run a washing machine.

Next, ask yourself what sort of care is required to maintain your loved one in either his or her own home or in your home or an alternative care setting. Who's going to provide this care? Will more than one family member be available to help? If you're reading this book, we assume that you are the person who has decided to provide most of the care your loved one requires.

Finally, using the information you've gathered, develop a schedule for your care plan. AD patients thrive on routine and may get upset when they don't know what to expect from one minute to the next. Performing each activity at around the same time each day gives shape and form to an AD patient's world and can help to settle his fears and make his behavior more manageable.

Over the course of the years that you'll be caring for your loved one, you will have many opportunities to take her around in your car — to a doctor's office, to pick up a prescription, to the grocery. NEVER under any circumstances whatsoever leave your loved one in a parked car, not even for a minute. She can get out and get lost, or, if it's a hot day, she can actually suffocate or have a heat stroke and die. ALWAYS take your loved one with you with you into a store or an office to run an errand. Or do these things while your loved one enjoys spending time with another responsible person or in a daycare facility.

## A sample daily schedule

This schedule presumes that your AD patient is ambulatory. Please note that naps are not included. Alzheimer's patients have trouble sleeping at night and naps can disrupt their schedules even further. This schedule is just a sample; adjust the schedule according to your loved one's level of cognitive and functional ability and your family's needs. A person with mild AD might have a schedule that reflects different interests or commitments; he or she may still be working or volunteering regularly. The important thing is to have a schedule and stick to it as nearly as possible.

7:00 to 7:30 a.m.: Get up and get dressed

7:30 to 8:00 a.m.: Eat breakfast, take medications, brush teeth

8:00 to 9:00 a.m.: Light activity such as walking, gardening, and so on

9:00 to noon: Activities away from home, such as doctor's appointments, shopping, beauty salon or an AD day program, or in-home activities such as simple games, television, listening to music

10:00 a.m.: Nutritious snack. Be sure to include this whether you're at home or out

Noon to 12:30 p.m.: Eat lunch, take medications if required

12:30 to 2:30 p.m.: Walking (to promote digestion), outdoor or community activity such as a trip to the zoo, botanical garden or museum

2:30 to 3:00 p.m.: Nutritious snack

3:00 to 6:00 p.m.: In-home activities, television, music, memory boxes, simple crafts

6:00 to 6:30 p.m.: Eat dinner, take medications if required

6:30 to 8:00 p.m.: Family time — simple games, songs, look at photo albums, watch home movies and videos

8:00 to 9:00 p.m.: Bathe, brush teeth, bedtime calming routine including music, gentle massage

9:00 p.m.: Bedtime

# Defining Practice Parameters and Standards of Care

In order to understand the type of medical care that is being provided for your loved one, you need to understand how doctors and other healthcare professionals decide how they are going to treat individual patients. In this section, we define Standard of Care. Then we define Practice Parameters, explain the difference between the two, and go over current Standards of Care and Practice Parameters for Alzheimer's patients. This information will give you a heads up on what to expect from your health care team and alert you if the care your loved one is receiving isn't what it should be.

Perhaps you've wondered how it is that doctors all across America, whether they're working in a 400-bed metropolitan hospital or a one-doctor rural clinic, all do pretty much the same thing when it comes to diagnosing and treating illness and injury. Whether they're presented with a case of the flu, a broken bone, a nagging cough, or a nasty burn, these doctors seem to have a good idea what to do about it, what tests to order, what medications to prescribe, and to know whether their patient should be admitted to the hospital or another care facility. How is this amazing synchronicity possible? Part of it is their education, of course, but what really keeps doctors on the same page are two things: Standards of Care and Practice Parameters that are clearly defined for each condition.

Doctors employ Practice Parameters before they decide upon a particular Standard of Care. However, we want to define Standards of Care first so that when you get to the section on Practice Parameters, you'll see how they work hand in hand with the Standards of Care.

*Practice Parameters* are guidelines for treating patients based upon proven and time-tested principles, meant to serve as both a reference and a screening tool to guide health care professionals in the diagnostic and treatment process, and to ensure that the decisions doctor's make are based upon the most current and reliable medical and scientific information and experience.

# Standards of Care

Standards of Care are the minimal levels of care, skill, and treatment that are recognized as appropriate and acceptable by the medical profession. Healthcare providers must adhere to these standards in order to provide an acceptable level of care for their patients. Standards of Care may include things like medications, tests, treatments, length of treatment, and anything else that could possibly impact the patient's clinical outcome. Standards of Care define how you may expect to be treated after you've been diagnosed with a certain condition.

Standards of Care may also incorporate values that are specific to an institution or individual doctor. For example, doctors and facilities that care for older patients may be concerned with their patient's dignity, social and emotional well-being, privacy, and safety as well as with their medical needs. So their standards of care will define the minimal acceptable standards in each of these specific areas as well as define expected minimal acceptable medical care.

Standards of Care can also be important in legal matters. Because these standards are published in medical journals and are so widely known and supported, when families are alleging malpractice against a doctor or a medical institution, often one of the first things their legal counsel will do is endeavor to show that the prevailing Standards of Care for that patient's condition were not followed.

# Practice Parameters

So, how are Standards of Care and Practice Parameters different from each other and why do we need both? Standards of Care define the care that patients with different illnesses and injuries should receive in order to have the best chance for good health and a good quality of life. Practice Parameters are clinical pathways that doctors follow to reach a diagnosis and decide upon a course of treatment. In other words, Practice Parameters help doctors select the appropriate Standard of Care to apply to each patient. And it's not a chicken and egg situation. Doctors employ Practice Parameters during their initial assessment of a patient and should be familiar with and adhere to them thereafter for the purposes of management. Standards of Care come into play after that initial diagnosis has been made. Both are critical in the practice of medicine.

# Putting Practice Parameters and Standards of Care to use

To better understand how Practice Parameters and Standards of Care are used in the real world, take a look at them in action. Say your child has the sniffles, so you decide to take him to the doctor for an examination. If your doctor finds only a runny nose and a slight feeling of illness and no fever, Practice Parameters based upon a body of evidence-based findings, hundreds of scientific observations performed over a course of many years would suggest to him that all he is looking at is a common cold. In this particular set of circumstances, no further testing and no prescription medications are necessary. Your doctor will then follow the Standard of Care for a common cold and probably tell you to give your child plenty of fluids and let him rest until he feels better.

However, if your child also has a high fever, chest pain, and is coughing up yucky stuff, prevailing Practice Parameters would require the doctor to perform a more extensive examination, and order some tests like a CBC, (complete blood count) and chest X-ray. In other words, each patient's symptoms help the doctor determine the clinical pathway she should follow to reach a diagnosis. Practice Parameters define the number and type of diagnostic tests that should be ordered for any given condition. After the diagnosis is made, the physician then applies the appropriate Standard of Care for that condition.

After your doctor has the results of the initial examination and the tests, Practice Parameters continue to guide him, to help him determine the next step in the course of treatment. Some test results may land your child in the hospital; others may send him home with a prescription for an antibiotic. The important thing to know is that your child, and every child in every pediatricians' office in the United States who visits the doctor with sneezing and sniffling, or coughing and fever, can reasonably expect to go through the same diagnostic procedures based upon the Practice Parameters for upper respiratory infection that every licensed physician should follow. These children can also expect to receive similar treatment based upon the Standards of Care defined for that particular illness.

Because Standards of Care inform healthcare providers as to what sort of care is usual and expected for any given condition, these standards help to ensure that patients receive a consistent and reliable quality of care throughout the health care delivery system. When institutions or individual health care providers fail to follow the minimal Standards of Care, problems may arise.

For example, if an elderly patient is injured after tumbling out of a hospital bed because the side rails of the bed had been left down, that falls below the acceptable Standard of Care, which clearly states that side rails must be up at all times for elderly, infirm patients, particularly those under the influence of medication. The lapse makes the hospital responsible for the patient's injuries. In contrast, if the rails were up and the patient still fell out of bed, the hospital could demonstrate that the accident took place despite the fact that they were following the Standards of Care.

Adherence to Practice Parameters and Standards of Care enhances patient safety and well-being, and greatly reduces the risk of treatment and medication errors, accidents, and opportunistic infections.

# Standards of Care and Practice Parameters for AD Patients

Although the Practice Parameters for diagnosing Alzheimer's Disease have certainly been evolving as new diagnostic tools and tests are introduced, they haven't changed nearly as fast as the Standards of Care. The introduction of cholinesterase inhibitors represented the dawn of a new era of care for people with AD. Good quality of life and a higher level of cognitive and functional abilities such as being able manage personal hygiene are being preserved for much longer periods of time than was previously thought possible, thanks to these new drugs. And even more effective drugs are on the horizon.

These developments have created a Standard of Care for Alzheimer's Disease that offers more hope for patients and their families than was ever thought possible in the past.

The Standard of Care for the treatment of Alzheimer's Disease is the administration of one of the three approved cholinesterase inhibitors — Aricept, Exelon, or Reminyl administered as prescribed. If you have any questions about the benefits of these medications, ask your doctor for additional information. The addition of 1000 I.U. of vitamin E given twice a day is becoming the standard of care.

When the cholinesterase inhibitors were first introduced, it was thought that they were effective only for a matter of months simply because the original clinical trials lasted that long. Now that they've been out a few years, doctors are discovering that in actual practice, these drugs, along with high-dose vitamin E therapy, are holding AD patients at much better levels of functioning for much longer periods of time than was thought possible.

The use of acetylcholinesterase inhibitors and/or vitamin E is not the standard of care for patients in advanced AD. There are some studies that would support the use of acetylcholinesterase inhibitors, but they are far from being conclusive to the point of being standard of care.

Although patients with advanced AD may not show the same degree of symptom stabilization as patients who started drug therapy earlier in the course of the disease, every AD patient should consider trying these medications, which may help maintain the activities of daily living, even for advanced AD. Sometimes, families don't realize a medication is benefiting their loved one until they stop it and it triggers an escalation of symptoms, resulting in guilt and regret for the caregiver and possible residential placement for the patient.

# Caring for AD Patients

You are about to enter a new world. The parent or spouse or sibling you've known all your life has been diagnosed with AD and is changing before your eyes; perhaps even changing into someone you don't understand or feel as close to as you would like.

Remember that your loved one has no more control over these changes than you do over the rising and setting of the sun. If you keep that in mind as you interact with him, you may find it easier to be truly compassionate, patient, and caring in your treatment of him. Simply maintaining a calm and upbeat approach can actually help keep an AD patient content and happy and, therefore, easier to manage.

If you're having trouble handling your loved one or find yourself becoming frustrated by her behavior, consider that your response may be triggering some undesirable behaviors or actually making the behavior worse. If you feel overwhelmed and out of control, you may not be getting the breaks you need. Remember to schedule regular respite care so you have time for yourself. In addition, it may help to give yourself some visual cues. Get a large marker and some 5 x 8 index cards and write one of the following words on each card: patience, tolerance, compassion, love, acceptance, gratitude, flexibility, and any other key word you think might help you remember your mission, which is to provide the best possible care for your loved one. Now tape the cards in prominent places around your house where they can remind you of your daily caregiving goals and keep you focused on the task at hand and away from negative thinking.

Even with the best possible care, your loved one's condition will progress and their symptoms and problem behaviors will increase. This is not a reflection of anything you may have done or haven't done, but if you take the blame on yourself and feel like you're incompetent or a failure as a caregiver, that can create more problems. Seek help immediately if you start to experience these negative feelings.

All the things we take for granted in the course of our day — taking care of our personal needs like bathing, going to the bathroom, preparing and eating a meal, running a load of clothes — can become monumental challenges for an AD patient as the disease progresses. So you will need to devise ways to help your loved one take care of his needs without demeaning him or triggering conflicts between the two of you. In this section, we discuss the various chores you may need to supervise and discuss ways you can help without seeming too pushy or intrusive.

You will need an extra dose of patience as your loved one's skills erode. Try to focus on the positive; as long as you're caring for her and trying to help her with the activities of daily living, you have an opportunity to continue your relationship with your loved one, even if it's very different from the relationship you had in the past. Remember . . . patience.

## Driving Miss AD Patient

The issue of driving is contentious; many AD patients see no reason why they shouldn't be able to keep driving indefinitely, while others want to drive only as long as it's safe. Only a few are willing to hand over their license and car keys right away. Transportation issues can become critical as AD progresses, so you should have some guidelines in place to help you make the decision about whether or not your loved one can keep driving and when they should stop.

Even among professionals there's disagreement on this subject. The American Academy of Neurology recommends that once diagnosed, people with AD not drive. The Alzheimer's Association recommends that cessation of driving privileges be decided on a case-by-case basis.

It's especially difficult to estimate an AD patient's capacity to drive because of the variability in their day-to-day functioning, not to mention the variations that can occur within the course of a single day. And neuro-psychological testing doesn't correlate to driving ability. When and how to intervene without risking demoralization of your loved one is a tough call.

Talk to your loved one soon after diagnosis and develop a strategy together. Discuss the issues — liability, safety, and peace of mind — that are important to both of you. Agree to abide by the results of a private driving evaluation. If the person administering the evaluation says your loved one can no longer drive safely, then take the keys. If your loved one passes the evaluation, repeat it every six to twelve months to stay informed about his actual level of driving skill.

This brings up a whole other issue — who's going to provide transportation for your loved one once he or she can no longer safely drive? At the same time you discuss when to end driving privileges, start recruiting volunteers to help you with transportation. Call your local Administration on Aging to see what sort of transportation services are available in your area, and check with senior centers and daycare centers to see if they provide round trip transportation as part of their service. Don't try to do it all yourself. Ask other people for help in driving; if you're the primary caregiver your plate is already full enough without taking on all the transportation duties for your loved one as well. The key is to not miss a beat; have a plan in place so that your loved one's schedule and social activities can continue without interruption.

Another solution is to consider hiring a private driver or paid companion who can also serve as a driver. Don't assume that your loved one will fight you on this; even though they may be loathe to give up driving, their real fear is giving up their freedom. If you provide another way for your loved to get to his appointments and activities, he should be agreeable to the new arrangement. They may be particularly happy to have the companionship of the new driver.

If you're still having trouble convincing your loved one that he should no longer drive, enlist the help of your doctor. You can also check out the Alzheimer's Association fact sheet on Driving and Dementia at www.alz.org/whatsnew/driving.htm.

The Hartford Insurance Company has an excellent brochure called A Practical Guide to Alzheimer's, Driving and Dementia that's chock full of excellent advice, guidelines and tips. You can read it at www.thehartford.com/alzheimers/.

Finally, if you're still having trouble facing this issue, ask yourself: "Would I want my child or grandchild to ride with my loved one at the wheel?" The answer will tell you what you need to do.

## Managing personal hygiene

One of the most challenging tasks for an AD caregiver is trying to establish and maintain a grooming schedule. An AD patient who insists on dressing independently may don plaid pants and a flowered top, or put her bra on over her blouse. She may try to leave the house without any shoes on, or minus some important piece of clothing. Understand that this type of behavior is no bid for attention like it might be with a rebellious teen; it's simply a reflection of the confusion they are experiencing. If a situation doesn't involve an issue of personal safety but is more like selecting poor color combinations you can choose to ignore it. Save yourself the stress of intervening and value the fact that your loved one can still dress herself and exercise self expression and free choice, even if you don't always agree with her choice of wardrobe. Of course, you can always limit her choices to make sure that comfortable situation and weather-appropriate clothing is selected.

Then we come to the difficulties with bathing and oral hygiene. You may have to face your own shyness about seeing your parent undressed. And even if you don't have a problem, your AD patient might, particularly if he was raised in a more modest era and retains that modesty despite his AD.

Many Alzheimer's patients do retain some ability to take care of their own needs (with supervision) for quite some time after their diagnosis, particularly if they're being maintained on one of the cholinesterase inhibitors. Others require much more help and supervision right from the beginning. In this section, you can discover ways to manage your loved one's hygiene and grooming while maintaining her dignity.

### Bathing

Patients in the early stages of AD are unlikely to require assistance with bathing, but as the condition progresses, they do need help. Bathing an AD patient can be a major challenge for a variety of reasons. If the patient is larger than you are, you need to figure out a safe way to get him into and out of the bath or shower. Some AD patients develop a morbid fear of running water or falling on their head, which means you may need to get a shower chair and use a hand-held shower or resort to sponge baths for the duration of that fear. Advanced AD patients may be frightened of mirrors, because they don't recognize the people they're seeing and can't understand that they're looking at a reflection and not a real person. Regardless of the severity of the disease, most people may not feel comfortable undressing in front of anyone, even a spouse or close relative.

But you can't simply give in if your AD patient doesn't want to bathe, because bathing is an important part of keeping the skin and the entire body healthy. Bathing is also necessary to keep the patient feeling fresh and free from unpleasant body odors, particularly for incontinent patients.

Be flexible about the number of baths your loved one must take. Even if you're from a family whose members bathe every day, it isn't necessary to force your loved one to take a full bath daily; you can get by with sponge baths as long as the genital and rectal areas are kept clean.

As with all interactions with AD patients, bath time will benefit from the use of a set routine. Schedules help AD patients feel grounded and secure, so if you establish a pleasant routine and patiently let your loved one work through any issues he might have with the type of soap you're using, or the color of the towels, you can minimize the difficulties of bathing him.

To minimize problems, set the bath time at the time of day your loved one has always bathed. For example, if he always showered first thing in the morning, don't change his bath time to right before bed. This helps maintain his historic routine and reinforces long-time habits.

### Safety first

Before you give your loved one a bath, first inspect the bathroom to make sure it's free from safety hazards that could potentially cause injury. Here are some things to look for:

- Is the tub or shower floor non-slip? If not, install a non-slip mat or decals.

- Is the floor level and non-slippery? Repair any damage that could cause a fall, and if the floor is slippery due to a wax coating, remove the coating.

- Have you installed safety rated grab bars in the tub enclosure and by the toilet? If not, install them or have a handyman put them in for you. Towel bars are too flimsy to support a falling person's weight, whereas a grab bar could help him regain his balance and prevent a fall. Grab bars are available at most home centers.

- Is the water temperature safe? If not, to prevent scalding injuries and burns to your loved one, set the water heater on low or at 120 degrees Fahrenheit. Also be aware that AD patients may not perceive temperature in the same way, so something that feels comfortably warm to you may seem much too hot to them. Be sure to test the water with your loved one to make sure they like the temperature.

- Is the tub spigot cushioned? If not, you can buy a foam cover to help prevent serious injuries in case of a fall in most baby departments or at a medical supply store.

- Is the floor clear and free from clutter or anything that could cause a fall?

- Can your loved one safely sit down and get up from the toilet? If not, install a raised toilet seat and grab bars (discussed earlier in the chapter).

- Are the faucets clearly and correctly labeled?

- Is the tub large enough to hold a bathing chair? Bathing or bath chairs are available at medical supply companies or online. Measure the interior dimensions of your tub, and then look for a chair that will fit. Bathing chairs help caregivers bathe their patients safely.

If you have a large, walk in shower with a seat, you're ahead of the game. If you have a bathtub, you need to make some accommodations to make the tub accessible for your loved one while minimizing the risk of a fall.

# Help with bathing

If your loved one is simply too big or too heavy for you to lift into and out of the tub, you can get something called a bath lift or another device called a slider chair. Although these items aren't cheap, costing as much as $2,000, they're less expensive than renovating a bathroom. These chairs can save a caregiver from injury and even save money over the long run because the caregiver doesn't have to pay someone else to bathe his or loved one if the loved one has a bath chair. Visit www.adaptivemall.com/asbat.html for a selection of bath chairs.

### Prep work

Get your supplies and equipment together before you start the bath — mild soap, tear-free shampoo, washcloths, shower cap, nailbrush, a plastic pitcher for rinsing, and towels. Play some soothing music or put some nice-smelling potpourri out to calm your loved one's fears. If she is frightened of running water, draw the bath before you take her into the bathroom, testing the water with your hand to make sure it is a warm and pleasant temperature.

### Tub time

Speaking in a quiet and encouraging tone of voice, gently lead your loved one into the bathroom. If he is concerned about modesty, buy him a terrycloth wrap or robe that he can cover himself with; even if it gets soaking wet, such a robe is easy to launder. To help him manage the soap, buy a soap mitt that has a pocket to hold the bar of soap. You may find it easier to use liquid bath soap, which is available in a number of fragrances.

Be sure to wash your loved one all over. If your loved one is uncomfortable with your help, find someone he or she is more receptive to. A father may not want his daughter bathing him, for example. If you overlook some areas for modesty's sake, your loved one can develop a rash or a serious skin infection, particularly if he or she is incontinent.

After he has soaped up, use a plastic pitcher to rinse the soap from his skin and also from his head if you have shampooed his hair. You can use a hand-held shower attachment to make this job easier if your loved one doesn't object. If you use a conditioner on his hair, try a leave-in conditioner that doesn't require rinsing. But be sure to do a thorough job of rinsing soap; soap left on the skin can cause rashes or itchy, flaking skin. Soap left in the hair makes hair look dull and lifeless.

Some people prefer to wash their loved one's hair over the kitchen sink, particularly if they have a spray nozzle attachment that makes rinsing easy. Your loved one may prefer standing up for this chore as well. Just be sure that you get the water temperature right so you don't scald her with a sudden burst of hot water on her scalp. Or better yet, make an appointment for your loved one at a barber or beauty parlor. This can serve two purposes; it helps with personal hygiene and it's a pleasurable activity that gets you and your loved one out of the house. In fact, if your loved one is used to going to a beauty parlor or barber, it's best to keep up his or her routine rather than try to care for his or her hair at home.

The use of bath oil in the tub or shower is not recommended as it greatly increases the likelihood of a fall. If your loved one likes bath oil, offer to massage it into his skin after the bath, or allow him to do that for himself.

According to the Consumer Product Safety Commission, more elderly people are injured while using the bathtub or shower than from any other household equipment, stoves included. On average, more than 26,000 older adults are injured every year from a fall in a bathtub or shower. Just as you would never leave a child unattended in a bath, never leave your loved one unattended either, not even for a second. If your loved one is in the early stages of AD, he or she may object to being monitored so closely while bathing, so just make sure you are available nearby to provide assistance if the need arises.

### Dealing with fear or stubbornness

If you're having trouble convincing your loved one to bathe, don't turn it into a battle. Try to distract her with another activity and then try the bath again 20 minutes later. Be willing to do sponge baths for a few days until she settles down, or try associating the bath with a reward to make the idea more appealing. For example, if your loved one enjoys a foot massage, get some nice lotion, and tell her, "Let's take a bath and then I'll give you a foot massage." Hopefully, she will begin to associate the reward with the bath and be more willing to bathe.

If you're dealing with someone who wants to "do it all herself," it helps to use simple, one-step commands to get her started. For example, "Here is the soap. Wash your arms." Take your time and be patient; don't overload your loved one with too many products or too much to do at once.

If your loved one is still adamant about not wanting a bath, you can try giving him sponge baths for a few days until he gets over his objections. Or you might try one of the pre-packaged personal bath cloths that are widely available at discount and drug stores. These "baths" can be gently warmed in the microwave and contain an emollient, skin-soothing formula. They make a good substitute for those days when your loved one just will not allow you to bathe him in a tub or shower.

## Modesty issues

A big reason AD patients may refuse to bathe is embarrassment over being seen naked. A daughter who had to care for her ailing mother came up with a modesty garment called Honor Guard that can be used to cover private areas during dressing and bathing. This product is getting high marks from both patients and caregivers and reduces or eliminates bath time troubles related to modesty issues. At $29.95 for the women's style, which has a top and a bottom and $19.95 for the men's style, it's very affordable. Call 866-242-1282 for more information or visit www.personalcarewear.com.

### Dressing

If you're not careful, you can get into some huge battles with your loved one over choice and appropriateness of clothing. Because most AD patients are not fully aware that their judgment is lacking, when you tell them the pink and brown polka dot Capri pants don't really go with the orange ski parka, they're likely to take loud exception to your opinion. Or, they could feel demoralized. Either way, it's not a particularly pleasant start to a day.

As AD progresses, AD patients may have difficulty selecting their clothing because they are easily overwhelmed by too many choices. Consider culling their wardrobe down to five to seven of their favorite outfits to help avoid confusion. If they like to wear the exact same clothing or outfit every day, get multiple sets

AD patients have trouble with buttons, zippers, and fussy clothing that's hard to get into. This can become a source of frustration and may contribute to incontinence if they can't get out of their clothing once they're in the bathroom. Opt in favor of comfortable fabrics like cotton knits and easy styles like pull-on pants with elastic waists and knit tops that close in the front. Anything you have to slide on over the head can present a problem, because it's hard for an AD patient to coordinate the complex movements required to get a pullover on properly. Rubber-soled shoes and slippers can help prevent slipping and falls.

Try to lay an outfit out the night before so that your loved one doesn't have to agonize about what to wear. Be aware that it's not helpful to give general commands such as, "Get dressed," because AD patients have poor ability to successfully complete complex chains of behaviors. If your loved one wants to get dressed herself, supervise the activity, handing her the outfit in the order it's put on — underwear first, then pants, shirt, and socks. If she seems confused, give her precise instructions in a pleasant tone of voice. For example, instead of, "Put on this blouse," you could indicate the sleeve and say, "Put your arm in here."

Dress your loved one appropriately for the season and make sure he feels comfortable. If he gets too hot, some patients with advanced AD may surprise you by peeling off their clothes, even in a public place. You can avoid such incidents by dressing your loved one comfortably.

You'll have lots of issues to work out with your loved one as her AD progresses, so don't waste too much energy trying to get her to look like a fashion plate, or being angry because you don't approve of her clothing choices. Your biggest fight may be getting her to change her clothing at all. She may latch on to one favorite outfit and swear solemnly every morning that she just put it on fresh, even though you know you've been trying to pry her out of it for the last three days. If your loved one does become attached to one particular outfit, buy two or three sets of it so that she can wear one while the other is being washed.

## Oral hygiene

Taking care of your loved one's teeth is not only difficult; it can be downright dangerous. Even if you've convinced him to open wide and allow you to put a toothbrush in his mouth, he can change his mind and clamp down at any moment, giving you a painful bite.

But you have to persist; oral hygiene is every bit as important to your loved one's health and overall well-being as regular bathing is. AD patients have many nutritional challenges and teeth that hurt or ill-fitting dentures can be a big part of what's keeping your loved one from eating properly. For more on this issue, take a look at the "Nutritional challenges" section later in the chapter.

Pain is one of the major triggers of agitation and violent outbursts in AD patients. Pain can result from cavities or gum infections that your loved one can't really tell you about. So be sure to maintain a regular schedule of daily oral hygiene along with annual trips to the dentist to check for hidden problems. Notify your dentist in advance that your loved one has AD so he or she can make any adjustments necessary to ensure a good visit. You should sit in the room with your loved one during the examination to help keep him calm and ask the dentist to play soft music and speak in a calm voice as he explains each step of what he is doing to the patient.

Try brushing your teeth together. Seeing you put a toothbrush in your own mouth can relieve some of the fear of the unknown an AD patient may feel when confronted with a toothbrush, particularly if you make toothbrushing an enjoyable game. If your loved one will allow you to floss between her teeth, that's good, but it may well be too dangerous to floss if she's unhappy about it.

What about using an electric toothbrush? Although electric toothbrushes certainly help you get your loved one's teeth cleaner faster, some AD patients may be frightened by the sound of the motor. You'll have to experiment to see what reaction your loved one has to an electric toothbrush. If he tolerates it well, it can make your job easier.

You can buy sponge-tipped swabs pre-loaded with toothpaste; swabbing may be easier than brushing when eating out.

If your loved one wears dentures, they must be cleaned every day. Check your loved one's gums for any signs of irritation; if you find reddened areas or sores, the dentures do not fit as well as they should. Take them back to the dentist for an adjustment. Ill-fitting dentures can have an adverse effect on an AD patient's nutrition because they make it harder for her to eat.

Schedule an appointment for a regular check-up and cleaning with your dentist at least once each year, or more frequently if oral hygiene becomes a chronic problem.

### Grooming

A caregiver can easily become frazzled over grooming issues, but be aware that they may not understand what you're asking them to do. AD patients may forget the norms and routines for proper grooming, refusing to comb their hair or bathe, mixing and matching awful combinations of clothing, refusing to wear shoes, insisting they have on clean clothes when you're looking at a tattered, stained, stinky outfit.

Keep hair and nails neatly trimmed and the hair preferably in an easy-to-maintain style that doesn't require a lot of fuss to maintain. Depending upon whether your loved one's scalp is dry or oily, you may have to wash his hair several times a week to keep him looking fresh or just once a week or less.

Shaving can be tricky, particularly with razors. Try to switch over to an electric razor to avoid the possibility of cuts. If shaving becomes a battle, just skip it. An older woman doesn't absolutely need to have her legs or underarms clean-shaven and an older man can easily sport a beard.

Pay attention to your loved one's nails, particularly her toenails. Both fingernails and toenails should be trimmed twice a month. While you're trimming the toenails, check for signs of corns, bunions, and ingrown nails. If you find anything that might be hampering your loved one's mobility, have her treated by a reputable podiatrist. Pedicures may be scheduled if your loved one enjoys this.

Grooming can be a struggle, but if you stick to the basics and try not to get too upset or embarrassed if things don't go exactly the way you planned, you should be able to accomplish most grooming chores with minimal hassle.

## Dealing with incontinence

Perhaps no problem causes families more distress than dealing with ongoing incontinence. AD patients may not even be aware they have a problem.

Or they may do their business in inappropriate places like closets because they confuse it with the bathroom, a fact you may only discover when you try to track down that awful smell that's been lingering in the air for the past week or so.

AD patients with advanced disease may become incontinent for two reasons:

✓ They suffer from an age-related condition such as weakened pelvic muscles that causes them to lose urine when they laugh or cough.

✓ They may not have any physical problems that cause incontinence directly, but are wetting and soiling themselves because they cannot find a bathroom or cannot get to a bathroom in time, or can't get their clothes off in time.

Don't ever scold your loved one for having a toileting accident. He may already be embarrassed and upset as it is. If he can no longer tell you when he needs to use the bathroom, watch for visual signs such as restlessness or tugging at the genitals. Schedule regular toileting times into your daily routine.

Don't withhold water from your loved one in an attempt to manage incontinence. She may become dehydrated, which can lead to a urinary tract infection, which in turns exacerbates the incontinence. However, limiting caffeinated beverages can be helpful, because caffeine stimulates the bladder.

### Rule out a UTI

Patients with any stage of AD may become incontinent at any time if there is an underlying medical condition like an urinary tract infection or UTI. Incontinence should be evaluated by a doctor to evaluate the cause. Get to know the symptoms of UTI and monitor your loved one for them. Symptoms include

✓ A strong urge to urinate that can't be delayed

✓ Pain or a burning sensation when urinating

✓ Scant urine

✓ Urine tinged with blood

✓ Complaints of pain or soreness in the back, sides, or lower abdomen

✓ Chills, fever, nausea, and vomiting if infection is not caught and treated early

UTIs are easily diagnosed with a urine sample so don't hesitate to take your loved one to t doctor if you suspect a UTI.

### Try a few tricks

Caregivers have several proven options for managing incontinence; although no one technique is foolproof, the following strategies do help to reduce or eliminate episodes of incontinence.

- ✔ **Scheduled toileting:** The number one intervention to reduce incontinence is to establish a toileting schedule. A prompted trip to the toilet every two hours to four hours will significantly reduce the frequency of incontinence episodes or eliminate them altogether.

- ✔ **Prompted voiding:** Check to see if your loved one is wet or dry. Ask, "Do you want to use the toilet?" Help him to the toilet if he needs to use it. Praise him for being dry and trying to use the toilet. Tell him when you will come back to take him to the toilet again.

- ✔ **Habit training:** Habit training takes advantage of the fact that most people have a fairly regular natural schedule of toileting. Watch your loved one to find what times she urinates. Take her to the bathroom at those times every day. Praise her for being dry and using the toilet

It may help to tape a picture of a toilet on the door of the bathroom to remind the AD patient what that room is used for or keep a light on in the bathroom to guide him. Also, keep clothing simple; avoid complicated things like zippers and buttons; opt instead for pull-on pants that are easy to slide off in a hurry.

Be patient. Toileting treatments take time to work. Treat the person with AD as an adult with dignity. He may feel bad about being wet and your inappropriate anger may only serve to make the problem worse or trigger an emotional outburst from your loved one.

### Incontinence supplies

A number of excellent supplies are available for dealing with incontinence, including adult diapers, panty liners, and bed pads. You will have to help with wiping and flushing; you may want to use one of the soft, pre-moistened cleansing towelettes that are now available so you can do a thorough job of wiping, particularly after a bowel movement. If you use adult diapers, be sure to check them regularly, and change them as quickly as possible when they're wet, to avoid skin irritation.

## Preventing bedsores

As people age, skin cells tend to flatten and lose their protective barrier of fat and collagen, and oil-producing glands become less active, making skin thinner, drier, and more sensitive to damage. In addition, as AD advances, your loved one may become less mobile. When you add aging skin to immobility, that's a recipe for a bedsore.

A *bed sore* is a skin ulcer that may develop when the blood supply to the skin is cut off for more than two to three hours.

Bedsores occur most frequently on people who are bed-ridden or confined to a wheelchair, but anyone who's sedentary and stays in the same position for long hours can develop a bedsore. They tend to form on areas of the skin that are under pressure for prolonged periods of time, such as the buttocks or the heels of the feet.

If your loved one is sedentary, bed-ridden, or spends long hours in a wheel chair, you should regularly inspect their skin for bedsores. The first sign is a red, painful area that eventually turns purple. If you don't intervene and treat the bedsore at this point, the skin can break open and become infected. These infections can be dangerous; once they work their way into underlying tissue like muscle, healing can be very slow.

If you pay good attention to the condition of you loved one's skin and take care to move them regularly, you can prevent most bedsores. Here are some tips to keep bedsores from forming:

- ✔ Turn or reposition your loved one frequently to keep pressure from building up in any one spot on the skin.

- ✔ Buy a special mattress cover (available at medical supply stores) designed to reduce pressure points across the body of a bedridden person.

- ✔ Add soft padding to any spot in your loved one's bed or wheelchair that seems to be putting pressure on his body.

- ✔ Keep your loved one's skin clean and dry and inspect it regularly for any signs of redness or breakdown.

Even with the most diligent care, people with AD can still develop bedsores, particularly as the disease advances and they become more sedentary. Here are some pointers for treating bedsores, but remember, any bedsore should first be evaluated by a physician who will prescribe appropriate treatments based on the severity and location of the bed sore.

- ✔ Eliminate all pressure on the affected area.

- ✔ If the bedsore is open, protect it with a wound dressing or medicated gauze.

- ✔ Keep the bedsore clean to prevent infection.

- ✔ Administer antibiotics as prescribed by your doctor.

If all else fails and a bedsore won't heal, your doctor may recommend an out-patient surgical procedure to transplant a patch of healthy skin to cover the bedsore and encourage healing.

## Nutritional challenges

You may have a tough time keeping your AD patient properly nourished, particularly as the disease advances. He may have problems with chewing or swallowing, or may be subject to episodes of choking, which can be very frightening for you (and for him!). Many AD patients lose weight because they just don't eat enough; their sense of taste and ability to smell may be diminished and that takes away two of the prime biological appetite boosters. A routine family dinner may be too chaotic for an AD patient; they may have problems selecting the food from the plate or in using utensils.

For other patients, memory problems may cause them to think they haven't eaten even though they've just completed a meal. They may demand another meal and gain weight as a result. If you're thinking, "How can my mom be hungry? She just ate!" remember that AD wreaks havoc with the senses and the sense of satiety, that lovely feeling that tells us when we're full and have had enough to eat, diminishes in AD patients along with the other senses. So do monitor the amount of food you give to make sure your loved one is not eating too little or too much.

In the following list we go over several tactics you can try to help boost nutrition:

- Schedule meals for the same time every day and make sure mealtime is a calm and pleasant event. Don't let the dinner table become a battlefield over eating; both you and your loved one lose out if you constantly fight over meals.

- Keep the surface of the table clean and uncluttered. Don't use tablecloths or table linens like place mats and napkins; these can be a source of distraction for the AD patient.

- Keep distractions to a minimum. That means no TV during meals!

- Keep knives and other sharp utensils out of reach in a locked drawer or cabinet. Serve food already cut up and ready to eat.

- Serve five or six small meals instead of three large meals. AD patients are easily distracted and you may have a hard time getting your loved one to sit still long enough to consume a large meal. Smaller meals composed of just one or two tasty, nutritious foods that are easily managed often bring better results.

- Focus on serving easy foods like sandwiches and finger foods like chicken or steak strips.

- Meals don't have to be served in the dining room or kitchen. If your loved one has a new "favorite room" or special nook in the house, serve snacks and small meals there

- Don't serve junk food. Avoid snacks and meals that are either too highly salted or loaded with sugar or artificial ingredients.

- ✔ Watch the food's temperature to make sure it isn't too hot or too cold.

- ✔ Don't rush. Allow plenty of time for your loved one to chew and swallow each bite before presenting the next one. If you try to hurry her, she may run the risk of a choking episode.

- ✔ Lock medicine and cleaning supplies away, or better still, remove them from the bathroom and kitchen.

### Poor nutrition

A number of factors can contribute to poor nutrition in an AD patient. Your loved one may have problems with his teeth or gums as mentioned previously in the section on oral hygiene. A medication may be reducing his appetite. Or he might not know what to do with his utensils or have mechanical problems such as not understanding how to get food on a fork or how to get the fork to his mouth. Finally, an AD patient may have diminished swallowing ability, which can lead to choking. After a couple of choking incidents, your loved one may be afraid to eat. Fortunately, we know a few ways to address these problems.

The Alzheimer's Association offers these tips to stimulate chewing and swallowing in AD patients who are having difficulty eating.

- ✔ Use rough-textured foods, such as toast or sandwiches made on toasted bread, to stimulate the person's tongue and encourage chewing and swallowing.

- ✔ The person with Alzheimer's sometimes has little sensation of food in the mouth. By gently moving the person's chin, you can get him to chew.

- ✔ Stimulate chewing by touching the person's tongue with a fork or spoon. By lightly stroking her throat, you can remind her to swallow.

Serve foods that are tasty and nutritious, yet easy to handle. For example:

- ✔ Cooked vegetables and fruits (may be mashed or pureed)

- ✔ Bite-sized pieces of meat or cheese (no larger than one-half inch in diameter)

- ✔ Scrambled eggs

- ✔ Fish sticks

- ✔ Small finger sandwiches

- ✔ Toast

- ✔ Pudding

- ✔ Nutritional shakes

Avoid foods that may cause choking (see the list in the "Choking" section, later in the chapter) Also avoid foods that are hard to chew, like tough cuts of meat, or hard snacks, like pretzels or taco chips.

As a rule, AD patients have an easier time swallowing thicker liquids like shakes and soups. They also seem to prefer soft foods and sweet foods but make sure the sweets you serve are natural. Don't load them up with too many artificial sweeteners or too much refined sugar.

If your loved one is having trouble swallowing, you should cut her food into very small pieces, or mash or puree it. Alternate bites of food with a sip of a beverage to help her swallow.

### Weight loss

It may be that despite your best efforts, your loved one continues to lose weight. If this happens, consult your doctor about adding a calorie- and nutrient-rich beverage supplement to the diet. A number of brands are available at most supermarkets and drugstores, but they are expensive and you have to be careful of high-sodium content. Because these products are liquid and taste good, they are usually easy to get down, but be aware that even with liquids, choking is always a possibility with an AD patient.

Even if your loved one is losing weight, try to stick to a regular meal schedule. If your loved one forgets that you served a meal just 15 minutes before and expresses an interest in food or tells you he's hungry, put out a plate of nutritious snacks like cheese cubes or scrambled eggs cut into small squares rather than preparing an entire meal again or denying him the opportunity to get some food down.

As your loved one progresses through the stages of AD, you may find it more and more difficult to get her to eat. She may lose interest in food entirely and refuse to open her mouth when offered food. This is just part of the process. Be sure to keep the doctor informed of any changes in nutrition and weight and ask for suggestions to encourage better eating habits in your loved one.

### Choking

Chewing and swallowing become less and less coordinated as AD progresses, making it difficult for your loved one to take in proper nourishment. Another problem that results from this loss of coordination is choking.

A number of things can minimize choking episodes. The first is to limit foods that are prone to trigger choking. Here are some examples:

- Hard candy
- Taffy
- Hot dogs
- Nuts
- Crunchy foods like chips or crackers

> ✔ Peanut butter
>
> ✔ Chewing gum
>
> ✔ Grapes or cherries
>
> ✔ Thin liquids if given too rapidly

Give liquids in a cup with a sipper lid or use straws to help regulate the flow of the liquid and prevent choking.

Choking can also happen when AD patients eat inappropriate things like dirt, glue, or pieces of fabric. You should try to keep the environment around your loved one as clean and clutter-free as possible to minimize the chances for this sort of behavior.

If your loved one does choke, don't slap him on the back as this could worsen the problem. The safest way to rescue someone who is choking is to perform the Heimlich Maneuver. For complete illustrated instructions, go to www.heimlichinstitute.org/howtodo.html#chokingAnchor.

You should review these instructions now so that you will know what to do should the need arise. Remember that an older adult is frailer, so be careful about the amount of force you use in performing the Heimlich Maneuver, or you could inadvertently crack a rib.

# Planning Activities and Exercise

You need to keep your loved one up and about. A good daily dose of movement and supervised light exercise can have many benefits besides the obvious physical gains.

If you develop a series of quiet and enjoyable activities for your loved one, you gain a few minutes of respite in your busy day. AD patients like things that keep them occupied, and respond favorably to activities that stimulate their senses in a gentle way.

## Entertaining activities

When you plan activities for your loved one, be sure to keep his current level of ability and his natural interests in mind. Choose entertaining activities that provide gentle stimulation. Avoid anything that's too complex, because that will only lead to frustration.

Here are some ideas for planning activities:

- If you have a well-trained pet that your loved one cares for, let the dog or cat spend a few minutes with her at around the same time each day. Some animals have an uncanny sense around ill humans and seem to know just how to conduct themselves to provide the most comfort. If your cat climbs onto your loved one's lap, curls up and starts purring, watch to see the reaction. If she accepts the animal and even start petting it or talking to it, then you've found a pleasant way to help your loved one occupy her time for a portion of each day. If, on the other hand, the animal's presence upsets or frightens your loved one, then this is not a good idea.

- Some AD patients respond favorably to stuffed animals or dolls, particularly female patients. Sometimes simply holding a doll or stuffed bear can calm an upset or agitation.

- Other AD patients respond favorably to photos of family members. Let him help you select the photos he likes and assemble them into a 4 x 6 album the can carry around and look at whenever he likes.

- Another good idea is to make a memory box. Cover a shoebox with bright contact paper and put in five or six of your loved one's favorite keepsakes from his past. For example, you might include a prom photo or baby pictures or a souvenir postcard from a favorite vacation, even a soft piece of cloth cut from one of his children's baby blankets. Include anything that you know has special meaning for your loved one, but don't include any sharp or breakable objects. Then, whenever he wishes, he can sit down and go through the box and enjoy the fond memories the objects bring back.

When planning activities, don't forget the great outdoors. Many AD patients seem to really enjoy a nice walk or a chance to dig in the garden.

You may be baffled when, without warning, an activity that your loved one has enjoyed for many weeks or months is suddenly refused. Remember that AD is a progressive illness, so something that worked yesterday may not work today because your loved one may not have the same abilities, memories, and knowledge today that he had yesterday. Don't let it upset you. Just devise some simpler activities to take the place of the one being rejected.

## Safe exercise options

Exercise helps to combat depression, improve circulation, lower blood pressure, and keep bones and muscles strong. It can improve balance, thereby reducing the risk of falls. It can also help AD patients sleep better and retain fine motor skills.

Of course, you can't just slap a bike helmet on an AD patient and send her packing down the street. You should select exercises that are suitable for her age and condition, like walking, dancing, or gardening. In fact, exercise is often more enjoyable for AD patients if you make it part of an activity your loved one has always enjoyed in the past.

If your loved one wants to participate in an activity you think is too danger- ous, like cycling, find a way to make it happen. You can find special bikes made for handicapped adults that are very sturdy and stable; some models even have seats for two. If your loved one wants to swim, fit her with a life jacket and jump in the pool with her. You can find creative ways to incorpo- rate almost every sort of exercise into an AD patient's life, but if your loved one asks you about mountain climbing or hang gliding, you might just have to pass.

Researchers at The Mayo Foundation for Medical Education and Research have found that exercising four times a week improves both the emotional and physical health of women who are caring for a relative with dementia. Study participants slept better, felt less stressed and depressed, and experi- enced a drop in their blood pressure, leading researchers to conclude that physical activity is beneficial for both the caregiver and the person he or she cares for.

Several Alzheimer's daycare centers offer exercise programs for seniors; check with your local providers — many do offer exercise classes separate from their daycare program. The YMCA also offers a broad range of classes for older adults and the one in your area may offer a special class for AD patients. If nothing is available nearby, consider hiring a coach or personal trainer to promote your loved one's activity. The coach can be an actual trainer or a paid companion; it doesn't matter as long as they supervise the exercise and perform it along with your loved one.

Start slowly and don't try to push your loved one to do too much to start. Ten to fifteen minutes is plenty to begin with. Remember, you're not training for a marathon. You're trying to help your loved one stay as healthy as possi- ble for as long as possible.

Always consult a physician before beginning any program of physical activity for your loved one or yourself. You can also hire a physical therapist to set up the exercise program for your loved one, either in your home or at a gym or exercise facility that has experience in working with AD patients.

If at any time during the exercise session, your loved one complains of dizzi- ness, shortness of breath, or any sort of pain anywhere in his or her body but most especially chest pain, stop exercising immediately and call 9-1-1 for medical assistance.

# Preparing for Bed

It would be wonderful if, at the end of a long and busy day, you could simply tuck your loved one into bed, say a prayer, turn out the light, and then go to sleep yourself. Unfortunately, that's rarely the case with AD patients, because many of them have trouble sleeping through the night.

 Physical restraints to keep an AD patient in bed at night and prevent wandering are not recommended, as they can increase episodes of agitation. Also, such restraints are dangerous because they make it difficult to evacuate the AD patient in case of an emergency situation, like a fire.

David Harper, a research psychologist affiliated with Harvard Medical School found that caregivers cite sleep disturbances as one of the main reasons why they decide to place AD patients in residential facilities. Take a look at the following list for several steps you can take to help make bedtime easier and give your loved one a better chance of getting a full night's rest. Instead of making bedtime into a combat zone, try to make it as pleasant an experience as possible.

- ✔ Restrict caffeine intake after noon. Caffeine takes a long time to pass through the body and can keep your loved one up and buzzing around for a full six hours or more after one little cup of coffee. Also, try to not let your loved one nap excessively as that can lead to additional difficulties in falling asleep at bedtime.

- ✔ As often as possible, put your loved one to bed at the same time each evening. Depending upon her needs, start the before-bed routine about a half hour to a full hour before bed. Help her into her night clothes and with her grooming and toileting. Speak in a soft and pleasant voice. When you have her dressed for bed, take her to her bedroom and help her into bed. Sit and talk with her for a few minutes until she begins to feel sleepy. Play soft music, turn on a night light, and use aromatherapy to help your loved one associate bed time with pleasant feelings. Offer an incentive if she settles down quickly, like a foot massage with her favorite lotion, or read her a story.

- ✔ You can't stay up all night long just to watch your loved one. If he has a habit of wandering at night, try installing some of the alarm devices described in the sidebar "Keeping track of an Alzheimer's patient."

Remember that sleep problems are part of AD. You must be patient with your loved one and try to understand that she isn't waking you up in the middle of the night with any malicious intent. When she awakens in a darkened room, she doesn't know where she is, and she becomes frightened and disoriented.

## What about sleeping pills?

Many families, exhausted by the nightly midnight ramblings of their AD patient, beg doctors for sleeping pills so the rest of the family can get a decent night's sleep. We don't advocate this course of action for several reasons:

- ✔ Sleeping pills can add to daytime confusion for AD patients

- ✔ Sleeping pills may increase the risk of falls

- ✔ Some types of sleeping pill can lead to physical dependence

- ✔ Sleeping pills can lose their effectiveness after a few days, requiring a larger dose to maintain the desired therapeutic effect

However, if you're desperate, your doctor may prescribe a week's worth of a mild, non-addictive sleeping pill to give you and your family members the chance to catch up on your sleep. Be sure to keep a close eye on your loved one the following day to see how he responds to the medication and report that response to the doctor.

# Making the House Safer

Alzheimer's Disease patients function best in a calm and well-structured environment. That means eliminating potential sources of trouble as much as you can.

Most of us take our homes and familiar surroundings for granted. If you've lived somewhere for ten years and you've completely adjusted to the little half step up into the kitchen where a tile has cracked and shifted, you probably don't think too much about it. Your foot just automatically hitches up that extra half inch every time you go into the kitchen.

According to The National Center for Injury Prevention, falls are the leading cause of injury deaths to adults aged 65 and older. One in every three older adults falls at least once each year. Falls account for 87 percent of all fractures in adults aged 65 and older, with the most common injury being a hip fracture. In 1999, hip fractures cost Medicare approximately $7.59 billion in reimbursements.

So remember: For an AD patient, that half inch step into the kitchen could be disastrous, leading to a serious fall and maybe even hospitalization. Earlier in this chapter, we went over ways to make the bathroom safe for an AD patient. In this section, we talk about making the rest of the house safe as well.

## Patient proofing your home

In addition to locking up knives and other sharp objects in the kitchen, you should lock up matches and lighters. You should also put a kill switch on your stove or remove the knobs so that your loved one can't accidentally start a fire. Put childproof latches on all your cabinets, and if you have any throw or area rugs in the kitchen, remove them. Throw rugs are real tripping hazards, even if you have them secured to the floor with carpet tape. Remove any electrical wires that run across open spaces to prevent tripping, and put childproof plugs in all your electrical outlets.

Walk around your house and look at each room with a critical eye. If you see something that looks like it could cause a problem for your loved one, remove it or secure it so that it no longer presents a hazard. Then you can rest assured that you have done your best to patient proof your home. Even with all reasonable precautions taken, accidents can still happen. Don't blame yourself. Seek treatment for whatever injuries your loved one may have and move forward.

Here are some more specific tips:

- If your loved one wanders, you need to secure the entire house and yard to keep him from getting lost. Install locks on top of entrance doors to keep your loved one from getting outside unsupervised. Install locks on windows and use childproof doorknobs to make it more difficult for him to escape. Put locks on your garden gates, and if your yard is not fenced, consider putting in a fence as soon as possible so that you can keep your loved one secure at home while allowing him to engage in normal, healthy outdoor activity. But remember, no fence is tall enough and no gate is secure enough to substitute for your supervision!

- Disengage the garage door opener. Install alarms at the exits to let you know if someone is trying to get out. You can use alarm mats that sound if someone steps on them, or alarms that sound if the door is opened. If you can't afford alarms, hang a bell on the door to alert you if someone is leaving (although this may not be enough to wake you from a sound sleep).

- Let your neighbors know about your loved one's condition so that they can alert you if he manages to sneak out despite all your precautions. You might even want to take your loved one on a nice walk around the neighborhood to introduce him to your neighbors, but remember, discuss your concerns either before or after this visit. As you might imagine, AD patients don't like to be discussed as if they were not standing right there.

- If you have a flight of stairs in your home, you must put gates at both the top and the bottom to keep your loved one from trying to go up and down unassisted. Mark the first step, top and bottom, with a wide, brightly colored tape so they'll be aware of where it is. Make sure the handrail is securely fastened to the wall and will support the weight of a falling person. If the handrail is flimsy, have it replaced.

- Install smoke alarms and don't use portable space heaters because they cause too many fires. Cover the fireplace and put cushioned corner bumpers on sharp edges of furniture to prevent injury in case of a fall.

## Keeping track of an Alzheimer's patient

No one knows exactly why Alzheimer's patients wander, but the reality is that a certain number of them do. If your loved one wanders, it probably scares you to death. To help make sure the wandering isn't a tragic experience, a number of programs are available to help find your loved one found and return him home.

Use iron on labels with your loved one's name, address, and phone number imprinted on all his clothing, even his socks. This could make a big difference between a speedy return or a lot of red tape if your loved one gets lost.

The Alzheimer's Association sponsors a program called Safe Return. For a one-time registration fee of $40, you receive an ID bracelet or necklace with the organization's 24-hour toll-free emergency crisis line. In addition, when you report your loved one missing, Safe Return faxes his picture and information to local law enforcement agencies. If someone finds your loved one, she calls the number and you can

be reunited. Call 1-800-272-3900 for complete information or visit www.alz.org/ResourceCenter/Programs/SafeReturn.htm to register.

Project Lifesaver is a digital tracking device that allows wanderers to be tracked and recovered within a matter of minutes. It's currently available only in certain Eastern states. Visit www.caretrak.com/lifesaver.html or call 1-800-842-4537 for more information.

If your loved one has medical problems in addition to Alzheimer's Disease, you should consider a Medic Alert bracelet. It provides important medical information that doctors or paramedics might need in the event of an emergency and it also has a special ID number and a 24-hour emergency line that rescuers call to tell Medic Alert that one of their clients has been found. Call 1-800-432-5378 for more information. Bracelets cost between $35 and $75 and they charge a $15 annual membership fee.

## Getting clutter out of the way

We have one last thing to address, something you may live with every day and not pay too much attention to, but it's something that can be very dangerous for your loved one. That something is clutter.

You may love your stacks of magazines and newspapers, and laugh when you open a cabinet and 20 plastic containers come tumbling down. But what seems cozy to you may present a real danger for your loved one. In his weakened condition with diminished ambulatory skills and impaired balance, it may be almost impossible for him to navigate around your treasures.

ADEAR offers a free booklet to help you "patient-proof" your home. You can download a free copy at www.alzheimers.org/pubs/homesafety.htm.

If you just can't bear to part with all your treasures or simply don't have time to deal with cleanup at the moment, gather your stuff up in boxes and cart it to a mini storage. But be careful about reorganizing your loved one's familiar environment too quickly and too drastically. Familiar spaces and old routines are the AD patient's friend; changing too much quickly can trigger undesirable behavior or cause anxiety or paranoia. These clutter tips are for YOU, not for your loved one.

## Considering remodeling

When you walk through and assess your house, you may come to the conclusion that certain areas are simply not going to work, no matter how much reorganizing you do. At that point, you might consider remodeling part of the house to accommodate your loved one's needs. You may be able to get money from your insurance policy or Medicare to help defray the cost of remodeling if you can prove that it is required for valid medical reasons.

Talk to local contractors. It might be more economical to build a small addition with a bedroom and accessible bath than to tear out an existing bath and walls to remodel. Whether or not you remodel will depend upon your financial situation and your loved one's needs. Perhaps by combining two households, you can find the capital to make the needed structural changes in your own home.

# Dealing with the Patient's Emotions

Throughout the process of caring for your loved one, you're going to be dealing with a lot of emotions — yours, his, and those of your other family members and friends. AD patients are particularly subject to frustration because it's so difficult for them to navigate their days, always looking for something, trying to remember something, worrying about something. It's a huge burden for any one person to bear.

A great deal of the successful management of an AD patient rests with the way the caregiver treats him or her. If you always try to respect the person's dignity, let him know you love him, treat him with courtesy, patience, and compassion, you can minimize outbursts. But even if you're so good and thoughtful and caring that you're about to be nominated for sainthood, the day may come when your loved one just pitches a tantrum or sinks into a spell of the blues. It's not a failure on your part — it's the disease advancing. Seek counseling and take your loved one for a checkup; if the change in his or her behavior is sudden, the reason might be a medical one.

## Managing mood swings

Wild mood swings can actually be one of the early signs of AD, but as the condition progresses, you may start to see more persistent tantrums or depression in your loved one (although the apathy of some AD patients is frequently misdiagnosed as depression). Other families have to contend with a loved one who always seems to be in a bad mood for no discernible reason. It's tough to deal with someone who is always finding fault and picking at you, but just try to remember why this is happening and separate the event from your feelings for your family member. He is not being difficult on purpose.

Caregivers and healthcare providers should look for possible underlying causes for these behavioral problems, including pain, psychosis (paranoia), medical conditions, and side effects of medications,

Doctors may be reluctant to treat psychiatric symptoms pharmacologically in AD patients because many psychiatric drugs, particularly the anti-psychotic medications, have undesirable side effects in older adults, causing fogginess, disorientation, and sleepiness that can contribute to a fall.

So what can you do if medications aren't appropriate? A good therapy for mood swings in an older adult is to get her out of the house and into some enjoyable and appropriate activity. Many families have found that enrolling their loved one in an adult daycare center, even for a half day, two or three times a week, can greatly improve dispositions all around.

## Depression and Alzheimer's Disease

If your loved one is not sleeping or eating well and seems sad all the time, or expresses negative feelings, she may be clinically depressed. In the early stages of AD your loved one's depression may result from her diagnosis and the realization that she will gradually lose her capacity to function.

Regular exercise can help an older adult feel better, both physically and mentally. Talk to your doctor about other therapies. If nothing you do seems to lift your loved one's spirits, you should schedule an appointment for an evaluation to determine if your loved one needs medication to help control the depression, or some other more appropriate therapies. Your doctor may also refer you to a specialist. Antidepressant medications may be helpful and are generally well tolerated. In addition, your loved one may benefit from counseling or participation in a support group designed especially for people with mild AD.

Your loved one may not be the only one battling the blues. Caregiving is one of the most stressful jobs in the world, so in the next chapter you can find some good ideas to help you cope while you're serving as your loved one's caregiver.

# Part IV

# Respite Care for the Caregiver

The 5th Wave By Rich Tennant

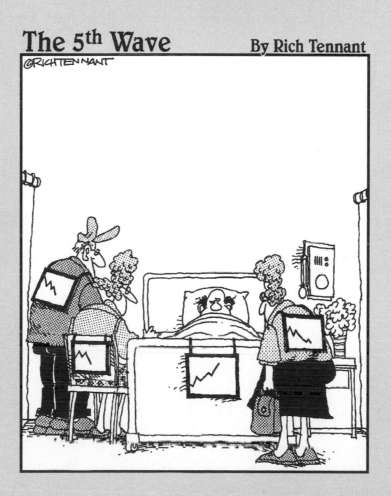

## In this part . . .

We present some ideas to help the caregiver manage stress and cope with the demands of caregiving. We help you take better care of yourself, maintain your own physical and mental health, and enlist help from family, friends, professional caregivers, and support groups. We even show you how to juggle work, family, and caregiving in a productive way. Finally, other family members can find out how to help the primary caregiver.

# Chapter 17

# Coping While Caregiving

* * * * * * * * * * * * * * * * * * * * * * * * * * * * * * * * * * * * * * * * * * * * * * * * * * * *

## In This Chapter

▶ Understanding that caregiving is hard work

▶ Looking at the emotional and physical costs of caregiving

▶ Keeping a positive outlook

▶ Asking for help

* * * * * * * * * * * * * * * * * * * * * * * * * * * * * * * * * * * * * * * * * * * * * * * * * * * *

*I*t's difficult to comprehend the mind- and body-numbing exhaustion a person can experience when confronted with the multiple responsibilities of caring for an Alzheimer's Disease patient. Caring for an AD patient can literally be a 24-hour a day job. If you don't develop a good support system early on, serving as a family caregiver can damage both your mental and physical health, divide your family, and even hurt your career. Caregiving has also been associated with increased mortality and lowered immune system functioning.

While serving as a family caregiver, it's easy to overlook your own needs and the needs of others who depend on you (but who aren't as dependent on you as your AD patient). You can get caught up in the cycle of endless demands and crises and lose sight of the other important things in your life, which may lead to burnout. You'll have days when you wish you could clone yourself because you don't know how you're ever going to get everything done. All this responsibility weighs heavily and can eventually exact a high toll. Caregiver burnout leaves everyone in the lurch and only adds to the feelings of overload, failure, and isolation you may be experiencing. Your burnout is also a source of distress for your loved one and can trigger or sustain his behavioral problems and frustrations.

In this chapter you discover the ways that caregiving can impact you and your family and some smart ideas to help you cope. You find tips for dealing with your fatigue and handling the situation if you or another family member becomes ill. We also cover the special considerations involved in caring for a parent or a spouse.

Finally, we talk about the importance of maintaining an even keel and a positive outlook, and the role that humor can play in helping you cope.

# Caregiving Is Hard Work

When you first take on the role of caregiver, you may have misgivings or you may feel confident that you can handle the job no matter what. After a few weeks of on-the-job experience, you'll probably see things more realistically. Even if you feel up to the job, you can't get around the fact that taking care of a cognitively impaired adult is one of the hardest things you'll ever do.

According to The Family Caregiver Alliance, an estimated 19 to 22 percent of American families are providing care for a cognitively impaired family member. Seventy percent of all AD patients, or about 2.8 million of the estimated 4 million cases in the United States, are cared for by a family caregiver for all or part of their disease.

Numerous studies point to caregiver attitude as a predictor of stress level and burnout. If you have a positive outlook and remain calm, you're less likely to suffer from depression and other health problems than caregivers with negative attitudes who see themselves as overburdened by responsibilities. Respite care isn't a luxury or an option; it's a critical part of good caregiving.

You can avoid caregiver stress, burnout and other potential problems if you take good care of yourself. Try the following strategies:

- Confront your feelings head-on and deal with them before they boil over.

- Be kind to yourself, get help, and schedule time off.

- Acknowledge that what you're doing is very hard work; don't try to pretend it's nothing.

- Acknowledge that it's not all sheer drudgery.

---

## Fast facts

A 1999 survey conducted by Caregiver Resource Centers found that

- 78 percent of caregivers lived with the person they were caring for.

- 18 percent quit their jobs to provide care.

- 42 percent cut back on the number of hours they worked outside the home to increase their availability to the person requiring care.

- 58 percent of the caregivers reported signs of clinical depression.

- Caregivers provided an average of 10.5 hours of care per day for their loved one, for a total of 73.5 hours of care per week.

If you can manage the balancing act, caregiving can pay off in a big way psychologically, giving you the satisfaction of performing a compassionate service for someone you love. Some caregivers report learning more about their own strengths as a result of caregiving. They may find that they are better problem solvers; have stronger organization and management skills; and are more flexible, tolerant, resilient, nurturing, and affectionate than they thought possible. Perhaps these attributes were always there but went unrecognized or unappreciated until the person became a caregiver.

# Caring for an AD Patient Affects You Emotionally

People react to AD behavior in many different ways. It can bring out your best or your worst. You may become angry and take your feelings out on your loved one. You may feel helpless and depressed. Or you may be brokenhearted, grieving for what you have lost, for what AD has taken from you and your loved one. Or you may feel strong and composed, burdened but not overburdened. In fact, you may feel all these emotions.

In a 1999 study published in the *Journal of Gerontology: Psychological Sciences*, researchers found that the more hours of care a person provides and the more problem behaviors her loved one demonstrates, the higher the caregiver's risk for depression and burnout. However, caregivers who had a good relationship with the person they were caring for, good emotional support, and a high level of confidence in their own abilities were less likely to experience burnout, even if their patients exhibited difficult behaviors.

## Dealing with negative emotions

Your attitude toward your caregiving responsibilities depends upon many factors, including the following:

- Your personality
- Your relationship with the person you're caring for, both in the past and in the present
- Whether you volunteered for the job or were recruited by circumstances beyond your control
- Who else is depending on you for support and care
- The amount of support you seek and receive

If you find yourself dwelling on negative thoughts or feelings, deal with them as soon as possible to keep them from spiraling out of control. If you do experience a crisis of control, it could seriously impact your own health and lead you to abuse your loved one in some way. The following sections give you tips for dealing with some specific negative feelings.

### Anger and frustration

Anger and frustration are usually a result of feeling put-upon, as if the whole situation were just plopped in your lap without anyone asking your opinion. A common source of anger for adult children of AD patients is the sense that the caregiving responsibilities aren't equally divided, they don't feel that their other siblings do enough. If you're angry, get those feelings under control because angry caretakers can trigger aggressive behavior from AD patients.

You're more likely to experience anger if

- The caretaking role was thrust upon you.

- You have or have had a difficult relationship with the person you're caring for.

- You're isolated and don't have the support of other family members or friends to help you shoulder the burden of caregiving.

- Your loved one exhibits difficult behaviors, such as irritability or repetitive questioning or if he resists your efforts to help care for him.

Here are some steps to take if your negative emotions start to overwhelm you:

- **Get help for your anger.** Talk to a therapist, enroll in an anger management course, or talk to your spiritual advisor. Don't let your anger fester and build until it explodes in a crisis situation.

- **Join a support group.** Joining a support group for AD caregivers gives you a healthy outlet for your anger and the opportunity to be heard and feel validated. Added bonus: Other members of the group are likely to have good suggestions for handling angry feelings based on first-hand experience. (See more about support groups in Chapter 19.)

- **Don't isolate yourself.** Caregivers with the angriest feelings are often those who feel cut off from the rest of the world because of their responsibilities. If you feel this way, ask a family member or friend to relieve you for a few hours on a regular basis. Use that time to connect with friends old and new —, attend a club meeting, a church social — anything that puts you in the company of other people you enjoy. Staying connected in this way keeps feelings of isolation to a minimum.

✔ **Take care of yourself.** Anger can also build when you're neglecting your own needs and not taking care of yourself. No matter how tough your situation, if you make it a priority from the beginning, you can and should find time every day to pamper yourself. Exercise, read a magazine, dig in the garden, pursue your hobbies — just make sure whatever you do is something that will relax and de-stress you, make you feel good, and take your mind off your caregiving chores for a while.

## *Depression*

Depression is a serious problem among caregivers. Depending upon which study you read, 30 to 50 percent of AD caregivers are depressed. Depression is more common among caregivers who have lower incomes, care for patients who exhibit more problem behaviors, feel overburdened, are female, and have had a bad relationship with the patient in the past.

You may be suffering from depression if you

✔ Feel tense or irritable

✔ Have frequent headaches or stomachaches

✔ Sleep or eat more or less than usual

✔ Lose interest in activities you once found pleasurable

✔ Have feelings of hopelessness

According to the National Mental Health Association, approximately 12 million women a year are clinically depressed in the United States — about double the rate of men. But 41 percent of the women surveyed didn't seek treatment because they were embarrassed, ashamed, or thought that it was normal for menopausal women to feel depressed. If you have any of the symptoms mentioned previously, you may be depressed. Get help! You don't have to keep feeling bad.

Many studies have shown that unresolved long-term depression can have a devastating effect on physical health, with higher incidences of heart disease, hypertension, and stroke in depressed caregiver populations than in control groups who are not caregivers.

To overcome depression, try some or all of the following strategies:

✔ Seek personal or group counseling.

✔ Ask your doctor whether an antidepressant medication is appropriate for you.

✔ Find regular relief from your caregiving duties to take care of yourself and your own needs.

✔ Avoid isolation; seek the company of your friends and peers.

✔ Enroll your loved one in a respite or daycare program, which is not only good for the patient's social well-being but is a key way for you to manage stress over time.

In other words, give yourself a break. Wallowing in the blues only makes them worse — seek help, and you can overcome depression.

### Grief

The odd thing about the grieving process and Alzheimer's Disease is that you're grieving the loss of someone who isn't dead. Because caregiving responsibilities can last for many years, the grief you feel can also last. You're not likely to be able to work your way through grieving unless you make a conscious effort to do so.

As with other negative feelings, the best relief for your grief is to seek appropriate counseling. Unresolved grief can not only negatively affect your ability to provide appropriate care for your loved one, but it can also damage your mental and physical health.

## Accepting altered relationships

We have unique relationships with each of the special people in our lives. One of the toughest aspects of dealing with an AD patient is watching that relationship change before your very eyes; all the things that made it so wonderful — the shared memories, the secret jokes, the facial expressions — can fade as AD continues its inexorable march.

It can be incredibly difficult for a caregiver when the person she cherishes begins to regard her differently as AD becomes more severe. Even if your loved one still recognizes you as a friendly face, he may not know exactly who you are or remember your familial relationship on a consistent basis.

### Losing your life partner

When the AD patient you're caring for is your spouse, you have an additional emotional burden because you're losing your life partner. As AD progresses, your loved one may lose most of your shared history, perhaps even forgetting that you had children together, and that loss can be very difficult to handle.

You can help recall old family memories by creating photo albums and memory boxes containing mementos of special times you shared and photos of your children, grandchildren, and even the family pets. Although these aides can help with reminiscing, they don't "boost" memory, so don't use them to quiz your loved one — quizzing may upset him.

## I can't bathe my mom!

Aside from the stressful emotions you may feel, you have practical matters to consider. For example, a son from a modest family may feel uncomfortable washing his mother's private area or wiping her after she uses the toilet.

Instead of stressing out, hire a home health aide who can provide those services for your mother. Or buy a modesty garment to preserve your parent's dignity while you're bathing her or helping her in the bathroom.

Your relationship with your spouse during her illness will be shaped by the relationship you've shared throughout your life together. It will also be impacted by the kinds of behavior your spouse displays over the course of the illness. Obviously, it's more difficult to care for an AD patient who has angry outbursts than it is to care for someone who sits quietly and smiles sweetly all the time and has retained the capacity to express appreciation.

If you have adult children, be sure to enlist their help. Don't try to handle all the caregiving chores by yourself. And take a few minutes each day to talk quietly with your spouse, recounting some favorite shared memory from long ago to reinforce your bond.

### Becoming a parent to your parent

Taking care of a parent can be a real challenge, even if the child is 50 and the parent is 72. Role reversal is never easy, and assuming the caregiving role is especially difficult if you're used to depending on your parent.

If you've had a difficult relationship with your parent all your life, you may not want or be able to provide care. Don't feel guilty. Hiring someone to provide care is better than forcing yourself to do it, because your negative feelings may build to neglect or explode in an abusive incident.

If you don't live in the same town as your parent and aren't able to be part of the caregiving team, you still have many ways to help your other parent or your siblings provide care. See Chapter 22 for ways you can help even if you live halfway across the country.

## Finding serenity

Although you can't control or change Alzheimer's Disease, you have control over how you handle your caregiving responsibilities, how you interact with your loved one, and how you let the situation affect you. As difficult as caregiving is, you do have choices. With wise choices that empower you and make you feel good, you not only survive the caregiving experience but thrive and grow as you rise to meet the challenges of caring for your loved one in new and creative ways. With bad choices, you end up feeling over-whelmed, over-burdened, burned-out, resentful, depressed, physically ill, and miserably unhappy.

Serenity is not going to find you; you have to actively pursue it. Make time for yourself, even if it's just 15 minutes. In 15 minutes you can

- ✔ Take a bubble bath
- ✔ Read a chapter in a book
- ✔ Read and answer e-mail
- ✔ Call a supportive friend
- ✔ Massage your feet with peppermint lotion
- ✔ Pick some flowers and arrange them in a vase
- ✔ Listen to your favorite song — several times!
- ✔ Make a fruit smoothie

Alaskan dog sledders have a popular saying: "The pace of the pack follows the pace of the leader." As an AD caregiver, you are your loved one's leader. If you're always crabby, impatient, snappish, angry, short-fused, and martyred, how do you think your loved one (and the rest of your family members) are going to react? But if you're patient, kind, loving, and compassionate, you'll find that you get an entirely different response from your family and your AD patient. The choice of how you act is up to you.

## Caregiving and Your Physical Health

You may find it hard to believe, but taking care of an AD patient can have a significant impact on your physical health. Whether your health is affected depends on how well you care for yourself while you're taking care of your loved one. If you let yourself go, overlook your own needs, eat a poor diet on an irregular schedule, and are constantly sleep deprived, the combination of physical neglect and increased stress can actually make you sick.

Caring for another adult is hard work. Depending upon the severity of your loved one's condition, you may be doing the work of an entire staff of an Assisted Living or AD Center, from director, business manager, head RN, LVN, aide, housekeeper, cook, and maintenance man to lawn boy. You may be con-stantly bending, lifting, twisting, and straining, which can lead to muscular injuries such as strains, sprains, or even skeletal problems resulting in back, neck, or knee pain.

Unrelenting stress constantly bathes your system in the stress hormone corti-sol. Although cortisol is quite valuable in normal concentrations, researchers at Stanford University found that caregivers had irregular levels of cortisol, which may raise their risks for heart disease and some types of cancer.

A study conducted at the University of California at San Diego concluded that mortality from all causes is 63 percent higher in spousal caregivers than in non-caregivers. A Stanford University study concluded that 40 percent of all AD caregivers die from stress-related disorders before their patient dies. The University of Pittsburgh estimated that 25 percent of nursing home place-ments are a direct result of caregiver illness or death.

Caregivers are also subject to higher rates of weight gain or loss, adult-onset diabetes, anemia, ulcers, high blood pressure, insomnia, and alcohol or drug abuse than non-caregivers.

All these undesirable effects can be negated by taking care of yourself. If you eat a balanced diet, exercise regularly, get support for your stress, sleep six to eight hours every night, take a few minutes every day to pamper yourself, and strive to maintain a positive outlook, then you should be able to bring your physical health risks back to normal. See the following sections for tips on how to take of yourself while taking care of your loved one.

## Taking care of yourself first

Although it may seem selfish, you absolutely must put your own health and sanity first. Why? Well, if you run yourself into the ground and end up in the hospital with a heart attack or stroke, or you're so tired you fall asleep at the wheel and have a bad car accident, who's going to care for your loved one then? When you have another human totally dependent upon you for every-thing, not putting yourself first can put them last.

By putting yourself first and making sure all your needs are met — physical, emotional, and spiritual — you are actually making yourself a better care-giver, not to mention a better spouse and parent. You're not only preserving your own well-being, but also sending a powerful message to the people around you: you're doing an important job, but that doesn't mean you will neglect yourself, so nobody else better neglect or marginalize you either.

Enlightened self-interest can have a whole host of unexpected benefits, so start practicing it today. Being your own advocate doesn't mean you always get the biggest steak or the cake with the most icing; it means that you care for yourself as much as you care for your loved one, and that you will not sacrifice your health or the quality of your life in order to take care of him or her. It means you understand that with some planning ahead, you can assem-ble a support team that will help you to have it all — a spouse, kids, a career, and still serve as a caregiver. It's not easy, but you can do it.

## Fighting fatigue and illness

Unless you're careful, the stress of long-term caregiving can lead to fatigue, and ongoing fatigue makes you more susceptible to illness. You can help yourself stay healthy if you pay good attention to your body's need for rest. If you feel yourself getting over-tired, do whatever is necessary to get a few nights of good sleep to relieve your fatigue. Here are a couple of ideas:

✔ Ask a family member to take over your loved one's care for a few nights so you can catch up on your sleep.

✔ If you don't have a relative nearby, hire a home health aide for a couple of days or check your loved one into an overnight respite care center.

# Using Humor to Cope

*"Against the assault of laughter nothing can stand."*

Mark Twain, The Mysterious Stranger, 1916

When you're at your wit's end and don't think you can take one more thing piled on your plate, take a few minutes to laugh. No, really. Why do you think someone made up that cliché: "Laughter is the best medicine"? When you're laughing, you can't be frowning at the same time.

Laughter takes your mind off your problems, if only for a few minutes. It increases respiration, relaxes tense muscles, and makes you feel good. Seeing you and other family members laughing also makes your loved one happy. It reminds him of good times from the past and helps distract him from his own worries and fears.

One of the best remedies for a bad mood is a good dose of laughter. According to a 1996 study, laughter lowers blood pressure, reduces levels of stress hormones, boosts immune function (by raising production of infection- and disease-fighting cells), and triggers the release of endorphins (Mother Nature's natural painkillers and mood enhancers). So grab a funny video and watch it with your loved one. You'll soon feel better.

Even if you couldn't make a living as a stand-up comic, you can find plenty of ways to inject a little humor into your day.

✔ **Find humor in some of the situations that arise because of AD.** Your loved one can say and do some pretty funny things. Just remember to laugh with them, and not at them.

✔ **Think of your all-time favorite comedies and buy a few on video or DVD.** Stay away from the heavy dramas — caring for an AD patient should provide about all the drama you can stand.

> ✔ **Subscribe to an Internet joke service.** Visit a few humor sites until you find one that matches your sense of humor. Some are risqué, some are corny, but only you know what makes you laugh. Here are some to try: www.jokeaday.com, www.laffaday.com, and www.laugh-of-the-day.com.
>
> ✔ **Watch a late-night talk show.** The best jokes are in the opening monologues, so you can grab a few laughs without staying up too late.
>
> If you have cable or satellite television, check out Comedy Central.

Lots of things can make you laugh. Find something that works for you and use it whenever you feel down or overwhelmed. A hearty laugh may be just what you need to get going again.

# Knowing When to Ask for Help

Even with the best routines in place and good stress management techniques, you're still only one person with one set of hands and 24 hours in your day. If after establishing routines, you find that you still can't get everything done, don't stress out — ask for help.

Early on, schedule regular time off from your caregiving chores. Having a few hours a day to yourself, at least 2 to 3 days a week, is critical if you plan to provide care for your loved one for the duration of his illness. If money to hire help is tight, ask local day care centers if they have scholarships available or have sliding scale fees based on financial need.

## Making a volunteer list

Make a list of everyone in your family, and close friends and neighbors. Beside each name, write an honest assessment of his ability to contribute to the care of your loved one. Hopefully, two or three people will stand out as those you can trust to help with your loved one's care.

Call each person and ask for help, or invite everyone to your home for a meeting. Lay out your schedule, explain where you need help, and ask for volunteers. Perhaps you can't get to the drycleaner to pick up your clothes, but your neighbor who uses the same drycleaner may be happy to get them for you. Maybe you don't have time to shop for groceries, but your sister is happy to get your order when she goes shopping.

If your loved one has special care needs such as incontinence, it's not fair to expect an untrained volunteer to manage that problem. When you need some time off, try an adult day care center or hire a home companion/caregiver.

# Getting help for abusive tendencies

The National Center for Victims of Crime estimates that 1 out of 25 elders is abused in some way every year. Although the incidence varies by community from 2 to 5 percent of the elderly population, the total number abused every year in the United States is between one to two million seniors.

Many situations can cause a caregiver to lose control and strike out physically or verbally at the person they're caring for. People who haven't spent much time around an AD patient in the later stages of the disease have very little understanding of just how maddening it can be to have to answer the same question 20 or 30 times a day, or be constantly accused of stealing, or clean up an incontinent person time after time. Add an isolated, overwhelmed rundown caregiver and a few financial, job or marital problems to this mix, and you have a recipe for abusive behavior just waiting to come to the boil.

If you don't deal with your anger, it can grow to the point where you may abuse your loved one. If you exhibit any of the following warning signs, get help immediately! Schedule emergency respite care for your loved one until you can get your angry feelings under control.

- You feel indifferent or angry toward your loved one all the time, not just occasionally.

- You blame your loved one for all your problems and negative feelings and don't accept responsibility for your own behavior.

- You isolate your loved one from other family members to retain control of the situation.

- You habitually exhibit aggressive behavior; for example, you shout, name-call, threaten, or insult your loved one.

- You feel a desire to hit or hurt your loved one.

- You have a history of alcohol or drug abuse that is getting worse.

If you do lose control, call your local senior center for information about anger management and stress relief classes. Join a support group, seek counseling — do whatever it takes to make sure it doesn't happen again. If despite your best efforts, you find yourself abusing your loved one, make other care arrangements to ensure her safety.

# Chapter 18

# Finding Support

· · · · · · · · · · · · · · · · · · · · · · · · · · · · · · · · · · · · · · · · ·

### In This Chapter

▶ Knowing what kinds of support are available

▶ Looking at support groups — do they really help?

▶ Finding a counselor or confidante

· · · · · · · · · · · · · · · · · · · · · · · · · · · · · · · · · · · · · · · · ·

Managing the care of your loved one without any support from others is like being Sisyphus, who was condemned by the Greek gods of Mount Olympus to roll a heavy boulder up a mountain, only to see it roll back down to the bottom again and again. Sisyphus is the symbol of endless labor. Unless you want to vie for his job, you need to find some support early on while taking care of your loved one.

Support can and should come in many forms — it can be a friend's voice on the phone, a strong neighborhood teen who comes to lift your loved one into bed every night, a church friend who cooks dinner one night a week, a sister who flies in from across the country every three to four months so you can have two weeks off, or even a group of strangers who are struggling with the same problems as you. The kind of support you seek depends on the kind of help you need. What form the support takes isn't important; what's important is that you have support. Taking care of an Alzheimer's Disease (AD) patient by yourself is an overwhelming job. Keeping yourself up to the task requires regular breaks, and that's where support comes in.

In this chapter, we discuss the kinds of support that are available for caregivers and help you tune in to local resources. You find out how to identify possible sources of support and figure out whether a formal caregivers support group is right for you. Finally, you discover the importance of seeking a counselor or a confidante to help you shoulder the burden of taking care of your loved one. This chapter focuses on emotional support and physical respite for the caregiver; if you need information about possible sources of financial support, see Chapter 14.

# Finding Out What's Available

AD is becoming so prevalent that even smaller towns are likely to have some support services available for caregivers within the area. Obviously, if you live in an urban area, your choices are more extensive. Even suburbs sometimes have a surprising array of support services available.

Support falls into two categories — formal and informal. *Formal support* is provided by governmental agencies, non-profit organizations, healthcare providers, and church and volunteer groups. *Informal support* is provided by relatives, friends, and neighbors.

## Formal support — enlisting the experts

Organizations that provide formal support for caregivers are the first places to turn to for help when taking care of your loved one. Because these groups specialize in offering support, the assistance they provide is usually on target and helpful. On the other hand, working with bureaucracies can be frustrating, and you may have to deal with delays. But if you are persistent, patient, and calm, you can usually get the help you need.

### Government agencies

A number of federal and state agencies deal with caregivers' and senior citizens' issues. The type of help you're seeking determines which agency you contact.

The Administration on Aging (AOA) provides services to older individuals who have economic, social, and health needs. They maintain offices in every state and many larger cities. An agency of the U.S. Department of Health and Human Services, the AOA was created in 1965 with the passage of the Older Americans Act (OAA).

The AOA is part of the National Network on Aging, which is one of the largest providers of home- and community-based care for seniors and their caregivers, providing services for about seven million people annually.

The AOA has a downloadable guide for caregivers available at www.aoa.gov/ wecare/content-pdf.html. The online version is available at www.aoa.gov/ wecare/default.htm.

The OAA funds six core services:

> ✔ **Support Services** provides information about local services and practical assistance, such as transportation to and from doctor's appointments, grocery stores, and drug stores. Support services also provide maintenance, handyman, chore, and personal services to enable seniors to stay in their own homes as long as possible.

✔ **Nutrition Services** provides hot meals for seniors, as well as the opportunity for seniors who are socially isolated to enjoy their meals and each other's company. Seniors who are house-bound can get a hot meal delivered daily. Nutrition counseling, health screenings, and general counseling are also provided at senior centers.

✔ **Preventive Health Services** educates seniors about making healthy lifestyle choices to prevent chronic disease through exercise, proper diet, smoking cessation, and health screenings.

✔ **The National Family Caregiver Support Program (NFCSP)** was created to help individuals and families who are providing primary care for a senior family member (or a disabled relative or grandparents caring for grandchildren). The NFCSP provides information about local services and helps in accessing those services. The program also offers information on counseling, support groups, supplemental care services, and caregiver training to help caregivers understand their roles, make good caregiving decisions, and solve their caregiving problems.

✔ **Elder Abuse Prevention** provides services to at-risk seniors and their families to help them recognize and detect elder abuse and consumer fraud. The program also enhances the physical, mental, and emotional well-being of elderly people by providing pension counseling, ombudsman programs to investigate and resolve complaints made by residents of residential care facilities, Medicare patrol projects, and projects to encourage the reporting of waste, fraud, and abuse in residential care facilities.

✔ **Services to Native Americans** provides most of the mentioned services in a way that satisfies the cultural and social traditions of Native Americans.

To find services and resources for caregivers in your community, call the AOA's Eldercare locator toll-free at 1-800-677-1116. The AOA coordinates caregiving information for a number of other agencies and organizations, both publicly and privately funded. All that information is available through this one number.

### Nonprofit organizations

The local chapters of the Alzheimer's Association and the Family Caregiver Alliance provide excellent resources for caregiving questions and crisis resolution. The Alzheimer's Association may have scholarship funds to cover the cost of their *Safe Return* program or defray the cost of hiring a paid companion or homemaker.

The Alzheimer's Disease Education and Referral Center (ADEAR), sponsored jointly by the National Institutes on Health (NIH) and the National Institute on Aging (NIA), offers education for families caring for an AD patient and sponsors support groups for both caregivers and AD patients.

If you need a quick answer to a question about AD, your role as a caregiver, or locating community resources, you can chat live online with an ADEAR Alzheimer's Disease specialist Monday through Friday from 2 p.m. to 4 p.m. Eastern time. Go to http://209.70.85.166/support/camden/index2.php for the link. Or you can call 1-800-438-4380 toll-free Monday through Friday from 8:30 a.m. to 5 p.m. Eastern time. Or email your questions by filling out the form located at www.alzheimers.org/contact.htm. The Family Caregiver Alliance has an AD fact sheet located at www.caregiver.org/factsheet.html. The alliance publishes an informative newsletter four times a year that is packed with the latest information about AD research, caregiving, funding, family issues for caregivers, and a host of other topics.

The National Family Caregivers Association (www.nfcacares.org/) is an advocacy group that supports caregivers and trains and organizes them to speak out at public meetings to raise awareness of family caregiver issues and promote political action to assist and relieve caregivers.

Many states sponsor Alzheimer's Caregiver Support groups online, which have chat rooms and message boards where caregivers can communicate. These sites usually have resource centers and some, like the University of Florida, offer excellent learning centers that provide professional quality online training for Alzheimer's caregivers.

In addition, the Alzheimer's Disease Centers (ADCs) offer valuable Web sites with information on treatment, research, and practical information on caregiving. Go to the ADEAR Web site for links to various ADCs and other important Web sites.

Many smaller organizations provide online support and fellowship for caregivers across the United States, and family caregivers themselves host some sites.

### Healthcare providers

If your loved one has an overnight hospital stay for any reason — even a bad cough — take advantage of a little-known service provided by hospitals called *discharge planning*. Discharge planning, overseen by registered nurses, social workers, and case managers, provides continued care for your loved one for a period of time after his discharge from the hospital. In the case of elderly patients, particularly those with dementia, discharge planners want to make sure the patient's basic needs are met after she returns home.

Discharge planners can connect you with community services — everything from counseling to meal delivery to support groups to caregiver training. Many hospitals provide free or low-cost round-trip transportation for seniors and disabled people who are visiting a doctor affiliated with the hospital and to people coming to the hospital to get tests. This service can be a tremendous help for caregivers who work because it keeps them from leaving work to provide transportation. Keep in mind though, that when your loved one has AD, you should be present at his or her doctor visits to ensure compliance with the doctor's medical recommendations.

### Church and volunteer groups

Although churches and volunteer groups may not have the vast resources provided by the federal government, many of them do offer valuable services for people struggling with caregiving issues. Ask your pastor if your church has volunteer sitters or respite care, and take full advantage of the program if it's available. Many of these faith-based programs are very affordable and may even be free for families with limited finances.

Many churches and volunteer groups also offer hot meal delivery for seniors and transportation services for doctor's appointments, shopping, and errands. Call your local senior center to see what volunteer groups are active in your area.

## Informal support — getting by with a little help from your friends

Informal support can come from a variety of people. Informal support doesn't even have to involve the care of your loved one; it can be someone doing something for you, such as running an errand so you can stay with your loved one and not hire a sitter. For example, perhaps a co-worker is willing to cover your desk for two hours once a month when your loved one has a doctor's appointment. Perhaps you have an understanding boss who allows you to take an hour off here and there or rearrange your lunch breaks to accommodate your loved one's needs.

Whether help comes from family, friends, neighbors, or people online you've never met, informal support helps you do a better job of caring for yourself and your loved one.

### Family

You may not think you have to ask family members for help; you assume they're just going to step right up to the plate and volunteer. But that may not always be the case, especially if they perceive that you've taken over and have things in hand. If you want help from a family member, be specific about what you want her to do and ask nicely; don't demand her assistance and don't try sending her on a guilt trip. A lot of stress, resentment, and anger among adult children providing care for a parent is caused by the perception that other siblings aren't doing their part. It's true that responsibilities are rarely shared equally; so many factors like work, family demands, distance, the quality of the relationship and how it affects the people involved, personal strengths and weaknesses, play a role that equal division is almost impossible.

The best way to get help from someone is to communicate clearly what you want him to do. Look him in the eye, and in a pleasant tone, tell him what chores have to be done. Instead of assigning chores, give your family member a choice of chores. Ask whether he wants to pick up the prescription or sit with your loved one for half an hour while you do it. Let him choose what he's most comfortable doing, and you're more likely to get his. Every person responds very differently to the news that someone she loves has AD. Don't push someone who is uncomfortable with the situation beyond what she's comfortable doing. (See more about family dynamics in Chapter 20.) If your brother is squeamish about bathing your mother, ask him to shop for groceries instead. Every chore is valuable and helps relieve you in some way. By being flexible and willing to accept help in whatever form it's offered (as long as it's a reasonable offer), you actually encourage people to help you even more. But if you're bossy, picky, and constantly nagging people to help and then criticize the way they do things when they do help, don't be surprised if they're nowhere to be found the next time you have a chore for them.

### Friends and neighbors

Friends and neighbors can sometimes be even more helpful than family members because they don't have the history and baggage of your family dynamics to contend with. They can just step right in and do whatever needs to be done. But like family, friends have to know that you need help before they can offer assistance. Let your friends know what your needs are, and you can have a veritable army of people running errands, cooking meals, and offering to sit with your loved one for a few hours so you can have a break.

### Online support

Oddly enough, the people who offer you the most emotional support may be people you never even meet. Members of online news groups and chat rooms who serve as caregivers for a loved one with AD know just how you feel, because they feel the same way. They're facing the same day-to-day problems, the same worries about money, and the same feeling of overload that you are. This shared experience can make for some very nurturing friendships.

## Looking into Support Groups

Many different organizations sponsor support groups for AD caregivers, including The Alzheimer's Association, Assisted Living residential care facilities, churches, and senior centers. Support groups provide a comfortable and accepting atmosphere where caregivers can talk openly about their concerns and problems and gather new information about AD and the caregiving.

If you're looking for a group in your area, call the local chapter of the Alzheimer's Association or ask your loved one's doctor or counselor for a recommendation. The local council on aging and senior center may also have some good suggestions.

Visit several groups before deciding on which to join. Some groups may appeal to you more than others. If one group has a bunch of whiners who dominate the discussions, that won't be much help and you probably want to keep looking. If you join a group and come away from the sessions feeling worse and not better, try another group. The ideal group is comprised of a nice cross-section of caregivers who exchange information and tips, listen compassionately to other member's problems, and offer reasonable suggestions.

The two main types of support groups are

- ✔ Groups led by a professional, such as a doctor, nurse, or social worker who has direct experience dealing with AD.

- ✔ Self-help groups led by someone who is currently caring for an AD patient or has cared for one in the past and has become a volunteer advocate for caregivers.

Depending on the type of group you join, meetings may be educational or emotional in focus or both. Educational meetings offer a variety of speakers on different topics related to AD care. One night a speaker who is a political activist and AD advocate may fill you in on the latest legislation affecting seniors or caregivers. Another night a nurse may tell you tips for basic self care and medication management strategies or a Web site with good resources and information for caregivers. A registered dietitian may give you nutritional tips and hints to get your loved one to eat well. Or you may hear a doctor involved in a clinical trial for a new drug telling you the latest news from the research front.

Groups that offer emotional support for caregivers usually have a less formal structure to the meetings. Members may sit in a circle and share stories, shed a few tears, hug each other, offer advice and solutions to specific problems, and allow each other to vent in a safe atmosphere.

If you have trouble getting out of your house to attend a meeting, dozens of online support groups are available — formal, moderated, and informal. Just enter "Alzheimer's caregiver online support" in any search engine and you get a huge list of sites. Check out several until you find one with people who are on your wavelength.

Support groups may be available for both caregivers and AD patients. Many centers schedule meetings for both groups at the same time so caregivers can relax and enjoy the meeting, knowing their loved one is in an enjoyable and secure situation at the same time. In some larger centers, the group for your loved one may be a true support group for people with mild AD, or a respite service offered to those with varying levels of AD so that the caregiver can attend his or her own support group meeting without worry.

# Finding a Counselor

Seeking the help of a professional counselor, such as a psychologist, psychiatrist, social worker, pastor, or doctor, may help you and your loved one make the most of your situation and stay on a more even keel. People in the early stages of AD can benefit tremendously from counseling. Just having a sympathetic ear really helps sometimes. If you don't want to see a counselor regularly, consider visiting one to help you through a crisis situation.

Ask your doctor to recommend a counselor who has experience working with AD patients and their families. Running your finger down a list of names in the Yellow Pages and ending up in an office with someone who specializes in truant teens isn't going to help you much. Call the counselor and ask about their experience in counseling patients and families dealing with AD.

Counseling provides many benefits, including the following:

✔ You can talk through your feelings about your caregiving role and express any doubts or fears you have in a safe, controlled situation to a person who is qualified and experienced enough to offer you real solutions.

✔ A good counselor teaches you better ways to cope with the stress of caregiving and teaches you proven stress reduction techniques

✔ Counselors help AD patients look at their situation in a more positive light, and can also encourage patients to take a proactive stance and work actively to maintain their health.

Remember, the best approach to managing your love one's care is to take advantage of ongoing education and support. Don't wait until a crisis arises.

# Chapter 19

# Taking Care of the Caregiver

*In This Chapter*
- ▶ Taking time out
- ▶ Treating yourself well
- ▶ Avoiding isolation
- ▶ Staying in touch with friends

*W*hen you're caring for an Alzheimer's Disease (AD) patient, it's all too easy to completely let go of your former life. Friends, hobbies, work, and even other family members can all fall by the wayside if you focus too intently on your caregiving role.

To stay healthy and keep yourself and everyone around you calm and centered requires a bit of balance. If you give all your time, energy, and attention to the care of your AD patient, you're neglecting other priorities, including your own needs. This tunnel vision doesn't make for a very happy caregiver. To borrow a wise old cliché, "If the caregiver ain't happy, then ain't no one gonna be happy."

Don't feel guilty for wanting to take time off from your caregiving duties to relax with your family, go off on your own to see a movie, or get a massage or facial, play a bracing round of handball or hand of bridge, or, even go on a vacation. If you've been a member of the neighborhood garden club for ten years and never missed a meeting, don't start missing them now. There's nothing wrong with wanting to go on with your life as it was. AD disrupts life enough — don't give it more power by neglecting yourself. Of course things change and it becomes more difficult to get away, but with advance planning, almost anything you want to do is possible.

In this chapter, you discover the importance of taking time for yourself and some good ways to lift your spirits when you're having a tough time. You see how isolating yourself from your normal support system can lead to trouble. You also find out how to rally other family members and friends to form your own personal cheering section.

# Giving Yourself a Break

Family caregivers provide an average of 70 hours per week of care for their loved ones. The number of hours can get even higher as AD progresses and care requirements become more demanding. Seventy hours a week is already almost double a normal 40-hour work-week. A week has only 168 hours. If you're working 40 hours and providing care for 70 hours, that leaves just 58 hours (which is a little over eight hours a day) to do everything else — sleep, prepare meals, eat, pay bills, interact with your other family members, and go out to see friends.

You may feel you can't possibly take time out to do things for yourself. How can you when you've got so many other things to take care of? Well, you can (and need to) take time out for yourself. In this section, we tell you how.

## Turning off the guilt

What are the reasons you don't take time out from your caregiving duties to do something for yourself? Do you feel guilty? Are you worried what other people may think if they see you out having fun when everybody knows you have a dependent family member at home? Do you just think you don't deserve to have a good time?

Whatever your internal voices are telling you, tell them to be quiet, because you're about to discover the vital importance of regularly taking time out for yourself. Taking time out for yourself isn't just a good idea; it's an essential idea.

Before you get started on ways to treat yourself well, try a little exercise to get rid of any lingering feelings of guilt you may have about taking some time for yourself. The American Association of Retired Persons developed a Caregiver's Bill of Rights for its members who are caring for a family member (see the nearby sidebar). Read through it, and if you have to, print it out and tape a copy in several places around the house — the bathroom mirror, the refrigerator, and the laundry room — to remind yourself that as valuable as your services are, you're much more than just a caregiver. You're an individual with unique needs and desires, and you have every right to take care of your needs.

## A Caregiver's Bill of Rights

**I have the right to take care of myself.** This is not an act of selfishness. It will give me the ability to take better care of my loved one.

I have the right to **seek help from others** even though my loved one may object. I recognize the limits of my own endurance and strength.

I have the right to **maintain facets of my own life** that do not include the person I care for just as I would if he or she were healthy. I know that I do everything that I reasonably can do for this person and I have the right to do some things just for myself.

I have the right to get angry, be depressed, and **express difficult feelings** occasionally.

I have the right to **reject any attempt** by my loved one (either conscious or unconscious) to manipulate me through guilt or anger.

I have the right to **receive considerations, affection, forgiveness, and acceptance** for what I do for my loved one as I offer these attributes in return.

I have the right to **take pride in what I am accomplishing** and to applaud the courage it has taken to meet the needs of my loved one.

I have the right to **protect my individuality** and my right to make a life for myself that will sustain me in times when my loved one no longer needs my full-time help.

I have the right to **expect and demand** that as new strides are made in finding resources to aid physically and mentally impaired older persons in our country, similar strides will be made toward aiding and supporting caregivers.

Reprinted by permission of AARP

Statistics tell us that family caregivers provide an average of 70 hours per week of care for their loved ones. That figure can get even higher as AD progresses and care requirements become more demanding.

According to The American Academy of Family Physicians, the value of care provided in the home by family caregivers averages $34,517 per family per year. In 1997, The Administration on Aging pegged the total value of family caregiving services at $196 billion annually, or 18 percent of the total healthcare expenditures in this nation. That number is expected to rise dramatically as the number of families providing in home care a relative is growing every year.

## Scheduling personal time

You may be asking, "Exactly where am I supposed to find four hours a week to keep up with my bowling league?" (or chess club, or poker with the boys, or standing hair appointment, and so on). The answer is that you make the time. Of the 168 hours in a week, you can't take time away from the 40 hours a week you spend at your job, and you can't really take any time away from the 58 hours a week you sleep and take care of your family and household chores. So, the logical place to find the time is among the 70-plus hours you take care of you loved one each week.

Decide what you want your weekly activity to be, figure out how long you need and when you want to do it, and make other care arrangements for your loved one during that time every week. Be sure to schedule enough time to comfortably complete your outing, including round-trip transportation, or the fun of a relaxing afternoon can be ruined by racing through traffic to get home on time for your sitter to pick her son up from school.

For example, if you go see a 90-minute movie and the theater is 20 minutes away from your house, you need 90 minutes plus 40 minutes of transportation time — that's a grand total of 130 minutes, or two hours and ten minutes. If you schedule your sitter for just two hours, you'd better bring your jet pack because you're not going to make it home in time without it.

You don't have to do the same thing every week. One week you may want to see a movie, and the following week you may want to have lunch with your spouse or a close friend. What's important is that you schedule regular breaks for yourself and then actually take them.

# Being Good to Yourself

Maybe it's that old Puritan ethic rearing its head, but something about the culture of the United States makes it difficult to put yourself first or to even think of yourself at all. But ignoring your own needs is a false economy; you may save an hour or so in the present situation but lose days or even weeks if you become ill or get injured. Because the incidence of illness and accidents rise dramatically when caregivers are overly stressed and aren't taking proper care of themselves, you need to schedule a little relaxation and recreation for yourself.

But how do you schedule time for yourself, especially when both time and money are tight? Look for small ways to bring a smile to your face — activities that help you forget your worries, if only for a few minutes.

## Treating yourself to a little pampering

Pampering yourself doesn't have to be expensive or time-consuming (although nothing is wrong with splurging now and then). Here are some ideas to get you started. Most of them can be completed in 15 minutes or less, and some cost absolutely nothing.

- ✔ **Watch the birds.** Buy a small Lucite bird feeder with a suction cup and attach it to a window where both you and your loved one can see it. The comings and goings of birds and all their little dramas as they fight for spots at the feeder, chase each other, and sing and chirp will bring a smile to your face. Added bonus: watching birds is a great activity for your loved one.

Cost with seed: $10 to $15

✔ **Try something fishy.** A 1999 study at Purdue University found that tanks of brightly colored fish curtailed disruptive behaviors and improved eating habits of AD patients. Another study from the University of Pennsylvania reported that watching fish in an aquarium reduced stress and lowered blood pressure of AD patients.

Cost: $30 and up for aquarium set-up, including filter, pump, and fish food; $10 and up for an assortment of fish.

✔ **Get private.** Take 15 minutes of absolute solitude to get yourself re-centered. Go outside, turn your face to the sun and soak up its warmth, or lock yourself away in your study with your journal or a good book. Set a timer for 15 minutes and let the tension flow out of your body.

Cost: nothing!

✔ **Burn an aromatherapy candle.** All sorts of wonderful fragrances are available. Even discount stores and drug stores have aromatherapy candles now, so you don't have to mortgage the farm to buy one. Select a fragrance you especially like, and light the candle in a protected place so your loved one can't get to it. In about 15 minutes, its soft fragrance suffuses an entire room. Remember that an open flame can be dangerous for a person with advanced AD, so don't use this suggestion if your loved one is in the severe or profound stage of the disease.

Cost: $3 to $5

✔ **Dream on.** If you want to pamper yourself at bedtime, the next best thing to your mom singing you a lullaby is a dream pillow. Dream pillows lull you into a better night's sleep using soothing blends of herbs proven to relax jangled nerves. Long Creek Herbs has the best selection available online at www.longcreekherbs.com/dream.html#pillows. They grow their own herbs, so the pillows are always fresh and highly fragrant.

Cost: $8.95 per pillow (plus shipping)

✔ **Try chocolate therapy.** When you're feeling stressed, indulge in some really tasty chocolate and eat one piece very slowly. Take the time to notice the chocolate's fragrance, color, and texture. Savor the delicious taste as it melts in your mouth. Why does chocolate make you feel so good? It's just science: chocolate contains a mood-enhancing chemical called *theobromine,* the same chemical our brains manufacture when we think we're falling in love. Don't eat chocolate more than once or twice a day, though, or you may have to buy *Dieting For Dummies.*

Cost: $1 and up per piece

TIP

## Scents and sensibilities

If you're afraid to light a candle around your loved one, set out a dish of potpourri or buy a fragrance diffuser that plugs into an outlet. Add a few drops of your favorite fragrant oil to a ceramic diffuser or buy diffusers with fragrance gels already packed inside. Can't make up your mind about which fragrance to choose? Lavender is very soothing and calming.

✔ **Dig in.** Plant some flowers in a spot where you can easily see them from the window. If you don't have a yard, buy a bouquet of inexpensive flowers from the grocery store or buy a flowering potted plant in full bloom, such as a geranium, miniature rose, chrysanthemum, or an African Violet.

Cost: $5 and up

✔ **Act like a baby and have a good cry.** No fooling. Many caregivers bottle up their feelings in order to stay focused on their tasks. But repressing emotions can have detrimental health effects or lead to depression, a lapse in care for your loved one, or even an explosion of anger or inappropriate behavior. Even if you're the sort who never cries, rent a tearjerker to get the old waterworks going. Lock yourself in your room and scream, cry, and beat your pillow to a pulp — do anything you have to do to get the emotions flowing. You'll feel better afterwards; your pillow, however, will probably feel worse.

Cost: nothing — unless you have to replace your pillow.

## *Pampering yourself macho style!*

Along about now, male readers are probably saying, "Enough with this girly stuff! How about some pampering for guys, too?" There's no reason why men can't light a candle or indulge in chocolate, too. But here are some ideas for ways men can pamper themselves:

✔ **Feed your face.** Order your favorite take-out food — Chinese, pizza, ribs, or whatever you like.

Cost: $10 and up

✔ **Putter around.** If you enjoy golf but rarely have time to get out to the links anymore, buy an indoor putting green and practice your putts in the den for 15 minutes. TriFli Sports has a good selection, starting at just $19.95 at www.walkinggolfbags.com/inputgreen.html.

✔ **Rock out.** Pop your favorite CD or cassette tape into your portable stereo, plug in your headphones, and listen to music. Or tune the radio to your favorite station. If you're really feeling ambitious, dance to the music. Dancing is a great way to relieve stress.

Cost: Portable CD player $40 and up. Portable tape player $20 and up. CDs $10 and up. Cassette tapes $8 and up. Radio $10 and up

✔ **Take a virtual trip.** Set your timer for 15 minutes, sit in your favorite, most comfortable chair (preferably a recliner or a rocker), and lean back and put your feet up. Look at a travel brochure or read through a magazine article about your preferred destination. Pay particular attention to the photographs. Now close your eyes and envision yourself at that place you've always wanted to visit — on the white beaches of Hawaii, climbing the Mayan ruins in Mexico, or the Eiffel Tower in Paris, photographing the Grand Canyon, or strolling through that museum downtown you've been meaning to check out. After your 15 minutes are up, you feel relaxed and refreshed.

Cost: nothing

✔ **Put up your dukes (or watch someone else put up his).** Order a favorite pay-per-view sporting event on television.

Cost: $15 and up

✔ **Whack some weeds.** Grab a weed whacker and mow down as many weeds as you can find in 15 minutes or trim the edges of your driveway, sidewalk, or patio.

Cost: $30 and up for a weed whacker

✔ **Clean up your act.** Remember to take a bath or shower every day. No, this tip isn't a joke. One of the first things caregivers do when they get overloaded is let go of their personal hygiene. Even if you have only five minutes for a quick shower, make that time special and associate it with renewal and re-energizing yourself. Get a nylon body scrubber, fill it with your favorite shower gel, and as you scrub yourself down, pretend you're washing away all your worries. Do this, and your bath cleans more than the outside of your body — it washes away the cobwebs from your spirit as well.

You can pamper yourself in many other ways, too. You're the best judge of what it takes to bring a smile to your face and help you feel more calm and more in control. Pampering empowers you to be a better, more dedicated (and less distracted) caregiver.

# Avoiding Isolation

Given the multiple responsibilities a caregiver must juggle, shutting yourself away in your house with your loved one and all your problems might seem like the simplest thing to do. In fact, self-imposed isolation is a common reaction among caregivers exposed to long-term stress. But isolation is bad for several reasons:

- ✔ Humans are social creatures, designed to interact with one another. Depriving yourself of the company of others and trying to go forward without any meaningful relationships has the same effect on your body as stress.

- ✔ If you keep to yourself to avoid stress, you're still stressing your mind, body, and spirit through the act of isolation.

- ✔ Interacting with others gives you a sounding board. Problems can seem worse than they really are if you don't have anyone to discuss them with. Talking through a particular situation with a sympathetic friend helps in many ways — you come up with different solutions, compare the advantages and disadvantages of each and ultimately realize you do have options.

- ✔ Self-imposed isolation keeps you from asking for other's help, which adds to your caregiving burden.

As your loved one's AD progresses and requires more care and attention, shutting yourself away becomes particularly easy to do. Even when caring for someone in the most advanced stage of AD, taking time out for yourself on a regular basis is important; otherwise your mental and physical health suffers. Staying connected to other family members and friends is one of the best ways to keep you primed for the caregiving role.

## Understanding why you really do need people

Keeping up friendships with people who can go anywhere they want any time they want is difficult, but you can do it. Some people are going to drift away after you tell them you're caring for your loved one. But many friends step forward and volunteer to help you in any way they can. Most gratifying of all, after you get plugged into the caregiving community, you find many new friends who are also caring for a loved one with AD.

Once you make friends with other AD caregivers, a world of new possibilities opens up. Perhaps you can share the cost of a paid caregiver for your loved one or enroll your loved ones in a daycare center together after they get to know one another. You can also alternate providing transportation to respite care.

TIP

## Talking to others who've been there

Looking for someone who really understands your situation and can lend a sympathetic ear? Join the message boards and live chat rooms available at www.alzonline.net/message board/index.html. You can meet other AD caregivers there — some who are looking for answers to specific questions, and others who are just searching for a good listener or a few minutes of understanding and sympathy. But remember you also need human contact. Online message boards and chat rooms are good in a crunch but are no substitute for direct human contact. Relying strictly on this sort of impersonal communication can be almost as isolating as never going out of the house at all.

No matter what your situation, you've no good reason to shut your friends out of your life just because you've become a caregiver. If you tell yourself that none of your other family members or friends can possibly understand your situation or how stressed and overwhelmed you feel, you're giving yourself an excuse for cutting others off and making your own fears about isolation come true. To avoid isolation, you must help you friends and family understand your feelings; they can't read your mind.

How others see you relates mostly to how you present yourself and your situation. If you play the martyr and reject help or are angry and blaming, then of course you're going to drive other people away — people who can offer real support and assistance if you just ask them for help. As your loved one's AD progresses and they require more care and attention, it's particularly easy to lose contact with other family members and friends. Even when caring for someone in the most advanced stage of AD, it's important to keep taking time out for yourself on a regular basis or your mental and physical health will suffer. Staying connected to other people you care about is one of the best ways to keep yourself primed for the caregiving role. Call, write, send them an e-mail — make sure they know you care about them and think about them regularly. Regular communication keeps your support network active.

Numbing your feelings to avoid the pain and frustration of dealing with an AD patient is another negative coping mechanism. By cutting yourself off emotionally, you also miss out on many joyful moments, like when your loved one smiles sweetly at you or remembers a funny story from the past. The other people in your life don't want you to be cold and remote either; they want the same warm, wonderful person they've come to rely on over the years. Don't lose yourself — caregiving is a demanding job, but by its very nature it's a temporary one.

## *Keeping good friends around*

Let your friends know that you need their love and support now more than ever. After news gets around that you're serving as your loved one's caregiver, a few of your friends will voluntarily step forward to offer assistance and a few others will fall away. Losing touch doesn't mean they're bad people; maybe they just don't know how to handle the situation.

If someone offers to help, don't be shy about accepting his offer. And don't be shy about asking for help when your responsibilities threaten to overwhelm you, either.

If you're not getting the responses you expect, check your own attitude. If you're ashamed or self-conscious about your loved one's condition, that sends a negative message to the patient and to others and they respond accordingly.

Relying on one friend or family member for all your assistance can overwhelm her and maybe swamp your friendship as well. If you have weekly errands to do, try getting two or three people to run them. Then, alternate weeks so one person isn't responsible for helping you out all the time.

Writing down the list of chores you need assistance with is helpful. Then, show the list to other family members and close friends and ask them which items they can be responsible for. When you're well organized, you make a more effective team leader. Your friends and family members may be only too willing to help you, but are waiting for you to ask them. You must mold your team in the ways that best serve your needs.

# Chapter 20

# Handling Work and Family as Caregiver

---

*In This Chapter*

▶ Developing routines to maximize your time

▶ Managing a job and caregiving responsibilities

▶ Harmonizing family and caregiving duties

▶ Finding special time for your family

---

People who hold down a job, take care of their families, and also care for a loved one with AD might argue in favor of human cloning. Sometimes you don't have enough hours in the day or enough hands to get everything done, and having two or three of you to pick up the slack would be nice. Michael Keaton cloned himself in the film *Multiplicity* with comically disastrous results. But some weary midnight when you're standing over a sink full of dishes while a load of clothes spins in the washer and another waits to be folded in the dryer, and you still have to pack lunches and finish a report for an early meeting at work, cloning yourself might seem like a brilliant idea.

Despite reports to the contrary, human cloning is still the stuff of science fiction, and household robots aren't economically feasible for the average homeowner. So, how can you juggle work and family while caregiving?

In this chapter, you find out how to enlist the help of your boss, co-workers, and family members — not just to help you care for your loved one, but also to help keep the parts of your life that don't revolve around caregiving on track. You may not mind putting your career on hold for a while, but you don't want to lose your job entirely.

The same goes for family. You may put off the trip to Disney World, but you don't want to put off weekend picnics in the backyard or snuggle time with your children (or spouse!) because you all need the closeness that makes you a family, now more than ever. But family dynamics can cause problems. Read on to discover the best ways to keep it all together.

# Understanding the Importance of Routines

With so many tasks to accomplish every day, caregivers can get overwhelmed easily; the work must be shared to prevent caregiver burnout. The best defense against drowning in a sea of to-do lists is to determine what you need to accomplish each week at home and at work. Then, make a schedule and stick to it. Although putting a schedule together takes time, knowing what you have to accomplish in any given time period more than makes up for the time you invested developing the schedule.

Make a chore schedule, divided into daily, weekly, and monthly chores. Hold a family meeting and ask your spouse and children to assume responsibility for a few of each. Let them choose what they prefer to do; if you "assign" tasks, they may feel some resentment. Be careful about overloading children with too many chores. Put family members' names next to the tasks they chose. For example, put your teenage son's name next to taking out the garbage or mowing the lawn — whatever he volunteers to do. Perhaps your spouse can cook dinner a couple of nights a week. By breaking tasks into manageable chunks and sharing the workload, you get a lot more done. Stay on top of your day-to-day schedule and days flow more easily. Problems develop only when you ignore day-to-day chores and let them pile up.

For easy-to-follow daily household routines, check out www.flylady.net/pages/FLYingLessons_Routines.asp

Routines help you stay on top of your job as well. Evaluate your workload and look at any recurring deadlines (such as end-of-month-close or sales quota periods) and factor them into your schedule. Compare your work and home schedules to avoid conflicts. For example, don't schedule a doctor's appointment for your loved one during a busy time at work. After you get in the habit of following routines, they become second nature. In the long run, routines save a lot of time and energy and let you squeeze the maximum productivity out of your days with minimal stress.

# Juggling a Job and Caregiving Responsibilities

How do you see your job? Do you work just to bring in a few extra dollars, or are you passionately committed to a particular career? A person who has slowly climbed the career ladder toward a long-cherished and just-in-sight goal may feel unhappier about reducing his or her workload to provide care for a loved one than a person who temps 20 hours a week just to earn extra money. Some people see their jobs as a respite from caregiving, but don't get caught up in this belief. If you're juggling multiple responsibilities, you must schedule regular, true respite breaks to keep from burning out.

It may be that you have no choice; your family absolutely needs every penny you earn, so you can't quit your job or reduce your hours. How do you cope in that situation? Here are some suggestions.

## FMLA to the rescue

Until 1993, overloaded employees juggling work responsibilities with caring for an impaired loved one were pretty much on their own. Employers didn't see the need to cut caregivers any slack: either you did your job and carried out your assigned tasks in a timely fashion, or you didn't. And if you didn't, you more than likely lost your job.

This standard changed with the passage of the Family and Medical Leave Act (FMLA) in 1993. The FMLA allows any employee who has worked for at least a year for a company with 50 or more employees to take up to 12 weeks of unpaid annual leave to address family emergencies, without losing medical benefits or his or her job. Companies that disregard this policy and fire employees who take family leaves face stiff civil penalties and open themselves up to lawsuits.

Although the FMLA marked a milestone and caregivers across the nation applauded it, this act didn't cover the other 40 weeks a year — weeks when caregiving requirements continue, in spite of work deadlines and important meetings. More needed to be done.

In December 2000, Congress approved the National Family Caregivers Support Program, which provides free services for millions of families through local Area Agencies on Aging. (To find the AOA nearest you, call 1-800-677-1116 or visit www.aoa.gov/eldfam/How_To_Find/Agencies/Agencies.asp.)

But as more and more employees entered the ranks of caregivers, employers began getting on the bandwagon, realizing it's more expensive to recruit and train new employees than to invest money and time in retaining experienced long-term employees going through difficult times in their personal lives.

## Throwing a rope: How employers help working caregivers

Businesses incur real costs when employees' work days are impacted by caregiving responsibilities — costs related to hiring temps to sub for absent employees, lost productivity due to workday interruptions and emergencies involving caregiving, and finding and training new employees to replace workers who quit to provide care, to name a few. Working with employees experiencing a caregiving crisis takes supervisors away from normal duties, slowing down the workflow. Employees who are caregivers and don't have good support systems in place also suffer more physical and mental health problems, meaning higher insurance claims for employers.

Most major companies have figured out their interests are best served if they have a reasonable and consistent policy to help employees who are caregivers. After all, the number of caregivers is growing. According to projections by the National Alliance for Caregiving, the total number of employed caregivers in the United States is expected to increase to nearly 15.6 million by the year 2007, which is roughly one in ten employed workers. While there are no consistent standards from company to company for dealing with caregiving issues for employees, most employers do recognize certain caregiver needs:

- ✔ The desire for a flexible schedule
- ✔ The opportunity to telecommute, if the job permits
- ✔ Long-term care insurance
- ✔ On-site adult daycare (still rare, but more companies offer it every year)
- ✔ Office-based support groups for caregivers
- ✔ Workshops and educational programs
- ✔ Family leave
- ✔ Stress management classes
- ✔ Employee Assistance Programs
- ✔ Flexibility when using benefits; for example, the ability to use accumulated sick leave as paid days off to provide caregiving services

Employers who offer understanding and flexibility to their employees who are caregivers reap benefits that they can see on their bottom lines. Bosses who are the most flexible about allowing employees to find creative ways to get their work done and provide caregiving services are rewarded with fewer work interruptions, better job performances, higher job satisfaction, and significantly lower turnover.

Larger companies with more resources usually offer more extensive support programs, but even smaller firms are willing to help valued employees however they can. Ask your benefits manager what help is available. Then, explain the situation to your immediate supervisor and explore solutions to help you keep up your job performance while serving as a caregiver.

When you find co-workers willing to help, be sure to thank them and offer to return the favor whenever possible. Everyone has days when they must leave work early or take an extended lunch to run an important errand. On those occasions, offer to help your co-workers meet their deadlines. If you can't do that, write a note of gratitude or buy small potted plants for their desks. How you do it doesn't matter; just let them know you appreciate their help.

## Grabbing the rope: Taking advantage of employee benefits for caregivers

Employers aren't mind readers. You have to let them know your situation and what sort of relief may be beneficial. You may not get every consideration you ask for, but even a good compromise is better than juggling too many responsibilities without support.

After you determine how your caregiving responsibilities may impact your job, figure out what accommodations you need to make your schedule work. Do you have to take time off to take your loved one to the doctor once or twice a month? Will you be 15 minutes late to work every day because the adult daycare center opens too late for your current work schedule? Write down your desired schedule and ask your boss for a few minutes to discuss solutions. By putting your needs in writing, asking for help, and asking your boss to be part of your team, you're giving yourself the best chance of getting the flexibility you need to make it work.

If your company is small and your employer isn't required to offer family leave, discuss other options. Perhaps your boss is open to a job sharing arrangement that allows you to work half days. If your boss agrees to this arrangement, offer to train the person who shares your job. Even if your boss considers you to be irreplaceable, remind him that he can either help you moderate your responsibilities and work schedule or face the prospect of replacing you. If you have an hourly or part-time position, explain your situation to your supervisor and tell her you may not always be able to work your normal schedule if your loved one has a crisis. Line up other employees who are willing to cover for you as needed.

Don't mix work and caregiving. If you're at your desk but spend most of the day on the phone with caregiving business, you aren't getting much work accomplished, and sooner or later, your boss will notice. Make personal phone calls during lunch or on your breaks and ask hired caregivers to call during lunch, except for emergencies.

Occasionally, you may come across a boss who doesn't budge an inch and refuses to even grant family leave. If you're eligible for family leave, gently remind him of the law's requirements. If you're still not getting anywhere, you may have to consider finding another job or quitting work. Keeping two full-time occupations at once — caregiving and your job — is simply too stressful without any scheduling and workload flexibility.

## What will caregiving cost you?

Businesses aren't alone in suffering economic losses from caregiving. According to a 1999 MetLife study about the impact caregiving has on work, employees who provide caregiving services for a relative take a major hit in the pocketbook as well. Here are a few key figures based on an average of seven years of providing care:

✔ $566,443 is the average amount of lost wages per caregiver.

✔ $25,494 is the average amount of lost Social Security contributions, resulting in a benefit decrease of $2,160 annually.

✔ $67,202 is the average amount of lost pension plan contributions, resulting in a benefit decrease of $5,339 annually.

✔ $659,139 is the average total lost wealth, directly attributable to caregiving.

## *Making a contingency plan*

Life is full of little and not-so-little surprises. A contingency plan helps you cover your bases when something unexpected comes up at work or at home. Write your plan on a sheet of paper and make copies for other family members, hired caregivers, your supervisor, and your co-workers. Include the names and phone numbers of people who can provide alternate transportation or be substitute sitters or temp workers who can sub for you on the job. Having an emergency plan in place saves time and energy because everyone knows what to do in a crisis situation. Try to cover all the bases and create a fallback plan for every potential crisis situation. Make a plan for every situation you might encounter: for your work, your home, the day care center, and so on, and give copies of your plan to a responsible person at each location.

✔ **For work:** Ask co-workers in your department who have similar job responsibilities if they can help cover your job if you have a crisis. Be sure to clear any arrangements you make with your supervisor.

✔ **For home — one-time emergencies:** Write out your loved one's schedule and share it with a trusted friend, family member, or hired caregiver. Ask if she can serve as your emergency backup in case something prevents you from picking up your loved one from the adult daycare center on time or if any other short-term emergency arises.

✔ **Ongoing crisis situations:** For situations that may be ongoing, make more permanent arrangements. The same neighbor you rely on to occasionally pick up your loved one from the daycare center can't be expected to step into a full-time caregiving role if you become incapacitated. If you're hospitalized, you need time to regain your strength before returning to caregiving. If you have surgery, you may not be able to safely lift again for months. To prepare for such an event, line up someone who can take over for an extended period of time; perhaps a sibling, your spouse, a member of your church, or a hired caregiver can take your place. Give the person a copy of your loved one's schedule and the duties you want him or her to perform. Plan ahead by identifying suitable paid respite options. Gather information from local agencies to determine which facility you'd like to use. Most can have someone in your house or admit your loved one within 24 hours or the day you call. If you've been using respite services proactively to ensure you get regular breaks, your loved one is already familiar with the paid caregiver or facility. If you do this, your crisis is managed and your loved one's routine is intact.

✔ **If you die:** The last contingency plan you must make is arranging permanent care for your loved one in the case of your own death. Although it's not easy to think about, and preceding your loved one in death is unlikely, making a plan and putting it in writing is vital so that everyone involved knows what to do if the unlikely event happens.

# Balancing Family and Caregiving

One of the your delicate balancing acts will be figuring out how to care for your loved one without shortchanging your family. According to a study by the National Alliance for Caregiving and AARP, 41 percent of caregivers have children at home. Tensions can spiral if your spouse or children think you aren't paying them enough attention, while you may think the last thing you need is more people leaning on you when you're already so pressed for time.

Your road is harder if you have young children, because they don't understand why their grandmother or uncle is acting differently. They have even less understanding about why it takes time away from them and your family life, and they may not understand how to express their needs. Your children may throw tantrums, misbehave, and act out — anything to take your attention away from caring for your loved one and set it back on them.

The *sandwich generation* refers to people who are sandwiched between the needs of their parents and their children, shouldering the responsibilities of caring for both at the same time.

## Smoothing things over with the kids

Try a bit of creativity to overcome problems with demanding younger kids. Explain to them that your older family member has an illness that requires a lot of care. Draw an analogy they can relate to, such as reminding them how you cared for them when they had chickenpox or a bad cold. Then tell them that's the sort of care you must provide for your older loved one.

Even very young children can help with light chores, and including them makes them feel important, helps them overcome feelings of isolation, and keeps them feeling connected to you. Also, pay attention to how your children interact with the person with Alzheimer's Disease. You may find that they relate well to your loved one, but in some cases, children aggravate AD patients.

Be realistic when estimating the time required for caregiving activities. Most caregivers underestimate the time their loved one requires by 10 to 20 percent. Underestimating your time can get worse as AD progresses, and the amount and complexity of care required increases.

## Making a schedule

Schedule individual time with your children and spouse every day. Even if you meet for 15 or 20 minutes, you may be surprised how much information you can exchange. You can read your child a book (at a leisurely pace) or ask your spouse about her workday. Put all thoughts of your loved one out of your mind during this special time. Really listen to your children and spouse, and express your appreciation for the support they're showing you. Ask if they have any issues they want to discuss or problems that need solutions. Make them feel special, and you will feel special as well.

Even with the best planning, caregiving often disrupts the rhythm in a family. Everyone misses the special family activities you shared in the past and the day-to-day comforts you provided. In the first few weeks of caregiving, you can easily overlook your family's needs, putting them on automatic pilot and hoping for the best. This approach creates problems. When making your weekly schedule, include special family time and getaways as a priority. Doing so avoids hurt feelings and the difficulties that may arise when a family member feels neglected or overlooked.

## Being creative

If camping in the woods every weekend is no longer feasible, find new activities for your family. Think of other ways to do the same activity. For instance, put a tent in the backyard and let your kids sleep there on weekend nights. You may even join them if you have a good ghost story to share.

Perhaps you all like the zoo but haven't gone for a while because of your caregiving responsibilities. Can you take your loved one along on a zoo outing? Call ahead to see what accommodations are available. If your loved one tires after a little walking or has a tendency to wander, rent a wheelchair and push him around the exhibit areas. You can do the same for the aquarium or children's museum. If you think creatively, you can find ways for the entire family to participate in an enjoyable outing.

If your loved one is too impaired to come along, or you want to spend special time with your spouse and children, hire a sitter. Spending regular quality time with other family members is vitally important. If your kids are young when your loved one comes to live with you, and your loved one stays for ten years, putting off family fun until your caregiving responsibilities are over means you have put off your children's entire childhoods. Do you really want your children to graduate high school and go off to college thinking of you as an overworked shadow that flickered in and out of their lives?

## Communicating

Even if you've always maintained positive relationships with your siblings and your marriage is successful, the strain of caregiving can create conflicts. Deal with problems head-on. Don't let difficult family dynamics derail you emotionally. Honest, open communication and flexibility help resolve conflicts fairly — negotiate, compromise, and ask everyone to lay their concerns on the table. Are your family members worried about your loved one's care? Do they disagree with the diagnosis or how you're handling the situation? Do they feel left out? Are they worried about being asked to pay a share of the costs of caregiving, or do they think that because you have the AD patient in your home, you get to scoop up the entire family fortune? Whatever the problem is, get it out in the open so you can address the issue together. Counseling can be helpful in resolving uncomfortable situations.

Perhaps you're the one with the problem. Maybe you feel like you're doing all the work and your siblings or spouse aren't doing enough to help. Don't play the martyr; express your feelings calmly and ask for help. Instead of whining or crying about being overworked, hand out printed copies of your schedule and ask for help with specific chores. For example, if your daughter's dance class makes it impossible for you to pick up your loved one from adult daycare one day a week, ask your sister if she can take over the driving on those days. Ask your husband if he can pick up prescriptions on his way home from work. And remember, you can't force anyone to help; some people in your family may refuse to offer any assistance. If that's the case, move on. No amount of nagging changes their minds, and your bad temper serves only to reinforce stereotypes about your family dynamic.

It's normal for siblings and other family members to have differences of opinion on caregiving issues — how and when to use respite care, when to consider assisted living or a nursing home, and so on. As the primary caregiver, you may have to override their opinions. Counseling can help you make sure your approach is realistic and not a knee jerk response to old family conflicts and resentments. For more information on enlisting support, see Chapter 18.

Don't ask the same person for help over and over. Try to build a team of helpers and rotate your requests for assistance among them. This approach circumvents burnout and saves friendships.

Keep your family members informed, ask for their help in planning and problem-solving, and share responsibility equally, and you may be able to avoid most problems arising from underlying family dynamics.

# Making Time for Your Family

By now, you realize that finding special time for your family is a matter of priority. Make family time important, and your family stays happy and strong. Ignore family time, and you add to the heavy load of problems you're already shouldering.

Don't expect your spouse to understand your situation indefinitely. Make a date night once a week to just enjoy each other's company and to get away from the house and all your responsibilities. Don't let anything interfere with this time. Be sure to involve your spouse in caregiving plans. He may have valuable ideas to contribute — ideas you won't hear if you shut him out. Ask for help and accept what help is offered. Discuss finances and worries you have concerning your ability to pay for your loved one's care. Make plans for family outings. In other words, go on with your family's normal life.

Involving your adult children in the caregiving process can reap multiple benefits: you get additional help, an increased understanding of the situation, and the opportunity for each child to develop and strengthen his or her relationship with the person with AD.

Tell your younger children the kind of behavior you expect from them. Make a list of house rules and explain why the rules are important. For example, your teen likes to listen to loud music, but has a bedroom next to your loved one's room. Instead of trying to get the volume down, buy a set of headphones so your teen can listen as much as she wants without disturbing your loved one. Look for creative solutions that preserve individual rights without upsetting other family members. Don't overreact to slip-ups or mistakes. Remind your children of the house rules and ask them to follow the rules for everyone's benefit.

You can give every member of your family the attention they crave, and you can do it without cloning yourself. Plan ahead, involve everyone in the planning stage, and stick to your plan.

# Chapter 21

# Helping When You're Not the Primary Caregiver

*Y*ou experience many different emotions when you hear that your loved one has Alzheimer's Disease (AD) — especially if you're living far away from your loved one. Part of you may want to give up everything and rush to your parent's or grandparent's side; another part may feel guilty about not being there when you're needed; and still another part may feel helpless,

Even when you're not physically there, you can help your loved one and the primary caregiver. You can participate in the planning stage, when you're evaluating care options or examining financial arrangements. You can attend important medical appointments, such as the initial medical evaluation, treatment planning, or annual follow-ups. Help research local services, medical scholarship programs, and buy books on caregiving and inspirational texts to share with your loved one and the primary caregiver. If your loved one is moving in with one of your siblings or into a residential care facility, perhaps you can arrange your schedule so you can help with the move. Offer ongoing emotional support via phone calls, letters, and e-mail. You can contribute money for care, talk to doctors, take a vacation week during a critical time to give the primary caregiver a break, and do lots of other little things that show you care and want to help, even though you're far away.

This chapter reveals smart ways to contribute to the caregiving process, even from a distance, and points out some things you shouldn't do if you want to keep peace in your family. You find out how to recognize the Monday-morning-quarterback syndrome and ways to overcome your desire to second-guess everything the primary caregiver does. You also find tips to make your visits more productive and satisfying, even if you can visit only once a year.

Being hundreds of miles away when your loved one is facing a crisis like AD isn't the ideal situation, but with a little creative thinking, you can figure out ways to share your love, keep in touch, and offer a helping hand across the miles.

# Understanding How Family Dynamics Affect Caregiving Decisions

Before you decide the best way to contribute to your loved one's care, think about your family dynamics. If your family members communicate well, get along together, and treat each other with courtesy and respect, your family will obviously have an easier time caregiving than family members who don't speak because they're engaged in a 10-year feud. When a family is fighting, making satisfactory caregiving decisions is almost impossible.

When you live in a different town or state than the rest of your family, you may feel left out of the loop when it comes to caring for your loved one. Don't let those negative feelings create an even more difficult situation. Part of what you're feeling is a sense of conflict; you want to stay where you are and go on with your life, but you also want to be at your loved one's bedside 24 hours a day. You may feel like you have no control over the situation or that no one values your input, when in fact, they do. You have to work with your family members to find ways to help and stay informed about your loved one's condition.

If you live closest to the person with AD, other family members may automatically assume that you will provide the bulk of the care, and this can be a point of contention. Or if you're unmarried, divorced, or childless, you may be expected to step up to the plate even if you live far away and would have to give up your job and your current life to move home and provide care. Maybe you have small children or a tough job, or your other obligations are so demanding that you just don't see how you can help in the ways you're being asked to help. Good communication is the only way to get all these unspoken assumptions and expectations out on the table and resolve them fairly. Everyone involved needs to be heard and everyone involved should be willing to compromise a bit to arrive at the best caretaking solutions.

If you've always been the family leader and decision-maker or if you're the oldest child, your relatives may automatically look to you for guidance and direction, even if you're not the primary caregiver. If you're a middle child, you may be sensitive about your input being overlooked, whereas the youngest child may be either rebellious or resigned to someone else calling the shots in the family. Be careful these old roles and feelings don't create new tensions in the family.

Even the nicest families may have a troublemaker — someone who thinks that grandma's infirmity presents a swell opportunity to move in and drain the old girl's bank accounts. If this situation is possible in your family, you and your other family members must do everything you can to protect your loved one from fraud or intimidation.

You may also have family members who insist on characterizing your loved one's problem as just "old age," and they reject the diagnosis of AD altogether and express anger at family members who accept it. Don't expect much help from these naysayers until they can accept the true nature of the problem. In fact, they may actively work against what other family members are doing.

What you can do to help depends on your own situation, your strengths and talents, your resources, and your position within your family structure. No matter what your position is within the family, the primary caregiver may resent any suggestions anyone else makes, no matter how benign. Sit down with the primary caregiver and assure her that you appreciate her hard work and believe she's doing a great job. Tell her your suggestions are a way for you to stay connected to the situation and aren't an attempt to micromanage things from a distance. Open and honest discussion can be mutually reassuring and serves to forge a vital bond to help carry you through the difficult times ahead.

Whatever role you played in the family growing up and whatever patterns of behavior dominated your family's interactions in the past are likely to re-emerge in full bloom under the stress of the situation, even if you thought those things were all in the past. Even if you're in your 50s, you may still be the baby of the family when it comes to family dynamics, unless you've planned ahead and are prepared to forge a new role for yourself. It's not easy to redefine your role within the family, but stay calm, stick to your agenda and don't let anyone pull you back into an old argument. Stay focused on the present and redirect everyone's attention back to the problem at hand if they try to waste time and energy on old business.

If one of the reasons you moved far away from home was because your parent or grandparent who now has AD has a difficult personality or because your family is combative and you got tired of the fighting, then you probably dread coming back into the fold at this juncture in your life, even if you're just visiting for a week. Don't wreck your own life and sacrifice your serenity under the misguided belief that the only way you can help is to be physically present. Instead of getting caught in the middle of all your family's drama again, think of other ways to be supportive that don't require your physical presence. (See "Learning how to help" later in this chapter for some creative ideas.)

## Staying in the loop

When you live in a different town or state than the rest of your family, you may feel left out of the loop when it comes to caring for your loved one. Although these feelings are natural, don't let your negative emotions fuel an already-difficult situation. The primary caregiver already has his hands full and isn't necessarily leaving you out on purpose.

Take responsibility for keeping yourself in the loop. Set a time for a weekly phone meeting and keep the tone conversational and light. Make it clear you're looking for information and feedback, not a fight. The primary caregiver may be sensitive to criticism, perceived or real, so try not to be the person who knows just how everything *should* be done, especially as you're not there dealing with the day-to-day reality. An I-know-it-all-from-afar attitude can be really maddening for the primary caregiver who is, after all, the real hero in the situation. Notice we didn't say the primary caregiver is the *only* hero — just the one who's most likely to get the Purple Caregiver's Heart for caring above and beyond the call of duty.

After you figure out how your family dynamics work and how those old roles may impact caregiving, you're ready for a family meeting to determine the new roles each person plays in the caretaking process.

## Getting together

Whether family members agree or disagree about how to provide care for an AD patient, a family meeting is a good way to get thoughts out in the open and give everyone a chance to express his opinions. If emotions are really running high, you might want to consider scheduling your meeting with a counselor who can help you sort out your priorities and find workable compromises. Draw up guidelines for the meeting. Everyone can express her thoughts and feelings openly, without fear of being judged. Shouting and screaming aren't allowed; intense emotions don't accomplish anything and are very upsetting to everyone, especially your AD patient. Be willing to accept compromise solutions.

Remember that caregiving is more than just changing sheets and preparing meals. Caregiving has a spiritual and emotional dimension as well, and this is an area where caregivers can often get overwhelmed, especially if they feel isolated and don't have anyone to talk to. Even though you're separated physically, you can help your family and the primary caregiver by regularly communicating and staying emotionally close.

After the care plan is chosen, assign jobs or responsibilities. Let each family member contribute in ways that suit his talents, finances, and availability. If no one can realistically take on the role of primary caregiver, you know that you must make other care arrangements.

Even if it's not physically possible for the whole family to meet for a planning session, you can arrange a telephone or Internet conference with all your family members who are directly involved. If that's not feasible, speak to everyone individually to discuss what needs to be done and how the work and responsibilities can be divided up equally. Be sure to include your loved one in these meetings if at all possible; having input in the decisions that affect her care and quality of life is vitally important for an AD patient.

After the meeting, write out a care plan outlining the responsibilities of each family member who's involved. Send a copy to everyone for comment; this provides another opportunity for discussion and compromise. Pledge to keep each family member regularly informed about your loved one's condition, either by phone, letter, or e-mail.

# Learning How to Help

When you first hear about your loved one's AD diagnosis, you feel a jumble of emotions. Your first instinct may be to pack a bag and fly to your loved one's side. Before using any vacation days you may need later, sit down and think about your options.

Trying to keep up with an AD patient from a distance? Put all correspondence, medical reports, legal documents, and anything else pertaining to your loved one's care in a portable file box. Keeping this information separate from your usual files helps you find it quickly when you need it.

Having young kids, financial or health issues of your own, or a demanding job constrains the amount of time and effort you can expend helping your loved one. Being in a structured situation, like college or the military, also limits what you can do to help and when you can do it. Take all these factors into account when trying to determine how you can help.

You probably want to make at least one trip to visit your loved one, meet with your other family members, and assess the situation firsthand. If you return for a visit during your vacation, coordinate your schedule with the primary caregiver to make sure the timing is convenient. The caregiver may want to take a break during your visit or may want to stay and visit with you, enjoying your help and your company. Let the caregiver decide how to spend her time and don't load her up with a lot of guilt.

Keeping in touch with each other is easier now than ever before. Cell phones and e-mail have made staying in touch quick and inexpensive. How you choose to communicate with your family doesn't matter — just do it. Regular communication is one of the best ways to show you care and want to be part of the caregiving process, even from a distance.

## *Helping the primary caregiver*

You can do a lot of things to make the primary caregiver's load lighter and strengthen your family bond at the same time. No one expects you to pull up stakes and move halfway across the country to provide care. That's just not realistic. But you can help in many other ways; the important thing is to make sure that whatever you're doing fulfills an actual need and doesn't add to the caregiving burden. You can express your love and support by offering to

- ✔ **Provide financial assistance:** Providing care for an AD patient is expensive. If you have the means to offer financial assistance, this can ease the burden for the primary caregiver. Perhaps it allows a home health aide to be hired once a week to give the primary caregiver a break or maybe it pays for a daycare program or needed home modification or maintenance costs.

- ✔ **Provide telephone support:** Even though you're not physically present, taking five minutes a few times a week to call your loved one and the primary caregiver to let them know you love them and are thinking of them can go a long way toward relieving the isolation and loneliness that comes with being a caregiver.

- ✔ **Talk to your loved one's doctors:** When you have an opportunity to visit, be sure to accompany your loved one to the doctor and introduce yourself. You will feel more comfortable and confident about the care being provided for your loved one after meeting her physicians.

- ✔ **Educate yourself:** Become knowledgeable about every aspect of AD: its diagnosis, prognosis, and treatment.

- ✔ **Help with record keeping:** AD patients have thick medical files and tons of paperwork to keep sorted. It's easy for caregivers to let paperwork slide, especially with all of the other tasks they must tend to. Offer to organize and file all the paperwork during a visit. If you have a particular area of expertise such as accounting, law, or healthcare, offer to review documents relevant to your specialty on an ongoing basis.

- ✔ **Provide emotional support:** Send regular letters or e-mails with support and encouragement and share funny stories, good news, your love, or anything to make your loved one smile.

- ✔ **Help gather information:** When you're a primary caregiver, the last thing you have time to do is gather information. As a distant caregiver, you can help the primary caregiver by gathering information about care facilities and costs, clinical trials, AD research, medications, hired and substitute caregivers, and durable medical equipment.

- ✔ **Be the family chronicler:** When a family faces a crisis like AD, communications not relating to AD and the patient tend to fall by the wayside. Maybe your niece is getting married, but all anyone talks about is the AD diagnosis. If you're good on the computer (or even if you're not), put together a family newsletter once a month and include all the positive news you can gather — births, engagements, weddings, graduations, birthdays, anniversaries, and job promotions. Also provide the latest update on your loved one's condition. Include photos, if possible, and send the newsletter via e-mail or regular mail to all your family members. Your newsletter will become very popular and help your family weather the difficult days of caregiving with hope and humor.

✔ **Arrange a surprise:** You know how hard the primary caregiver works. To show your appreciation, arrange a surprise day or an evening out to recognize a special occasion like a birthday or anniversary. Enlist the help of other family members to hire a sitter and make reservations for a favorite restaurant. Depending on the caregiver's interests, throw in some movie or sporting event tickets, a few games of bowling, or a round of golf; make it something he really enjoys or doesn't get to do often because of his caregiving duties.

You can help from a distance in many other ways, in ways that are perhaps unique to your own family's situation. Be consistent, be persistent, and your family will feel your love and concern, even across the miles.

## Offering financial assistance

Sometimes when you can't realistically do much else, you may feel better throwing money at the situation. Although providing financial support is fine if you can afford it, don't compromise your own financial well-being just to assuage your guilt for not being with your loved one all the time.

Money is tricky. Talking about finances is never easy, particularly if your family is close-mouthed about financial issues. But in order to make good decisions, you need all the facts, so ask whether a caregiving budget is in place. Don't make a big deal if there is no budget; simply offer to help draw one up. Compare resources against needs and determine whether there is a financial shortfall. (For complete information on how to assess the resources, see Chapter 14.) If the primary caregiver is sensitive about money issues, assure him that you only want to help, not take over.

Talk to the primary caregiver and your loved one about what is needed, what resources are available, and any anticipated shortage of funds. For example, if your loved one's adult daycare costs $600 a month and she can contribute just $200 a month, offer to split the remainder with the primary caregiver and any other siblings or relatives, if you are able.

If you're substantially better off than most of the members of your family, they may look to you to foot most of the bills. You need to figure out how you feel about this. If you're glad to help, that's one thing, but if you're going to act like a martyr, that's quite another. The help that you offer should be given freely with no emotional land mines attached. If you don't like the idea of shouldering the bulk of the financial burden, you better figure out another way to help.

If you're in worse financial shape than your other family members, they may try to get you to shoulder your portion of the burden by supplying services like sitting and transportation, which, of course, you can't do because you're so far away. Try some of the suggestions listed in the preceding section instead.

# Dealing with Out-of-Towner's Guilt

No matter what you do, you may find yourself swamped with out-of-towner's guilt — the awful feeling that you could and should be doing more, if only you could figure out what. Feeling guilty is a normal part of the grieving process that accompanies a diagnosis of AD; you think you should do more, and the fact that you're physically distant only exaggerates your feelings. Deal with guilt in the same way you handle other negative, non-productive emotions — head-on. Bring your feelings out in the open, try to figure out what's making you feel this way, talk it through, and then let it go. If you've tried and can't get out from under your guilt and keep thinking that you really need to be with your loved one, try a few counseling sessions to see if that helps. If it doesn't, consider the practicality of moving. If you're retired, moving may be a logical consideration, but if you have kids in school or a high-powered job, relocating may not make sense.

Look at your schedule and resources to determine how much time you really can spend with your loved one and make the most of your visits. Don't let guilt drag you down. Remember, you've got a life of your own, and your loved one wouldn't want you to give up everything you've worked for to come sit and hold his hand. You can contribute to your loved one's care in other ways, so figure out what works for you and ditch the guilt complex.

# Part V
# The Part of Tens

The 5th Wave        By Rich Tennant

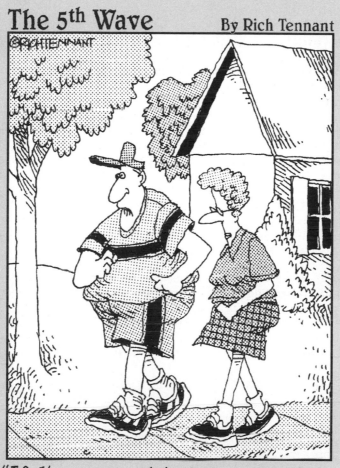

"If I'm supposed to be so over the hill, how come it feels like I'm still going up one?"

# In this part . . .

Every *For Dummies* book ends with top-ten lists, and this one is no exception. We tell you ten ways that caregivers can get a break, and we list more than ten invaluable resources for Alzheimer's Disease caregivers.

# Chapter 22

# Ten Tips for the Alzheimer's Caregiver

*E*very caregiver needs regular breaks from caregiving duties in order to remain healthy, happy, and capable of continuing to provide care. Caregivers can actually give themselves two kinds of breaks — good and bad — so we thought we'd give you five good breaks and show you the five bad breaks that can result if you overlook your own needs.

## Good: Ask for Help

Back injuries account for 46 percent of all caregiver injuries. If that figure seems a bit high, try to picture a 98-pound woman lifting her 200-pound impaired husband in and out of bed, in and out of the bath, and up and down from the toilet several times a day, day after day for years. Even if you're a champion weight lifter with muscles on top of your muscles, that type of repetitive strain eventually wears down even the strongest and most fit person, making them more susceptible to injury. Back injuries take a particularly long time to heal and sometimes mean that the caregiver can no longer provide care.

So give yourself (and your back) a break. Either buy a lifting machine, or, if your loved one still has some capacity to bear weight, a standing aid to help the person lift himself. Sturdy standing aids are available for around $300, but lifts can cost $1,000 (basic floor lifts) to $5,000 or more (fancier floor lifts or basic ceiling lifts), depending upon the system you select. Some lifts are available with custom ceiling tracks that enable you to carry your loved from the bed to the bath to the den, wherever you want the person to go, without having to do any lifting yourself.

Medicare may help with the less-expensive lifts but will not reimburse for the fancier units, which are considered luxury items. If your loved one is a veteran, the local chapter of the VFW may donate a lift.

If you can't afford a lift, consider hiring someone with more muscle than you have. And if you absolutely, positively can't get any help, at least learn the proper way to lift to minimize the risk of injury. Instructions for proper caregiver lifting are available at the Family Caregivers Online Web site at www.familycaregiversonline.com/body_mechanics_7.html.

# Bad: "I'd Rather Do It Myself"

If you insist on trying to heft your loved one in and out of bed all by yourself, and you don't know the proper way to lift, chances are you'll end up with a back injury. Not only will you be sidelined for weeks or even months and have to spend an average of $10,000 on treatment and rehabilitation, but if your injury is serious enough, you may no longer be able to care for your loved one.

# Good: Modesty Garments

Movies, television, and magazines include so much nudity and near nudity these days that people have become blasé about a little skin showing. But people raised in earlier generations tend to find nudity shocking and discomfiting. In fact, one of the main reasons that so many AD patients strongly resist bathing and toileting is that they're reluctant to expose themselves, even to a close family member like a spouse or a child, or don't understand the reason you want them to remove their clothing Or they could be cold, or frightened if you are moving too fast.

A modesty garment for your loved one can completely eliminate the problem. Available in models designed specifically for both males and females, modesty garments cover private areas but still allow easy caregiver access for bathing and toileting. They preserve the patient's dignity and greatly reduce problems with personal hygiene related to modesty concerns. They're inexpensive but worth their weight in gold for preserving the comfort and dignity of AD patients who need help with personal hygiene. See the "bathing" section in Chapter 16 for a link to additional modesty garment information.

# Bad: Birthday Suit

If you insist on stripping your loved one down to her birthday suit for personal hygiene chores, don't be surprised if she resists you mightily or starts claiming that she's already bathed or toileted when you know that she hasn't. A little bit of consideration for modesty goes a long way toward securing cooperation. Ignore it and you'll have a fight on your hands every time.

# Good: Ask for Volunteer Assistance

Many community resources are available for AD caregivers, including local agencies on aging, senior centers, church groups, caregiver support groups, and respite care agencies, so there's no reason to go it alone. If you have a problem, reach out and ask for volunteer assistance. Most of it is either free or very low cost.

# Bad: "I Don't Need Help from Anyone"

They gave out the martyr awards last week, so you're a little late. Why don't you want to take advantage of the many wonderful programs available to help caregivers just like you? Pick up that phone and call for help . . . right now.

# Good: Cook Once, Eat Twice

Lots of good recipes in magazines and cookbooks and all over the Internet show you how to cook double or even triple portions of a meal such as chili, soup, lasagna, or stew and then freeze the leftovers for a quick, nutritious, microwaveable meal for those insanely busy nights when you don't have time to prepare a meal. If cooking isn't your thing, see whether you can sweet-talk another member of your family into doing some bulk cooking for you once a month or so. You buy the ingredients, someone else cooks, and you freeze the meal. End result? You chill, instead of sweating dinner or resorting to fast food.

# Bad: Fast Food Bingo

As the demands of caregiving increase, many caregivers find themselves resorting to fast food meals. Not only is this expensive, but most fast food is high in unhealthy fats and sodium and low in nutritive value, which isn't good for anyone.

## Good: Remember to Laugh Daily

A little good humor can go a long way toward defusing tense situations and helping you maintain your perspective about your role. Read your favorite comic strip in the morning paper, watch your favorite scene from your favorite comedy, read the joke of the day — whatever you have to do to get the corners of your mouth pointing in an upward direction. Laughing releases good chemicals in your body that help bust the not-so-good chemicals released when you get stressed. So laugh!

## Bad: Wallow in Your Misery

It's hard to believe, but some people actually enjoy their own misery. Good for you, but did you ever stop to think how you're making the people around you feel? If you're feeling that unhappy and resentful about your role as a caregiver, it would be best for everyone if you arranged for another care plan so you can get back to being miserable all by yourself.

# Chapter 23

# More Than Ten Internet Resources for Alzheimer's Caregivers

*In This Chapter*

▶ Accessing information about the disease

▶ Finding online support for caregivers

*I*solation is a common problem among Alzheimer's Disease caregivers because the demands of their caregiving responsibilities on top of the day-to-day demands of their lives leave very little time to socialize. That's where the Internet can help. It not only gives you the opportunity to meet other caregivers and discuss problems and concerns with them but also gives you an invaluable tool to research information about Alzheimer's Disease.

If you've really just had about all the news about AD you can stand, you can shop for anything on the Internet, play games, read the news and movie reviews, or make hotel or plane reservations. In fact, you can find just about any kind of entertainment, education, or relaxing pastime you can think of on the Internet.

None of this helps much if you don't have a computer or an Internet connection. If ever there was a time to take the plunge, this is it. Many caregivers consider the Internet their virtual lifeline. Invest the time to learn how to use it; you'll be glad you did.

Don't want to mess with a computer? Try WebTV, where your Internet connection comes right through your regular television screen. A laptop keyboard lets you type messages, surf the Internet, and send and receive e-mail. If you can't access the Internet any other way, visit a nearby public library. All modern libraries now offer free Internet access for their patrons. Some even offer free classes to teach the basics of Internet use.

In this chapter, we introduce you to several invaluable Internet resources for AD caregivers. We provide the URL, or Internet address, as well as a brief description of what type of information is available on the site. You can also look for information yourself by going to one of the popular Internet search engines, such as Google (www.google.com), and entering keywords. The search engine looks through thousands of Web sites for your keywords and, in a matter of seconds, delivers an entire list of relevant sites. The more specific your search terms, the better your results. For example, if you want information on Alzheimer's caregiving but just enter "Alzheimer's Disease" as your keywords, you'll get back hundreds of thousands of sites pertaining to AD, but you'll have to search through them to find specific information on caregiving. However, if you use "Alzheimer's caregiving" as your keywords, your results will be much more relevant.

# ADEAR (Alzheimer's Disease Education and Referral)

The National Institute on Aging maintains an excellent Web site (www.alzheimers.org) with a vast store of information about every aspect of Alzheimer's Disease, from symptoms and causes to diagnosis and treatment. You can sign up for its newsletter, *Connections,* and order a copy of a terrific full-color book complete with CD, *Alzheimer's Disease: Unraveling the Mystery.* The site also has information about current clinical trials and AD research centers. ADEAR experts man a variety of live question-and-answer formats that are available to the public Monday through Friday from 8:30 a.m. until 5 p.m. Eastern Standard Time. You can reach them by e-mail, instant message, or the toll-free number, all listed on the home page of the Web site.

# Administration on Aging

Don't tell our editors, but you're getting a bonus here; we're counting the Administration on Aging as only one resource even though it offers several Web sites.

## Alzheimer's Disease information

One of the most comprehensive Alzheimer's Disease information sites on the Web, the AoA Alzheimer's Program site (www.aoa.gov/alz/carefam/carefam_disease.asp) offers a wealth of information about the disease and about caregiving for both the patient and the caregiver. It also includes links to valuable resources for families and caregivers.

## Eldercare Locator

Enter your zip code on this site (www.eldercare.gov), and you get help locating eldercare resources close to your home.

## Caregivers Guide

This site (www.aoa.gov/wecare/default.htm) is an excellent and truly complete online manual that answers just about any question that caregivers might have. If you prefer a printed version, the file is available as a PDF that you can download and print.

## State Agencies on Aging

This site (www.aoa.gov/agingsites/state.html) lists contact information including physical addresses, telephone numbers, and e-mail addresses for all the federally sponsored state Agencies on Aging. Just click on the first letter of your state's name, and you'll be taken to the correct spot.

## National Family Caregiver Support Program

This advocacy site (www.aoa.gov/prof/aoaprog/caregiver/caregiver.asp) helps caregivers track down the resources they need. It also offers them the opportunity to participate in advocacy projects and national policy making concerning caregiving issues.

## AgeNet Eldercare Network

This site (www.caregivers.com) offers a variety of informative articles and a chat room and also contains links to merchants who specialize in products for caregivers.

## Alzheimer's Association

The Alzheimer's Association maintains a vast and comprehensive Web site (www.alz.org) for Alzheimer's Disease patients and their families. It has up-to-date information about research, clinical trials, diagnosis, treatments, caregiving, and advocacy. Enter your zip code, and you get contact information for your local chapter. The site also offers resources in Spanish, Korean, and Chinese and a link to the Alzheimer's Association in the United Kingdom.

# Alzheimer's Caregiver Support Online

Sponsored by the University of Florida, this site (www.alzonline.net) offers a lot of information of interest to caregivers, and an excellent online training class for caregivers called Positive Caregiving. The site also includes a message board, chat room, and a reading room with a variety of excellent articles for caregivers. Also available is a Resource Center that offers forums presented by Alzheimer's experts.

# The Alzheimer's Foundation of America

The Alzheimer's Foundation of America is dedicated to improving the quality of life for both AD patients and their families. Visit their Web site at www.alzfdn.org/ for a wealth of information about the disease, its diagnosis and treatment, current research, and breaking news. They also provide links to education and social services resources and supports professional development for individuals who have dedicated their careers to Alzheimer's Disease research, treatment, and caregiving.

# benefitscheckup.org

The National Council on Aging maintains a Web site at: www.benefitscheckup.org/ to help people age 55 and over find programs that may pay part or all of their cost for prescription drugs, health care, utilities, and other services. Just fill out a short questionnaire and the site will let you know what programs are available in your area and if you qualify.

# Caregiver.com

This slick Web site offers information about a variety of topics that affect caregivers, including depression, nutrition, and how to handle a patient's incontinence. The Alzheimer's Channel at www.caregiver.com/channels/alzheimers/index.htm offers specific information for AD caregivers and hosts a discussion forum and a live chat on Tuesday and Thursday nights.

# CareSsentials

This site (www.caressentials.com) is dedicated to self-care for the caregiver. It offers a free subscription to a well-written free monthly newsletter called *Caregiver Tips.* You may sign up for the newsletter on the home page of this site. It also sponsors Caregiver Connection, a weekly free telephone support group for caregivers. Sign up early for this; each session is limited to 25 participants.

# Family Caregiver Alliance

The Family Caregiver Alliance maintains one of the very best sites for caregivers on the Web (www.caregiver.org). It has loads of statistics regarding caregivers and excellent, in-depth fact sheets for a variety of conditions that require a caregiver, including Alzheimer's Disease. Its quarterly newsletter, available online, contains information and advice about a variety of topics of interest to caregivers.

# The Leeza Gibbons Memory Foundation

The Leeza Gibbons Memory Foundation is the manifestation of Leeza's vision for a better standard of care for patients and caregivers affected by Alzheimer's disease and related memory disorders. The Leeza Gibbons Memory Foundation, through its signature program Leeza's Place, seeks to educate, empower, and energize both caregivers and the recently diagnosed. Leeza's Place integrates educational approaches, connective social activities, emotional support, and intergenerational programming to help those in need when the "diagnosis bomb" goes off in their family. The Leeza Gibbons Memory Foundation is dedicated to supporting the day-to-day needs of caregivers and those just diagnosed, with an equally strong commitment to a realistic and coordinated national strategy for finding a cure.

For more information about Leeza's Place or how to start one in your community contact The Leeza Gibbons Memory Foundation, www.memoryfoundation. org, telephone number 1-888-OK-Leeza.

# Long-Distance Caregiving

The American Association of Retired Persons maintains an excellent site (www.aarp.org/confacts/caregive/longdistance.html) with lots of good advice for long-distance caregivers. It offers everything from suggestions about what assistance you can contribute, even from a distance, to tips about how to keep peace in the family.

## National Family Caregivers Association

The National Family Caregivers Association (www.nfcacares.org) was created by caregivers for caregivers to share information, promote education and self-care for caregivers, foment advocacy, and offer mutual support. The group supports research into caregiver issues and works with legislators to promote bills to support the growing community of family caregivers.

## Needymeds.com

Many older Americans live on limited budgets and have trouble finding the money to pay for the medicines they need. Needymeds.com is an information source that links people who need help paying for medication to scholarship and charitable programs that pay part or all of the cost of their prescription drugs. Programs are available for all three widely used AD medications, including Aricept, Exelon, and Reminyl. The site is easy to use and very informative. For complete information, visit www.needymeds.com/.

## Medlineplus.gov

The National Institutes of Health and the United States National Library of Medicine maintain this comprehensive site with information on more than 600 health topics, including the latest information about Alzheimer's Disease. You can also find information about both prescription and over the counter drugs and a medical encyclopedia and dictionary to help you understand some of the jargon your health care providers may throw at you. There's also a directory to help you find a healthcare provider near you and a breaking news section to help you keep up with the latest information.

# Index

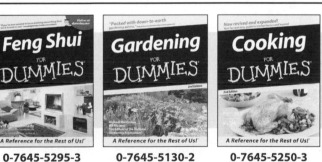
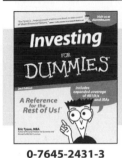
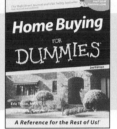
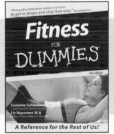
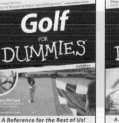
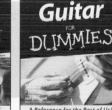
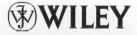

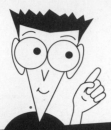

# FOR DUMMIES®

## A world of resources to help you grow

---

## TRAVEL

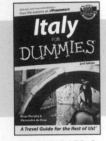

**0-7645-5453-0**

*Italy For Dummies*

**0-7645-5438-7**

*Hawaii For Dummies*

**0-7645-5444-1**

*Walt Disney World & Orlando For Dummies 2003*

**Also available:**

America's National Parks For Dummies
(0-7645-6204-5)

Caribbean For Dummies
(0-7645-5445-X)

Cruise Vacations For Dummies 2003
(0-7645-5459-X)

Europe For Dummies
(0-7645-5456-5)

Ireland For Dummies
(0-7645-6199-5)

France For Dummies
(0-7645-6292-4)

Las Vegas For Dummies
(0-7645-5448-4)

London For Dummies
(0-7645-5416-6)

Mexico's Beach Resorts For Dummies
(0-7645-6262-2)

Paris For Dummies
(0-7645-5494-8)

RV Vacations For Dummies
(0-7645-5443-3)

---

## EDUCATION & TEST PREPARATION

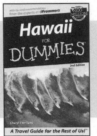

**0-7645-5194-9**

*Spanish For Dummies*

**0-7645-5325-9**

*Algebra For Dummies*

**0-7645-5249-X**

*U.S. History For Dummies*

**Also available:**

The ACT For Dummies
(0-7645-5210-4)

Chemistry For Dummies
(0-7645-5430-1)

English Grammar For Dummies
(0-7645-5322-4)

French For Dummies
(0-7645-5193-0)

GMAT For Dummies
(0-7645-5251-1)

Inglés Para Dummies
(0-7645-5427-1)

Italian For Dummies
(0-7645-5196-5)

Research Papers For Dummies
(0-7645-5426-3)

SAT I For Dummies
(0-7645-5472-7)

U.S. History For Dummies
(0-7645-5249-X)

World History For Dummies
(0-7645-5242-2)

---

## HEALTH, SELF-HELP & SPIRITUALITY

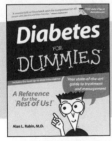

**0-7645-5154-X**

*Diabetes For Dummies*

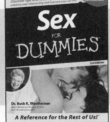

**0-7645-5302-X**

*Sex For Dummies*

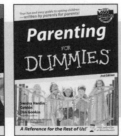

**0-7645-5418-2**

*Parenting For Dummies*

**Also available:**

The Bible For Dummies
(0-7645-5296-1)

Controlling Cholesterol For Dummies
(0-7645-5440-9)

Dating For Dummies
(0-7645-5072-1)

Dieting For Dummies
(0-7645-5126-4)

High Blood Pressure For Dummies
(0-7645-5424-7)

Judaism For Dummies
(0-7645-5299-6)

Menopause For Dummies
(0-7645-5458-1)

Nutrition For Dummies
(0-7645-5180-9)

Potty Training For Dummies
(0-7645-5417-4)

Pregnancy For Dummies
(0-7645-5074-8)

Rekindling Romance For Dummies
(0-7645-5303-8)

Religion For Dummies
(0-7645-5264-3)

---

**Available wherever books are sold. Go to www.dummies.com or call 1-877-762-2974 to order direct**